Living with Periodic Paralysis

by
Susan Quentine Knittle-Hunter
B. S. Special Education
B. S. Psychology

&

Calvin Hunter
M.S. Information Technology
M. Ed. Special Education
B.S. Psychology
B.S. Behavioral Science

First Edition
Periodic Paralysis Network, Inc.
2013

**The lower case 'L' on 'living' on the cover of this book is not a typo or error but used intentionally to signify that the term 'living' is being used very loosely in terms of this medical condition; patterned after the style of the poet and author E. E. Cummings.*

Living with Periodic Paralysis

by
Susan Q. Knittle-Hunter
&
Calvin Hunter

Periodic Paralysis Network, Inc.
Sequim, Washington U.S.A.

Living with Periodic Paralysis
by
Susan Q. Knittle-Hunter
&
Calvin Hunter

First Edition
ISBN-13: 978-1484062241
ISBN-10: 1484062248

1. Andersen-Tawil Syndrome 2. Periodic Paralysis 3. Hypokalemia 4. Hyperkalemia 5. Normokalemia 6. Hypokalemic Periodic Paralysis 7. Hyperkalemic Periodic Paralysis 8. Medical Malpractice 9. Rare Diseases 10. Potassium Channel Myopathies 11. Inspiration 12. Muscular Dystrophy 13. Voltage-Gated Potassium Ion Channel 14. Ion Channelopathies 15. Self-Help 16. Mineral Metabolic Disorders 17. Metabolic Acidosis

Printed in the United States of America.
2013-Reprint 2021

Notice-Disclaimer

The ideas in this book are based on the authors' personal experiences with Periodic Paralysis, and as such are intended to provide only educational information on the covered subject to the reader. This book should not be used as a medical manual, nor should this book be used as a diagnostic tool for Periodic Paralysis. The reader should consult a qualified health care professional or physician with expertise in Periodic Paralysis.

The names of persons and places were changed or omitted in some cases and any similarities to actual persons or places are merely coincidental.

By Susan

This book is dedicated to my children Tammy, Sandy, Jeff and Shari and to my grandchildren Connor, Tia, Cassie, Aaron and Carson and to my great grandchildren, yet unknown to me. May they live healthy lives.

This book is also dedicated to my mother, Lahlee Duggins, my great-uncle Edward Duggins, my brother Raymond "Butch" Knittle. Your struggles will not be forgotten. You are an inspiration to us all.

By Calvin

This book is dedicated to everyone who has the courage to question authority and follow the dictates of heart and mind. My heartfelt gratitude goes to Rosie, Laurel and sister Julie for your support in our moments of greatest need. Your trust, kindness and professional dedication will never be forgotten.

Table of Contents

Part Three: Managing Periodic Paralysis

Part Four: Psychological and Social Expectations

Also, by

Susan Q. Knittle-Hunter

Sandy's Story "I Wanna Go Home"

Cerebral Gigantism: Soto's Syndrome

Also, by

Calvin Hunter

Blue Sky Mountain:

Building a Home in the Uinta Mountains

Foreword One

In December 2008 I met Susan Hunter when her doctor referred her for counseling for anxiety. Susan was struggling with her mother's illness and impending death and was puzzled by the unusual symptoms her mother exhibited. Four years later Susan understands that her beloved mother probably suffered with the genetic disorder that runs throughout their family.

After multiple medical tests, misdiagnosis, and medication that threatened her own life, Susan found information on the Internet that led to a correct diagnosis of Periodic Paralysis. This extremely rare genetic disorder is practically unknown in the medical community but has now been confirmed by her doctors.

I had the privilege of walking alongside Susan and her devoted husband Calvin as she grieved the death of her mother, was misdiagnosed, and nearly died several times from inappropriate medical treatments. Doctors often thought she was malingering or suffering from anxiety or conversion disorder. It quickly became evident that her symptoms were real and very dangerous. It was heartbreaking to see Susan in paralysis and near death several times both in my office and at her home.

Susan and Calvin Hunter have the education, compassion, and research skills to put together this amazing book. It is well written, easy to understand and full of information about this difficult-to-diagnose Periodic Paralysis and related syndromes. Patients with these symptoms will find life-saving advice. Every medical school should have this book. It will be invaluable to every PCP, neurologist, cardiologist, renal specialist and MS clinics.

I'm delighted to see Susan manage her symptoms with rest,

diet, and no medication. She and Calvin have followed their dreams and moved to a home in the forest of Western Washington where they continue to educate through their website and this amazing book.

Rose M. Watne, MSW, LCSW Grants Pass, Oregon 2012

Foreword Two

I marvel at how modern medicine can miraculously save one person yet be deadly to the next. Clearly, there is still much to be desired when it comes to each individual's health and well-being. I met the Hunter family while working as a phlebotomist in southern Oregon. It was easy to recognize the signs that Susan and her husband Calvin were not getting what they desperately needed: Answers from their doctors and specialists.

Let me be clear; I value sound medical advice and professional expertise. It has saved many in my own family. However, no one ever has all the answers. Many times, we are faced with premature goodbyes, because of medical mistakes or misdiagnosis. Susan found herself in this very situation. Not only was her ailment nameless, but she also faced life threatening paralysis without warning. No solution or treatment was in sight. My job was to draw the blood for testing during these scary episodes that came out of nowhere. We had instantaneous rapport even though it was a stressful situation. Due to the seemingly inexplicable symptoms Susan experienced, doctors refused to listen. Tragically, Susan and Calvin were ridiculed and marginalized by the very people they trusted to help them get well! Susan pressed forward to find solutions and answers. Calvin was always at her side. I applaud their brave persistence to discover and create their own treatment plan. I feel privileged to know such modern-day pioneers.

This book is their story. It has not been easy for them. It has taken courage to be fully accountable for finding effective solutions without the guidance and aid of traditional medicine. This information may very well prove to be invaluable to you or someone you love who struggles with Periodic Paralysis.

Laurel Keith, PBT Grants Pass, Oregon 2013

Author's Preface
by
Calvin Hunter

There are many reasons why Susan and I wrote this book. My involvement since the beginning has focused on keeping Susan alive. In July of 2009, Susan had her first major episode of paralysis. She was sitting in a chair and suddenly was unable to move. I helped her to the floor where she lay until the paramedics arrived. She appeared to be semi-conscious but unable to move her arms or legs. The paramedics took her to the local hospital by way of an ambulance and our journey into the darkness began.

The book includes a culmination of activities and events that happened mostly between July 2009 and early 2012 written in essay and narrative form. The accounts include descriptions of events involving hospitals, medical professionals, family and friends, research and life-saving discoveries. It includes some harsh criticisms of the medical community, food and pharmaceutical manufacturers, insurance providers and governmental agencies set up to protect consumers. Many life-saving discoveries were made about diet, nutrition and medications. Life as we know it is at risk of extinction not by some asteroid or alien invasion but by the effects of an increasingly acidic environment.

Most of the information and ideas contained within this book came about as a result of taking medical vitals, Internet research, and creative thinking. Conclusions were formed after many hours of experimentation with nutrients, supplements, and other medical devices and interventions. It was and continues to be a laborious process with one success for every two failures. Throughout the process we have accumulated an array of at-home medical devices and medical testing equipment. Also included is information about interpreting medical labs, charts to record findings and graphs for reference.

There is no way for anyone to prepare for this type of situation. The thing that drives me to continue the uphill battle is my love for Susan. Watching the person I love take a downward spiral with very little hope of recovery, motivated me to take the necessary action to keep her alive. In the beginning the medical community gave no help and in fact they led us astray with misdiagnosis and a bag full of prescription medications that turned out to be the partial cause of Susan's highly acidic condition and paralysis.

The story began with an episode of paralysis and continued as medical providers misdiagnosed and misprescribed Susan's condition. Susan came close to death each time one of these providers prescribed pills, pumped foreign substances into her veins or inserted devices under her skin. It was through these near-death episodes that we gathered more information, which confirmed what we knew was at the heart of her illness and disease. We learned to question everything we were told by medical providers and even question the accuracy of medical test results.

This book shares information about the causes of Periodic Paralysis of which most medical providers have very little understanding.

Acknowledgements
by
Susan Q. Knittle-Hunter

I would like to thank my late mother Lahlee Duggins for showing me how to handle adversity, illness, pain and disability with dignity, bravery and a sense of humor. To my father William J. Knittle, thank you for your unconditional love, understanding and support. Thanks to my husband, Calvin, for saving my life and all you do to keep me alive and for your love, patience, and caring. Thank you also for your never-ending research and for your help with formatting and editing of this book. Thank you, Julie, for taking care of me and for wiping my tears when I could not. I want to thank Rosie, my therapist, for your constant faith and support and believing us when no one else did. Thank you Laurel, my lab technician, for your special help, understanding and support by coming out to the car to take my blood at those critical times and for your professional advice and friendship. I have a special thanks for the staff at Lincare in Grants Pass, Oregon, especially Carol and Tim, for saving my life by listening when no one else would. I would like to thank the specialist who believed me and finally diagnosed me. To the doctors and medical professionals who believed me and now see me and learn from us about Periodic Paralysis, thank you. For my children Tammy, Jeff and Shari and her husband Tom, thank you for your love and understanding and for being there for me always. Thanks also to my brothers, Butch and Brud, for your love and understanding. I am so sorry we share this disease. I hope the things in this book will help you to find a better quality of life. Thank you, Cousin Linda for all the information you provided me about your father, my uncle that helped in my diagnosis. Also, thanks to a few of my family members for sharing medical information with me as I traced our medical genealogy, especially my cousin Shari. Finally, thanks to the few family members who believe me and support me.

Acknowledgements
by
Calvin Hunter

There is one person who gave us hope during our darkest hours. Rosie Watne is the one provider who believed in Susan and believed in me. We will always be grateful for her wisdom and support. Thank you, Rosie, for listening and believing in the personal power each person has contained within the outer shell. You will never know the depth of my appreciation for being there during the times of our greatest needs. You are a gifted healer who understands the true meaning of the word healer.

The oxygen providers at Lincare also have our undying gratitude. You also were there in one of our darkest hours and listened to what we were saying. You took the time to properly administer tests and took the results of those tests directly to a medical provider who previously refused to listen. You persisted until that medical provider has no other choice other than to listen. You understood the critical nature of Susan's condition and helped save her life. Your services continue to help Susan get the most out of every day.

One other person who showed remarkable caring and support was Laurel, Susan's phlebotomist. Time after time she went the extra mile to accommodate our unique and unusual circumstances. She was in constant peril of losing her job for doing more than was prescribed by her employer. Her efforts demonstrated to us another example of a rare individual who meet their responsibilities in a very serious manner and treat the people they encounter with the utmost respect and care.

We also thank all the other professionals who came to our home on many occasions and provided Susan with the care she needed. We will always be grateful to Susan's physical therapists and home healthcare nurses.

Introduction
by
Susan Q. Knittle-Hunter

"I wake up nearly every morning totally paralyzed. I cannot move in any way. I cannot open my eyes. I cannot speak. My mouth is open and dry. I have urges to swallow but I am not able to so there is choking and an unusual sound in my throat every few minutes. My heartbeat increases and decreases intermittently and beats irregularly. As this happens, my blood pressure also increases and decreases, and my breathing may become labored and sometimes stop. These attacks may last from about forty-five minutes to several hours. During these episodes I am awake, and I am aware of and can hear everything going on around me.

At any time during an episode, I may have an irregular heartbeat, or I may go into cardiac arrest and/or respiratory arrest and die. Due to this knowledge, each episode can be frightening and frustrating and at times I cry. I can feel the tears running down my cheeks but can do nothing to wipe them away."

I have an extremely rare, hereditary, and progressive disease called Periodic Paralysis.

They say, "Invention is born out of necessity". *Living with Periodic Paralysis* was "invented" or written out of necessity or an urgent need. The fact is there are no other up-to-date books written about Periodic Paralysis (PP) and information found on the Internet is scattered and sketchy at best. There is an urgent need to educate those with the different forms of Periodic Paralysis and their family members on all aspects of the disease including how to manage and alleviate their symptoms. There is also an urgent need to educate the medical professionals dealing with those individuals, and their families, to learn to recognize, diagnose and properly treat their patients in a timely manner.

After a lifetime of illness, misdiagnoses and medical mistreatment (some of which caused irreparable damage), two years ago at the age of sixty-two, I finally discovered the name of the progressive disease that left me totally and permanently disabled with weak muscles throughout my body, intermittent periods of total paralysis, along with heart problems, breathing problems, blood pressure problems and exercise intolerance. Years of testing had ruled out all of the commonly known neuromuscular diseases. I had to look for the "zebra", as one of the over thirty doctors I had seen over the past six years had called it. I had to do it myself.

One day while on the Internet, I came across a disease called Periodic Paralysis. The symptoms were exactly what I had been dealing with. I was shocked and the more I read, the more I knew Periodic Paralysis was the disease that was affecting me. I wanted to know more about it. I wanted to know the what, when, where, how and why of it.

I wanted to know so many things. What type of disease is Periodic Paralysis? When was it discovered? Where can I find more information? Why did I get it? How can I get diagnosed? Is there medication or treatments that can help ease the symptoms? What type of doctor should I see? What is the cause? Is it a hereditary disease? Is it acquired? Where can I find a doctor who can treat my symptoms? What type of doctor do I need? How did I get it? Is it reversible? Are there different types of PP? What can I expect for my future? Am I dying? Are there others like me? Where could I find them?

I had great difficulty finding the answers to these questions. I found bits and pieces of information scattered throughout the

Internet, enough, however, to be able to understand some basics about Periodic Paralysis. I discovered one website with two discussion boards monitored by a few doctors. One was strictly for individuals who had a diagnosis and a patient needed to have permission to participate on it and another one was for anyone else who may have Periodic Paralysis or who wanted to know about it. I was shocked to be met with rudeness, a lack of assistance, non-responsiveness of the doctors on the board, and resistance due to the fact that I did not have a diagnosis yet. I eventually did find a few people who were willing to talk to me via email about Period Paralysis and who answered many of my questions.

I became painfully aware that there was very little information and very little help to be found for people in my situation, that is, having definite symptoms of the disease but no diagnosis. My husband Calvin and I began to research Periodic Paralysis and began to pull together every bit of information we could find to answer my many questions and to get a diagnosis. We hoped that a diagnosis would bring the opportunity for proper medication and treatment.

We discovered that very few medical professionals know about or understand this disease, including those who are supposed to be the "specialists" and "experts" in the field. We were met with resistance, rudeness, anger, apathy, intolerance, arrogance, disbelief, and mistreatment at every turn.

Based on the information we were able to find, Calvin put together a kit of medical equipment needed to monitor my symptoms, including a cardy meter to measure potassium levels, a blood pressure cuff, an oximeter to measure oxygen levels and heart rate, a meter to measure sugar levels and a pH reader to measure various levels of acidity. He also created a form to track the data as he painstakingly recorded it before, during and after my episodes. Over a two-year period of time, we experimented with various forms and amounts of potassium. We experimented with some medications. We experimented with diets. We experimented with oxygen therapy. We experimented with physical therapy and my tolerance for exercise.

Armed with our documented results, my medical records and with the cooperation of a few open-minded doctors, I eventually received a diagnosis. It was discovered that I have a very rare form of Periodic Paralysis unique to my family, which is progressive. There is no name for it at this time, there is no cure, there is no medication I can tolerate to treat it, there are no doctors who can help me, there is no known cause and I do not know what to expect for my future.

What we do know now, is there are several forms of Periodic Paralysis. We also know the causes of the paralysis, how to monitor and record the symptoms. We have been able to use all of the information we gathered to nearly stop my paralytic episodes from several a day to one or two a month. We discovered how to lessen the severity of the episodes. We discovered most of the things that trigger my episodes of paralysis and how to discover them. We discovered how to manage my breathing, blood pressure, potassium levels, pH levels and heart problems without medications. We created methods for finding a doctor who may be sympathetic, for getting a diagnosis and for how to discuss the disease with medical professionals, doctors, family members and friends.

Using the above information and the skills we learned as special education teachers, we created a website and discussion board for others who have symptoms of PP and cannot get help anywhere else. The Periodic Paralysis Network was created to provide a hands-on approach to understanding the disease, getting a proper diagnosis, managing the symptoms, and assisting caregivers and family members. We discuss issues relating to Periodic Paralysis in practical language. This book is an extension and culmination of our website.

After a lifetime of experience and taking over two- and one-half years of experimentation, detailed research and tremendous study to write, *Living with Periodic Paralysis* answers all the questions of what, when, where, how and why of Periodic Paralysis and unravels all the mysteries of this rare condition. Part One contains an account of my medical issues from birth until the present, in hopes of creating a scenario for which doctors and patients alike may be able to recognize the disease in its early stages. Part Two of the book covers every aspect of Periodic Paralysis. It is written in an easy-to-understand format. Each chapter is written with brutal honesty, and contains what the other books, discussion boards or medical sites about Periodic Paralysis on the Internet will not tell you. It is based on my experiences and what we learned through them. Part Three discusses the natural methods and technical information used to manage the symptoms based on years of research and experimentation. Part Four deals with the again brutally honest emotional, psychological and social aspects related to living with Periodic Paralysis for the patient, caregiver and family not found anywhere else.

Living with Periodic Paralysis may be read from cover-to-cover, section-by-section or by searching through the index for a particular subject. An appendix contains charts, data, photos, and lists. A "Works Cited" section and "Bibliography" contain over 200 references used for the research of each subject covered.

It is our hope that individuals suffering with any of the forms of Periodic Paralysis, whether diagnosed or not, may find the answers you are searching for in this book. We hope everyone reading this book will have a better understanding of Periodic Paralysis. If you have a form of Periodic

Paralysis, we hope you can improve the quality of your life by following our natural and common-sense plans and advice. If you do not have a diagnosis, we hope our ideas will be instrumental in helping you to get a diagnosis. If you are a doctor or health care provider, we hope you will be able to recognize, diagnose and treat individuals with Periodic Paralysis correctly, in a timely manner. If you are a social worker, therapist, caregiver, family member or friend, we hope you will be able to offer the understanding and support needed to your patient, family member, or friend who has this condition with your newly gained information. We especially hope you will know that you are not alone.

Part One
My Life with Periodic Paralysis

Chapter One

Alone in the Dark

"It is early morning when I awaken. I am lying on my back with my head slightly elevated on my pillow with my arms crossed and my hands on my abdomen. I attempt to open my eyes, but they will not open. I try to move my arms and legs, but they will not move. I try to speak, but my mouth is open and will not move. My tongue is thick and dry and will not move. I am breathing very shallow breaths in and out of my mouth. My heart is beating very quickly and every few beats I feel palpitations. Occasionally, my throat attempts to swallow but cannot and I choke making a gurgling sound as my head thrusts back against my pillow.

Oh no. It is happening again. I am afraid. What is this? What is happening to me? Will I stay this way this time? Will my heart slow down? Will the palpitations get worse? Will I choke to death? My breathing has stopped. I cannot take a breath. Am I dying? Dad, Mom, Sandy, are you nearby? Please help me get through this. A few seconds go by and finally I feel a little air enter my lungs; a shallow breath, then another. Thank the gods. Does Calvin know this is happening again? I cannot tell him. I am unable to wake him up because I am not able to speak, nor can I move. But I need him to listen to my heart, to watch my breathing and to make sure I don't choke. I am so afraid.

What time is it? How long have I been like this? How long will it last this time? I have an itch on my face but am unable to scratch it. Oh no, my breathing stops again. A few more seconds go by, finally another shallow breath. My eyes begin to sting, and I feel tears run down my face toward my ears. I am so alone. I have never felt so alone; been so alone. Please, please make this stop.

Why is this happening to me? Should I go to the hospital? After all, I am paralyzed. I thought doctors take care of people who are paralyzed. I wish Calvin would wake up and call an ambulance, but at the same time I am afraid to go to the ER. They treated me so bad the last 3 times I went. They treated me like I was faking these episodes. Why would I do that? Once they told me that I was having seizures. Another time it was possibly my heart. The last time they gave me a medication that almost killed me. I immediately went unconscious. Calvin had to remove me before I was discharged before they could do it again. What would happen if I went again to the hospital like this? I am afraid to go too but I want help. I need help. There has to be someone who can help me...

My eyelids are still closed. I am unable to move yet. My heart still races, and my breathing remains shallow. I am lucky to be able to hear. Calvin is softly breathing as he sleeps next to me. The heater clicks on. A bird is singing outside the window. Our cat scratches in his litter box. Life is continuing around me.
I am alone in the dark. (June 2010)"

Most books start at the beginning. This book must begin at the end. I do this to emphasize my desire that others will not find themselves as I have, totally disabled. It is my wish that with the use of this book, others will be diagnosed in a timely manner and will be able to manage their symptoms using the natural methods outlined in the following chapters.

I am a 64-year-old woman. I am totally and permanently disabled with weak muscles throughout my body including those involved with my breathing, heart, vision, and digestion. I have no energy to expend and cannot exert myself in any way. I am attached to an oxygen machine 24 hours a day. The electrical workings of my heart are defective. I have had a heart loop monitor inserted in my chest to monitor the tachycardia and arrhythmias, which include long QT interval beats. I have intermittent episodes of partial and total paralysis. I spend my days in a recliner, unable to walk farther than across a room. I must use a motorized wheelchair for anything farther. If I did not have the help of my husband, I would have to live in an assisted living program.

Over the last several decades I have progressively declined with a steady weakness and disability without knowing what was happening to me. I have been diagnosed and misdiagnosed with diseases from MS to Inherited Peripheral Polyneuropathy. I have been tested and studied for diseases from Friedreich's Ataxia to ALS and Parkinson's. Mitochondrial diseases, myopathies, and neuromuscular diseases have been ruled out. I have endured decades of costly testing which included painful laboratory studies, x-rays, MRIs, Cat Scans using harmful dyes, EKGs, EMGs, a muscle biopsy, and a sleep study. I have been hospitalized five times. I traveled to other states to see "specialists".

Each incorrect diagnosis brought mistreatment and improper medications, which caused irreparable damage. Each negative result or misinterpretation of testing brought humiliation for me. The doctors did not know or understand what was happening to me. Many doctors were frustrated, some were unsympathetic and a few of them were actually cruel and diagnosed me with psychiatric disorders, although I continued to decline physically.

Three years ago, after a lifetime of illness, misdiagnoses and mistreatment and progressive weakness and disability, my periods of muscle weakness became frightening episodes of full body paralysis as described in the passage, Alone in the Dark. I was unable to move in any way, unable to speak or open my eyes. However, I was able to hear and was aware of everything going on around me. These episodes lasted anywhere from fifteen minutes to seven hours, and I had several of them in a day and at night in my sleep.

About 6 months after they began, I finally discovered the name of the extremely rare form of a seldom seen and virtually unknown, progressive, incurable, hereditary disease, which had plagued me for nearly 50 years. I was diagnosed on February 7, 2011, with Periodic Paralysis.

Periodic Paralysis is a rare, hereditary disease characterized by episodes of muscular weakness or paralysis without the loss of sensation or consciousness. It is a channelopathy, a disease involving dysfunction of an ion channel for potassium, sodium, chloride and calcium. There are three types: Hypokalemic Periodic Paralysis, results from potassium moving from the blood into muscle cells in an abnormal way. It is associated with low levels of potassium during paralytic episodes. Hyperkalemic Periodic Paralysis results from problems with the way the body controls sodium and potassium levels in cells. It is associated with high levels of potassium during paralytic episodes. In Andersen-Tawil Syndrome (ATS), paralysis results when the channel does not open properly; potassium cannot leave the cell. This disrupts the flow of potassium ions in skeletal and cardiac muscle. During paralytic episodes, ATS can be associated with low potassium, high potassium or shifts in the normal ranges of potassium. Long QT heartbeats accompany it as well as certain skeletal abnormalities.

The form I have is ATS-like, because I go into paralysis when my potassium shifts low, high or within the normal ranges. I experience long QT heartbeats and have subtle skeletal abnormalities associated with ATS. However, in a genetic study, no genetic code was found for ATS, so the type I have, has not been named yet. The doctors believe it is form unique to my family and me.

Although, I have become totally disabled, most people with the condition will not. With an early diagnosis and proper medical treatment, most forms of Periodic Paralysis can be managed and controlled fairly well. By educating ourselves and with much trial and error, my husband, Calvin and I have discovered and compiled a set of activities, tasks, and steps which have helped me to finally control the episodes of paralysis. The components of the tasks are addressed and expanded upon in this book.

Chapter Two

My Childhood and Teen Years

As I contemplate the early signs of Periodic Paralysis in my life, I remember a time when I was nineteen and very ill during my second pregnancy. My father reminded me I had always been "sickly" growing up. I had never thought of it that way, but he was correct. I remember having every childhood disease that existed: measles (both types), mumps and chicken pox. I had tonsillitis at least two or three times a year and the stomach flu, with vomiting and diarrhea, and strep throat as often. I remember the fevers, the penicillin shots, and the delirium that followed. I remember holding a thermometer in my mouth, or worse yet, the embarrassment of having it done rectally. There were the enemas at the first sign of an illness. I was given crushed aspirin mixed into a spoonful of jelly. Watkins Mentholatum was rubbed on my chest and throat and then a flannel rag was wrapped and pinned around my throat. There was the 7-Up to soothe the tummy. Milk toast was a staple in our home. It was the only thing I was allowed to eat as I recovered. Recurring bladder infections began at age seven, and I wet the bed until I was twelve. Yes, he was right; I had been a "sickly" child. I obviously had been born with a poor immune system.

I was also born with some odd characteristics. My left foot and lower leg turned in. (Later in life, it was also discovered that I had an extra bone in my left foot.) I had severe fallen arches often called "flat feet". As a result, I had to wear extra sturdy shoes that were always different from everyone else. I was born with no eyeteeth or wisdom teeth. My second and third toes were partially fused or "webbed". An x-ray revealed I had been born with spina bifida occulta; part of a vertebra was missing. My little fingers curved inward. Most of these anomalies are seen in a form of Periodic Paralysis called Andersen-Tawil Syndrome (see appendix).

It was not just the childhood diseases or oddities, however, which affected me. I had horrible cramping or "growing pains" in my lower legs, mostly my calves. Periods of numbness in my feet legs, hands and arms, we called "going to sleep". I often woke with my neck or back stiff and in pain. We called that either "sleeping wrong on it" or a "cold in it". The muscle cramping and numbness continued into adulthood and the present, definite symptoms of Periodic Paralysis.

I was unable to keep up with the other children in many ways. I could not climb the monkey bars or do anything with my hands above my heads. I had difficulty climbing or walking uphill. I was weak and clumsy and poor at almost all types of sports. I was uncoordinated and tripped often. One time I climbed a tree but then could not get down. I just did not have the strength. My legs and feet hurt when I skated. I could not jump the gymnastic horse. After jumping on a trampoline for a few minutes, I was in extreme pain and weakness for days. These may have been some of my first experiences with exercise intolerance.

At the age of ten, it was decided that I would have my tonsils removed. My younger brother and I had it done the same day at the hospital. It was my first time to have any medication other than penicillin or multivitamins. The gas or anesthesia given to me caused me to be very ill after the surgery. I had a problem awakening after surgery and was nauseous and vomited several times. My brother did not have the same problems. Problems with anesthesia have been a problem for me with every surgery I have experienced. I have difficulty awakening, blood pressure issues and paralysis.

One Sunday morning when I was eleven, I was kneeling in church during Mass. I felt very strange and the next thing I knew I was waking up on the floor with everyone looking at me. This happened another time shortly after that, only I was on the end of a row and fell right in front of a priest walking up the aisle. The doctor believed these episodes were related to puberty issues, so rather than performing any testing in search of an answer, I was given a book about menstruation. It is probable that these were my first episodes of Periodic Paralysis in the form of syncope.

Besides passing out, I had periods of time in which I felt like I was going to pass out but did not. I also had periods of time in which I became "spacey" for a few seconds of time. I found myself staring straight-ahead and unable to move my eyes. I was often nauseous, especially in the mornings. I always got "carsick" when traveling any distance. These were probably early fleeting episodes of potassium shifting.

When I was about twelve, while walking in the country with my brothers and cousins, I slipped down a small cliff. Anyone else could have climbed up the incline, but I could not. My father and uncle had to come and "rescue" me with ropes and helped me walk back to my uncle's home. This may have been after a release of adrenaline from the fall. Adrenaline can cause a shift in potassium causing weakness or paralysis. Or, it may also have been exercise intolerance after having walked a distance.

Although I had many problems, as a child, I did lead a fairly normal life. I played with my three brothers, usually running from them. I spent time with my numerous cousins. I had school friends and friends in the neighborhood. I took music and accordion lessons, craft lessons, dancing lessons, tumbling lessons, swimming lessons, attended Girl Scouts, went camping and traveling like other children. I was a good student and got good grades.

There were a few areas in which I had some success physically. Depending on the move, I was able to do few things in tumbling. I could do cartwheels and backbends with help, but nothing else. Swimming was an activity I could do well and enjoyed. I could not run distances, but I could sprint. I walked a mile home from school every day and most everywhere else as a child and teen, including at times, almost two miles to the beach and back. The problem was that afterward I was very tired and had pain in my feet and legs and sometimes my back and neck.

High school was a difficult time for me when it came to physical education classes and sports. I was not able to keep up with my peers. No matter what the game or activity, I did not have the endurance the other students had. I was always the last student picked for any game and the first one out. I did not seem to have the strength or coordination the other kids had. I once was given an "F' in PE class due to not being able to keep up.

So, I was not only "sickly" as a child, but I was also often in pain, weak, uncoordinated, numb, clumsy, slightly overweight, spacey and nauseous. This followed through my teens and into adulthood.

Chapter Three

Babies and Young Adulthood

At the age of seventeen in 1965, while still a child myself, I gave birth to my first child. My first sign of being pregnant was passing out when I was about six weeks along. It happened a few more times before I went to the doctor, and it was confirmed. I experienced morning sickness nearly every day of the nine months, and it lasted through most of each day. The usual things affected the pregnancy, like acid reflux, hemorrhoids, and backaches. I also experienced severe lower leg and feet cramping every night.

I gave birth after twelve hours of labor without complication. I do not remember any problems with the saddle block (feeling numbed in pelvic region) I was given. I was not given anesthesia.

It was the second pregnancy in 1967, when I experienced complications. My husband had just arrived in Vietnam when I discovered I was pregnant after passing out. I hoped to continue working as long as I could. I switched to graveyard shifts in order to take care of my small daughter during the day, so I did not have to pay a babysitter. My parents had her in the late afternoon and evening, when I slept, and through the night.

This lasted only about a week, before I became extremely ill. I became very weak and fatigued. I was very nauseous, more so than normal morning sickness. I also experienced the severe lower leg and feet cramping every night. I had to quit my job as a phone operator. I lived with my parents and needed their help in taking care of my child. I remained this way for the much of the remainder of my pregnancy. At seven months along, I began to have terrible pains in my back and abdomen. The doctor gave me a shot in my back to stop early labor.

A month later, I went into labor again. I labored for twelve hours as before, but this time, there were complications, I was delirious and in and out of consciousness. As I look back now, I assume it was from the medication they gave me when I first arrived at the hospital. I know little about that time, except that I was told later that the baby and I almost died. She was not moving and had to be turned inside of me. I luckily gave birth without needing a c-section on Christmas Day. I had problems with the feeling returning to my legs and back after the local anesthesia. It took longer than it should have. I was extremely weak.

The next day I discovered that my new daughter was born with problems. She was diagnosed at the age of 4 with Soto's Syndrome a very rare genetic condition that causes rapid growth the first years of life, as well as other problems with all stages of development. She also was born with a deformed hip socket, turned in legs and feet and she was a floppy baby. She died at the age of five. These issues are common for children born with ATS.

I have written a book about her life and death and Soto's Syndrome, called *Sandy's Story "I Wanna Go Home" Cerebral Gigantism: Soto's Syndrome.*

Raising my girls and dealing with continual health and medical problems with my youngest daughter dominated the next few years. However, I began to experience some medical issues as well. The leg cramps would come and go. I began to experience numbness and tingling in my legs and feet. My hands began to cramp up when I would hold a pan to serve food for my girls. It was painful and took a few minutes to ease. They also became numb and tingly occasionally. I experienced pain in my breastbone area that was diagnosed as costochondritis an inflammation of the connective tissue. I had episodes of dizziness and sudden weakness.

In 1969 I was involved in an accident in which our car was rear-ended. I suffered whiplash and was in a great deal of pain in my neck and back. The doctor gave me muscle relaxers to ease the pain. For the next several days, I was in and out of consciousness, flat on my back with extreme weakness while attempting to care for my girls. I had them in the bed with me and can remember very little. I had no one near to help me. Once I stopped the medication, I was able to get back to my 'normal'.

I became pregnant again in 1970. Discovered it after passing out. This pregnancy was much as the first two times. I experienced morning sickness everyday with weakness, fatigue and muscle cramping. Taking care of my two girls was not easy. I gave birth to my son without the previous complications and in only 3 hours of labor, but the doctor did some reconstructive surgery after the birth. Recovery was slow and painful.

In 1972, while on the way to a medical appointment for my disabled daughter, I was involved in an auto accident. My youngest daughter was thrown from the car and seriously injured, and my oldest daughter was injured slightly. I had a broken nose. I ignored it for days while sitting with my daughter in the Intensive Care Unit.

I became extremely weak, dizzy, and fatigued. I had to go home. I grew worse and ended up in the hospital. While there I had to have surgery on my nose. I woke from the surgery in severe chills, shaking and unable to move or talk. Doctors and nurses surrounded me and seemed stressed as they attempted to awaken me and raise my severely low blood pressure. I had obviously had a reaction to the anesthesia.

I slowly recovered and Sandy also recovered after surgeries, broken bones, casts, and a long hospital stay. However, she passed away a year after the accident. She died of overwhelming sepsis, which is poisoning throughout her blood system from an unknown infection or metabolic acidosis. This is another indication that she also had Periodic Paralysis.

I was given a prescription for an antidepressant to help me deal with Sandy's death. I began to have weakness, dizziness, low blood pressure and passing out. I stopped taking the medication after a short time.

A few months later I was surprised to discover I was pregnant once again. The pregnancy went without many problems other than my usual weakness, leg and foot cramping, numbness, etc. Near the end I experienced a great deal of back pain and a few false labors. The birth was normal after about twelve hours of labor. The results of the saddle block were as before. It took a longer time than normal before getting back all feeling.

After giving birth, I did not bounce back right away. In fact, that happened with each pregnancy. I had great difficulty attempting to take care of my new babies and myself. I was extremely weak, fatigued and had problems with low blood pressure, and passing out, etc. I slept a lot and felt a buzzing in my head and heard it in my ears. The more I pushed myself, the worse it got. Eventually, I did recover to my "normal" self with help.

Over the next few years my physical problems continued. My religion at the time prevented me from using birth control, though I did use the pill several times. Each time I became very ill. I was flat on my back, nauseous, weak and had problems with low blood pressure and passing out. The other methods used did not work and I again became pregnant in 1975. I began passing out and became so ill that I was bedridden. I could not eat. I could not walk and had to crawl with much difficulty to the bathroom and back to bed. I do not remember much about that time because I was in and out of consciousness. Since it was summer, my oldest daughter took care of her siblings and me during the day.

I finally went to the doctor. He did not know what was wrong but told me that I would die if I did not have an abortion. This was not a difficult decision for me, but it was a problem for my family due to our religion. I did have the abortion and immediately I began to feel better.

Not long after that I had needed a medical procedure to scrape my uterus. The doctor also told me I needed a tubal ligation to prevent any further pregnancies since I could not tolerate the pill. Against the wishes of my religion and family I decided to have the surgery.

After both procedures, on an outpatient basis in which anesthesia was used, I did not recover from the anesthesia in a timely manner. I could not wake up and remained in and out of consciousness with low blood pressure and the inability to move. I stayed in the hospital overnight and into the next day before going home. Recovery was slow at home.

My normal problems continued along with recurring bladder infections and bouts of severe low back pain and neck pain. I also began to experience body wide pain in the muscles near my major joints. Antibiotics, muscle relaxers and pain medications left me weak, fatigued and gave me low blood pressure, passing out spells and a fast heartbeat.

Although I know now that the anesthesia and medications given me over the years caused those symptoms and much more, I did not know what was causing it at the time, nor did the doctors suspect it. I have had to piece all the information together after getting my diagnosis.

Chapter Four

Physical Problems Begin

My late twenties and early thirties brought many positive things to my life and some new medical challenges. Moving to a new home, with a pool, near the mountains in another state gave me the opportunity to swim and hike all summer and ski and belong to a health club in the winter. I was very active with my young and growing children with school, sports, crafts, music, dancing, scouts and church activities. We did a great deal of camping and traveling. I also worked full time as a special education paraprofessional.

I had a little difficulty at times keeping up with a busy schedule. All the previous things continued as well as monthly female problems. I awoke every morning with nausea and had periods of weakness and dizziness often. For days at a time, I would become weak and unable to get out of bed. I assumed I was having bouts of the flu.

I went through a series of medical tests. One of those tests was to determine if I had low blood sugar or hypoglycemia. After fasting overnight, I was given glucose over a three-hour period and blood was taken every hour to look for drops in my sugar levels. At the beginning of the fourth hour, the doctor sent me home. I picked up my children and headed to the airport to pick up a friend flying in for a visit. About 6 hours after the first dose of glucose, I was driving and suddenly began to shake uncontrollably and became weak and dizzy. I pulled the car over. We were in front of a restaurant. One of the kids ran in and got some water and crackers for me. After drinking the water and eating the crackers, I rested for a few minutes. The shaking stopped and I was able to resume my drive to the airport, though I remained weak.

The doctor believed I may have had a delayed reaction to the glucose and diagnosed me with delayed hypoglycemia. I began to follow a diet to manage the hypoglycemia. This may have been one of my first episodes of muscle weakness due to Periodic Paralysis.

One doctor believed I may have a problem with my electrolytes and gave me salt tables to take. They made me extremely ill, so I stopped taking them. Nothing else obvious showed up in any of the testing. This doctor may have been on the correct path, but I would not know for many, many years.

After I joined the health club, I attended a few group sessions with specific routines. I was not able to keep up with the others, I would have to stop after a few minutes of exercise, out of breath, my heart racing, my face flushed and in pain. I had I chose to do my own individualized program. I could never do the amount of time or the number of reps in my plan. I would always be weak and in pain the next day or two. I continued to go anyway, believing it was still the best thing to do for my health.

As a family we learned to ski and enjoyed spending the weekends on the slopes. I was, however, only able to ski for a short time, before my lower legs and feet began to cramp, and my back would ache. I pushed myself to keep up with my family despite the pain and despite the resulting days of weakness that followed.

There were many wonderful trails to hike in the mountains and canyons nearby. We spent our summer days swimming in our pool and hiking the trails. I wanted to spend as much time as possible in the forest. We packed lunches and hiked a certain distance then ate our lunch by a cool stream, falls or meadow and then hiked back down. I had a great deal of trouble going up the trails and pain in my legs and hips and back but did not let it stop me. And, by the time we got home, however, I could hardly move, like all my other activities.

No matter what the activity or how often I did it, my body

never seemed to get used to it, even if I did it every day. I still experienced weakness, fatigue, cramps, flushing, being out of breath, rapid heartbeat and pain. I just grew to anticipate it and expect it.

After my youngest child was born, she began to have episodes resembling small seizures. A great deal of testing ruled them out and anything else obvious. As an adult she now has the symptoms of Periodic Paralysis and is working on being diagnosed. She was ill much of the time during those years. At the age of seven, she became ill with salmonella and had to be hospitalized. She developed sepsis and nearly died. After 6 weeks in the hospital, she recovered after being treated with a "last resort" medication. She obviously had developed metabolic acidosis as had Sandy. As time went on we realized she also had learning disabilities and severe vision problems.

During this time my mother had a stroke. My grandmother had also had a stroke by the age of 50. I wanted to avoid ending up the same way. I became very conscious of my health and that of my family. I exercised and ate right. I did not smoke or drink. I had discovered that if I drank, I would fall asleep after just a few sips. I did not drink anything with caffeine either. It caused me to get weak and have tremors. I reduced my salt intake. I began to avoid any medications including aspirin.

Chapter Five

College and Building a Cabin

By 1981 I was divorced and had experienced a great deal of stress and many changes in my life. I lost my home and almost everything else I had. I was, however, lucky enough to meet and marry Calvin and once again, life became more stable and predictable for my children and me.

We bought a piece of property in the mountains about ninety miles from where we lived and decided to build a home. We hoped to live there full time eventually. We spent our summers and every weekend in the mountains working on building our new home. We also fished, hunted, cut wood, hiked and backpacked.

Calvin was completing his education in psychology and education. He encouraged me to return to college and become the special education teacher I had dreamed of for many years. So, I began to go to school full time, as I worked full time and built our beautiful home in the mountains. I did all of these things while raising my children and slowly progressing into a wheelchair.

Despite living a healthy life of good food, exercise and avoiding medications, taking a multivitamin and calcium tablet each day, all the health problems persisted, and new ones developed.

Once while rushing around the classroom, I hit my knee and fell to the floor, hitting my head, unconscious. I ended up in the hospital and after testing for various reasons, nothing out of the ordinary was found. This happened once again while Calvin and I worked on the sub flooring of the home we were building. Passing out occasionally or nearly passing out for no known reason continued.

I discovered that while working on aspects of the building, I was unable to help Calvin if it involved holding my hands and arms above my head. On projects involving my hands, they would painfully cramp and were unable to open easily or my hands and wrists collapsed if I held anything heavy. If I did anything on my knees, my knees would hurt and then my legs went numb. My back and neck would go out often and I found myself lying on the floor for days at a time until it would ease. After working on the house in the mornings and eating lunch, I became so fatigued and weak that I could not walk and had to lie down, and I usually fell asleep. I would wake up with my hands and legs numb and tingly.

During those years, I got the shingles. Bladder infections increased and became severe at times. Heart problems began to develop. I had periods of time with my heart racing or sudden fluttering or flip-flops in my chest, I discovered I had basal cell carcinoma (skin cancer) on my face. Hot showers, baths, hot tubs and steam rooms began to make me extremely weak. My doctor ordered a routine colonoscopy. I had problems once again with anesthesia. I was given the normal medications and the doctor began the procedure. Only a few moments passed when my blood pressure dropped into serious levels. I passed out. They stopped right away, and I woke up in a recliner. I stayed there for a few hours before my blood pressure rose to a normal level, and I felt well enough to leave. I never rescheduled another appointment.

One morning I woke up with chest pains, my heart racing, having trouble breathing and weakness. After beginning to feel a little better, I decided to go to work. I did have the chest pain, though not as bad, the rest of the day as well as weakness and trouble breathing. That evening we went to the ER, but the doctors could find no reason for it.

Six years passed. We finally graduated from college and we both secured teaching positions in the same school district in a small town thirty miles from our home in the mountains. By that time, we were able to live in the partially completed three-story house we called the "cabin". We spent much of our free time on finish work. We were breeding and raising

Australian Shepherds and Llamas. The kids had grown up, graduated and each had entered the military.

Chapter Six

Teaching

My first year of teaching severely disabled students, brought new awareness to my medical issues. It was a very physical job with a great deal of lifting and working on the mats with my students. I did not have the strength to do it and needed a great deal of help from my assistants. Sometimes I would get so weak, I would nearly collapse. I experienced overwhelming fatigue. I had to change the following year to teach students who were learning disabled, and behavior disordered to avoid the physical issues.

In 1990 at the age of fifty-two, I woke up one Saturday morning unable to move or speak. After a few hours, I finally was able to move a little but not enough to walk and could only speak as if I were a ventriloquist. This lasted about two days as I gradually came out of it. At that time, it was determined by the doctor that I had had a transient ischemic attack (TIA), a small temporary stroke. But I know now it was the first episode of full body paralysis I had that I was aware of.

I began to wake up during the night with my hands and arms numb; this progressed to include my legs and feet. I woke up each morning or during the night, if I needed to get up, unable to walk. I needed to hold onto the wall and furniture to maneuver my way around the house. This usually eased after a short while. I know now that I was having episodes of paralysis in my sleep and waking up totally or partially paralyzed at that time.

After sitting for a while at my desk or riding in a car etc., I began to have trouble getting up, standing and walking. My legs would be numb or had no feeling at all. I would try to take a step and trip or stumble. I learned to wait for a minute or two, and then walk in order to avoid falling.

Standing and waiting in line while shopping became more difficult. After walking a little, my legs got weak. I would have to shift from leg to leg. Sometimes one of my feet would start to drag.

I was sent to a neurologist who over a two-year period tested me for everything possible. I had EMGs, brain scans, MRIs and two spinal taps. Unidentified bright objects (UBOs or lesions) showed up on the MRIs. The EMGs indicated the beginning of peripheral polyneuropathy. His conclusion was possible Multiple Sclerosis (MS) although the lesions were not in the normal place for MS and the spinal taps were clear.

At the same I was diagnosed by a rheumatologist with fibromyalgia, due to the body wide pain I was experiencing. Heart problems continued and testing indicated I had mitral valve prolapse and benign irregular heartbeats called PVCs and PACs. Lab work indicated I had high cholesterol. Medication was prescribed for these issues including a statin and muscle relaxers. Both created problems for me including muscle cramping in my lower legs and low blood pressure.

X-rays revealed degenerative disk disease in my spine at all levels. This was undoubtedly the cause of much of the pain in my back and neck for many years. I was given pain medication to use as needed.

A routine bone scan showed osteopenia, the beginnings of osteoporosis. This was disheartening considering I had been taking calcium every day since I was in my thirties.

At night, as I was falling asleep, my legs would begin to jump and jerk. Sometime this lasted many hours. It was very uncomfortable and kept me awake as well as my husband. Soon, it started to happen in the evening when I would begin to relax from the day. This was diagnosed as restless leg syndrome. I was given several different medications to help ease it. None of them worked or they caused side effects that I could not handle so I stopped taking them.

I had problems sleeping partly due to the restless leg

syndrome so the doctor prescribed medication to help me sleep. The first night I took it, I was wide-awake the entire night. This is what is called a paradoxal effect. That means the opposite effect can happen. I later discovered that this is a common symptom that happens to people with Andersen-Tawil Syndrome.

I also began to experience fasciculations or muscle twitches in various parts of my body, but mostly my legs and feet. They were very annoying and could be seen under the skin. This usually happened as I relaxed or was stressed. It happened in my eyelids quite often.

One spring, I lost all feeling in my left arm and hand. It went numb and tingly. I was unable to use it for a month. The feeling came back suddenly one day. It has never happened again.

In 1998, I was teaching at the high school and had to climb a set of stairs to get to my classroom. As the new school year began, I found it more difficult to walk upstairs each morning carrying my books and teaching supplies and each time I had to use them through the day. After a few steps, my legs did not want to work. I had to pull myself up by my hands and arms. By the time I reached the top of the stairs, my entire body was shaking and felt like it was burning. I was in horrible pain and could not walk. I had to lean against the wall. After a few moments I was able to take a few steps, but my legs were weak, I had trouble making it to my classroom. I found I could not walk straight. I veered to the side.

Upon reaching the door, I fumbled with my keys to unlock it and had great difficulty grasping the doorknob and turning it. The door felt so heavy I had difficulty pulling it open and walking through it. It took me awhile to recover each morning. I discovered we had an elevator and began to use it until I could no longer teach.

I know now this was instant fatigue due to exercise

intolerance brought on by potassium shifting into my muscles. At the time I assumed it was due to the possible MS.

Bladder infections became so severe that before I felt any symptoms, I was urinating blood. I had to get to the doctor's office right away. He gave me antibiotics each time. I began to notice that each time I got a bladder infection, my symptoms got worse. I would be unable to walk or had great difficulty walking. We assumed that the infections were aggravating my MS conditions. I know now that it was the antibiotics that were creating metabolic acidosis and affected my muscles. This was related to the Periodic Paralysis.

I did have other times when my symptoms would increase, but I could not always understand what the causes were.

At this same time my heart problems were increasing. I was given a medication to help regulate it. My symptoms got worse, and I reached a point when I could no longer work. I went home in the middle of the school day due to severe weakness and a rapid heart rate on April 9, 1999. I was never able to return to the classroom. I was unable to get out of bed, could not eat and had difficulty speaking for many weeks. My teaching career ended after only ten short years.

I did not understand at the time, nor did the doctors, that it was probably the new medication and all the others I was on that had made my condition worsen and given me new symptoms for which more medications were prescribed. Later, I was able to understand that this was definitely a characteristic of Andersen-Tawil Syndrome.

Chapter Seven

Giving Up Teaching and Becoming Disabled

I saw some improvement over the following months by stopping some of the medications I was taking. However, Labor Day of 1999 was a day that changed my life forever. I woke up very weak and my legs felt like I was wearing very tight tights. I was off balance and had a great deal of trouble walking. We went to visit family for the holiday, but I needed help walking and then had to lie on the couch until we left. My mother gave me one of her canes and I have never walked unaided since that day, nor have I recovered from that day.

My legs never returned to normal, and the unsteadiness has never left me. The weakness and inability to walk became intermittent. These symptoms looked like Multiple sclerosis (MS) so my doctor believed it was probable MS. He ordered a lightweight wheelchair with wheels that easily popped off for me to use during the times my legs were too weak to walk. My upper body at that time was still fairly good so I was able to get the chair in and out of my car or truck as needed by myself and I was able to wheel myself around for shopping, etc.

I was sent to physical therapy with the hopes that my legs could recover some of the previous strength. After each session, I would wake up the following morning in terrible pain in my legs or whatever muscles I was using during the therapy. Sometimes I would begin to have pain while I was in the middle of the exercises and had to stop. I eventually stopped going to therapy before my prescribed time was up.

I had a few episodes where my legs lost feeling and I fell to floor when I stood up and would begin to walk. I saw the neurologist again for this and the excruciating pain I had begun to experience in my legs and hips. The neurologist believed this may be from the peripheral neuropathy and gave me a medication called neurontin. I began to take it and at first it helped. After a while, the pain began to increase. The more I took of it the worse my pain got. I had to stop taking it. This was the paradoxal effect again and of course, the fact that I did not need the medication to begin with.

In 2000, I had severe hemorrhoids and was referred to a surgeon. He wanted to do a colonoscopy as well as surgery to remove the hemorrhoids. I was nervous about it after the previous attempt years before had ended so badly, but reluctantly agreed.

At the colonoscopy, the moment they administered the medication to calm me before the procedure, I passed out. I woke up in the middle of the procedure feeling pain. I heard them discussing what they were seeing. When they realized I was awake, they quickly put me under again. I had trouble waking up and had to stay in the hospital for several more hours than expected. The scope revealed diverticulitis in twelve different spots in my colon.

I was very afraid of the surgery for my hemorrhoid removal. After the experience a few weeks earlier, the anesthesiologist was very concerned and very careful about the amount of anesthesia to administer to me. Things went as planned, until it was time for me to wake up. I woke up with the doctor, anesthesiologist and nurses surrounding me on the gurney. I was told that I had taken a long time to wake up and that my blood pressure was low, and they were very concerned. They got even more concerned when I could not talk or move in any way. It was quite a while before I was able to speak or move. Again, I had to stay in the hospital for many more hours before being released.

After going home, I had complications and was very ill with nausea and vomiting and severe weakness for days. I was in and out of consciousness. I know now it as due to an adverse reaction to the anesthesia and the pain medication. The doctor told me when I saw him for follow-up that I should never have surgery or anesthesia again, although he did not know why. I know now that it was due to the Periodic Paralysis. Anesthesia and most medications are triggers for potassium shifting into my muscles and paralyzing me.

After three attempts, on August 25, 2000, I was awarded disability through the Social Security Administration. It was determined I had been disabled since April 19, 1999. The determination was based on the following impairments considered to be "severe": Pain disorder, depressive disorder, fibromyalgia, degenerative disk disease and possible Multiple Sclerosis.

Over the next four years, I stayed busy despite my weakness and pain. When I was able, I wrote my first book. I knitted, sewed, cooked, baked and did crafts. I took care of the grandchildren and spent time with my mother. I drove to town to shop and run errands. We raised and trained llamas. We hosted parties for family and friends. We continued to work on the cabin.

I tried to go for walks when I could, and I used my wheelchair when I needed it. However, I had a continual, gradual decline with periods of total body-wide weakness and partial paralysis. Walking up the stairs in the cabin grew more difficult for me. Carrying and holding my grandchildren became painful and my arms grew too weak.

Calvin had become sick with several conditions and keeping up with living in our home in the mountains was becoming more difficult. We had snow for eight or more months a year. He had to clear it in order to get in and out of our property. He had to cut the wood in order to keep us warm. He was in pain a great deal of the time. It was sad for us, but we decided to sell our home and move to Oregon, which had a much better climate.

Chapter Eight

Moving, More Diagnoses and Doctors

The move in 2005 was difficult, but we were very happy once we got settled. We bought a small home on top of a mountain in the middle of five acres with a beautiful view of the valley. We were about 10 miles outside of the nearest town. We were at a much lower altitude, so it seldom snowed and melted quickly if it did. We enjoyed the warmer weather. We grew a garden and canned and dried our own food.

I continued to do the things I wanted when I was able. I drove to town and shopped using a motorized cart. I ran errands and used my wheelchair as necessary. My insurance paid for me to join a health club, so I joined the local one and began to swim and work out a little a few times a week. As time progressed my trips to the club became less frequent.

My mother lived with us, so I spent a great deal of time with her. She had many medical issues (she also had Periodic Paralysis although we did not know it at the time) so much of the time was spent taking her to doctors and getting her the help she needed.

From 2005 to 2009, my mother was in and out of the hospital and had seen specialists in every field of medicine. She recovered enough from her stroke at the age of 50 to be fairly active, except for some weakness on her left side. However, something else had been happening to her since that time. She became weak on her right side also and in general she had progressively declined to the point she could do very little for herself. She had always been a "sickly" person. It was too much for me to take care of her, so we finally placed her in assisted living.

She was a smoker and had COPD. She had congestive heart failure, severe osteoporosis, degenerative disk disease, diverticulitis, macular degeneration, seizure-like episodes, curved spine, fibromyalgia, prolapsed bladder, arthritis of the spine and other areas, and she fell and broke her arm in 2006 and it never healed. She was on twenty-five medications by the time she passed away in 2009.

During one of her seizure-like episodes I was shopping with her. I had never seen her have one before but had heard about them for years. She suddenly could not speak or move and slumped in her wheelchair. I called for an ambulance, and she was taken to the hospital. The doctors monitored her for a day or two as usual with no idea of what it was. She told me when I first arrived at the hospital that she "never wanted me to see her have one" because she knew it would frighten me. I have no doubt in my mind, now, that this had been an episode of Periodic Paralysis and that she had been having them for years. The doctors called them seizures and had been treating her with anticonvulsants since her stroke.

While dealing with my mother I was also seeing doctors to deal with my own declining health and strange episodes of weakness with heart, blood pressure and breathing problems. I could not find a medical doctor who would take Medicare when we arrived in town, so I had to settle for a nurse practitioner for my Primary Care Physician (PCP). He also saw my mother.

The nurse practitioner had several family members with MS and believed that is what I had based on my medical records and my symptoms. During the time I was under his care he referred me to nine doctors and a physical therapist. Due to pain in my left foot, I saw a podiatrist who diagnosed a stress fracture and found an extra bone also in the same foot. I was put in a walking boot cast and wore it for the next year. I was sent to a rheumatologist. He agreed with my previous diagnosis of fibromyalgia and gave me a medication, mirapex, which actually helped me, especially with the restless leg syndrome. The neurologist I saw, did not know what was wrong but suggested I be seen at major medical center in Portland. (I did not discover this for a few years, he never told me.) A surgeon diagnosed reflux esophagitis and a hiatal hernia, after a scope of my upper GI tract.

The cardiologist ran tests and told me some irregularities had shown up on a recent echocardiogram, ST segment and T-wave changes and I had a small heart that was overworking. He prescribed nitroglycerin for the chest pains I had been experiencing. The dermatologist diagnosed rosacea on my face. The gynecologist discovered arthritis and severe osteoporosis in my spine and hip. She referred me to an endocrinologist to treat it. He also ran a series of tests to rule out more conditions. He put me on a medication for the osteoporosis. I had to give myself an injection in my thigh every night.

We were shocked to discover I had severe osteoporosis considered to be at the "bone crush stage". I had been taking calcium every day since I was in my thirties. Research has led us to understand there is a connection between Periodic Paralysis and osteoporosis. A small percentage of people with PP can develop early bone loss in relation to the potassium shifting out of the bones and other organs as it shifts into the muscles.

I was also sent to physical therapy because of weak muscles and pain I was experiencing. He evaluated me to decide how he could help me. I was shocked and so was he when he told me that my legs had the "weakness of an eighty-year-old man". I began to go to therapy three times a week. Like before, I was always in pain and weak the day after therapy.

My nurse practitioner and I had a great deal of difficulty communicating about my care, my medications and my diagnosis. He continued to prescribe medications for the different symptoms and conditions I had including high cholesterol. Each statin that he gave me caused extreme pain in my calves. This was rhabdomyolysis, a potentially fatal condition. I had to stop taking them.

On each visit I would tell him I could not tolerate the

medications. He would get angry with me and once threw the pencil he was writing with. I had to find a new PCP and was lucky enough to find a young woman doctor willing to take me.

One morning, not long after seeing her, I woke up early and I went to my computer. I was sitting quietly checking my email when I began to feel the familiar symptoms with pain in my chest. The pain continued to increase and radiated to the right side of my neck and jaw. I had never felt chest pain like that before.

I slipped a nitroglycerin tablet under my tongue and waited. It did not help so took a second one. By the third tablet, I made my way to the bedroom to tell my husband. I had to crawl because I could not walk. Calvin called for an ambulance. It seemed like an eternity before the ambulance arrived. I was evaluated and placed in the ambulance. I was hooked up to oxygen and an IV. I was asked to sign my name on a document but could not write.

The ride to the hospital was a long one. I tried to tell the paramedics my history the best I could without being able to move my lips.

Once at the hospital testing began and Ativan, morphine and Zofran were administered as well as more nitroglycerin. According to the hospital records, I was experiencing episodes where my heart was beating a little fast and then jump to 120 beats per minute (bpm) then slow down again. My blood pressure was 138/56. My creatinine (CK) and D-dimer levels were elevated. I was admitted in order to rule out an ischemic cardiac event.

During the night I had another episode, and more medication was given to me. By morning I was doing better. The doctors believed it was likely related to reflux esophagitis and my hiatal hernia. I was discharged later that day. I was given a prescription for reglan for the reflux and told to continue the nexium I was already taking.

That night I took the reglan and had a horrible reaction. I could not fall asleep, and my restless leg extended through my entire body. I tossed and turned and kicked uncontrollably and never rested all night. It finally eased and I refused to take it again. My new doctor told me she believed I had a reaction called tardive dyskinesia.

I know now that the chest pain was a result of potassium shifting probably from one or a combination of the medications I was taking. Then the nitroglycerine made the episode worse and put me into full body paralysis. The IV I was given is a known trigger for episodes of Periodic Paralysis, as are ativan and morphine. I was lucky to get out of the hospital alive.

About a week later I developed phlebitis, an infection in the vein, in my arm from the IV. I had to get an antibiotic. It cleared up but returned a few weeks later. Another antibiotic finally got rid of it.

My doctor suggested that I begin to see a therapist to help me deal with my mother's impending death and my own health decline. I began to see a licensed social worker once a week. She was wonderful and caring person. She helped me a great deal and was with me through all the things I had to endure the next three years.

I continued to have bladder infection after bladder infection and blood in my urine even without infection. I was sent to a Urologist who diagnosed interstitial cystitis. I then saw another specialist. He ordered a kidney x-ray. A dye was injected into my arm during it. I suddenly felt very strange, then hot and started to tremor. My heart was beating extremely fast. I was unable to speak or move afterward. I had to be put in a wheelchair. We did not know it at the time, but the dye was a trigger for the paralysis. After that we refused to do the procedure planned to expand my bladder because he was going to use anesthesia. I have never returned to a urologist for that problem.

It was in June of 2009, and I had just finished my morning routine of swimming in the warm saline water pool. I drove to the grocery store. I walked from the car into the store and grabbed a cart. As I began to walk, my left leg felt like I was dragging it. Then I felt strange, and my body started swaying and to move all over. I felt a slight tremor through my body. I believed that I must look like a drunken sailor. I was very embarrassed and maneuvered myself as quickly as I was able through the store.

I was not sure what to do but got help with my groceries and made my way to the car. As soon as I sat down behind the wheel of the car, it all stopped. I drove home and told Calvin, about it. We attributed it to my diagnosis of probable MS and were concerned that I was entering a new phase of the disease.

One morning in mid July 2009, I went swimming and then hurried to an appointment with my endocrinologist. I walked the few steps from the car into the building, got on the elevator and rode it upstairs. I got out and walked a few steps to the office. Suddenly, I felt like I had just run a marathon and began to tremble all over. The same symptoms began as in the store when I shopped. I was escorted to the doctor's room to wait, barely able to walk, with only the aid of my cane. This continued as the doctor walked in.

I explained what was happening but that was difficult because my mouth was unable to form words. I had to speak as a ventriloquist does. He was extremely concerned and went quickly to get my primary care doctor, who was in the same office, to see me in this condition.

She did not come to see me but told him she had seen me as I walked past her office. She told him that she was already making plans to send me to see a specialist in Portland,

Oregon because she was sure something else was going on besides MS. They both dismissed me, and I was left alone to leave the office in that condition. I walked past the office workers, and no one offered to help me. I made it to my car, and it did not stop.

I took out my cell phone and called the "ask-a-nurse" from my insurance company. After explaining my symptoms, she told me to call an ambulance. I called Calvin first and he told me to do what I thought was best, so I made the decision to drive home because I was beginning to feel a little better. I made my way home very slowly and carefully on back roads.

Upon getting home, I was much better. Calvin had once again, missed seeing me in that horrible and frightening condition.

This happened a few more times over my next several visits to the grocery store or shopping. This lack of coordination of my walking muscles was ataxia. I began to need to use two canes to hold myself up and walk. My doctor was concerned with my stability on the canes and ordered a walker for me. She was worried about the possibility of falling and breaking bones due to my severe osteoporosis.

She referred me to OHSU in Portland, Oregon to be seen in the MS Clinic. After a five-hundred-mile round trip visit, it was determined that I did not have MS. A new MRI of my brain was ordered. It revealed a condition called small vessel ischemia or changes in the white matter of the brain. I need to note here that this issue has never been addressed.

Upon my follow-up visit to my PCP, she told me that she was leaving town to pursue her career in another state. She was very apologetic. I was devastated since I felt I finally had a doctor who really cared, understood and was trying to figure out what was really wrong with me.

I had to find yet another new doctor. The first doctor I chose to see told me that I was "too sick," and he refused to accept me a patient. The second doctor I saw accepted me but wanted me to cut back on some of the medications I was taking. Since I was on about fifteen at the time, I was happy to do that.

Chapter Nine

The Big "Seizure"

July 27, 2009 was a day that changed my life and Calvin's life forever. I had a regular morning and then began to not feel very well. I decided to lie down and fell asleep for a few hours. I woke up just in time to take a shower and get ready to go to my physical therapy session.

I took a shower and as I began to dress, I began to feel very odd with severe weakness and a slight tremor. I made my way down the hall to our office to tell Calvin that I would not be able to go to therapy. By the time I got there, I was weak, had difficulty walking and made my way to the chair. I began to tell Calvin how I was feeling, but I did not finish before I slid to the floor, unable to move and found I could not talk. Like other episodes, my mouth would not work. Calvin sat on the floor and held me. I was able to whisper without moving my lips that I needed help. He grabbed the phone and called for an ambulance. I continued in that state for about five minutes. When the ambulance finally arrived, I was extremely weak.

The paramedics evaluated me and decided it was best to take me to the hospital due to my blood pressure, heart arrhythmia and inability to move and the difficulty I was having speaking. I was hooked up with an IV and oxygen as I lay in the ambulance in the driveway. We sat there for quite a while before we left for the hospital. It was a long, slow ride to the hospital because we lived in the mountains about 10 miles outside of town.

During that trip, as we were driving out of the driveway, one of the paramedics gave me some glucose by mouth. He told me my sugar levels were low. Within a few minutes, my body was jerking uncontrollably, especially my legs and feet. They were beating against the back door of the ambulance. By the time I got to the hospital, I was worse than when the ambulance arrived at my home.

The saline in the IV had triggered new potassium shifting and the glucose had apparently raised my sugar levels. We know now that when potassium shifts into the muscles when the sugar levels are high that the sugar moves with the potassium into the muscles. This can cause muscle contraction, cramping and pain. The total paralysis as well as the muscle contractions throughout my body, made it look like I was having a seizure.

Upon arriving at the hospital my heart rate was over 150 bpm, so I was given ativan. I was initially able to answer some questions but continued to go in and out of paralysis. It was noted in the records that at times my strength was normal and at other times I was nearly flaccid. At times speaking was difficult. Calvin had to do most of the talking for me.

After a while, I fell into unconsciousness, obviously from the saline, glucose and ativan. I remember becoming aware of my husband discussing my situation with the doctors. He was very concerned and wanted them to keep me. They felt I should go home. They told him I was having seizures and that they did not treat seizures. So, Calvin was made to take me home with some new medications.

I do not remember how he got me home or much of anything over the next two days. I was in and out of consciousness. Calvin, being concerned, called my new doctor and asked if there was any way I could be readmitted to the hospital because he could not feed me or take care of me without help. After a few phone calls and my counselor getting involved, I was readmitted to the hospital. An ambulance was called to take me back.

I was treated well by the nurses and the hospital doctors, but my new PCP treated me horribly. The doctor was very angry and treated me horribly and wrote falsehoods in the record. The nurses were disgusted with him and everything he said and did. They were disgusted with how he treated me. Basically, he told me I needed to see a psychiatrist because I was obviously faking. He accused me of being suicidal because I had an assistive directive. He accused me of being a drug addict and took all my medications away and gave me antipsychotics and other more serious medications in their place. Calvin fired him after getting him to agree to home health care and physical therapy at home for me.

Calvin called his sister in another state and had her fly in to help him take care of me. He took me home expecting to get home health care and therapy for me right away. After phone calls and waiting, they never came. His sister stayed with us for several weeks.

Calvin continued to give me the medications the doctor prescribed. I was in and out of consciousness for days and in and out of seizures day and night. I finally stopped taking the medications the doctor ordered and I began to do a little better. The hallucinations and seizures stopped, but I was unable to walk or do anything for myself. Calvin and his sister bathed me, helped me with a bedpan and fed me. I had to be in my wheelchair. I began to have problems with not being able to sleep.

Calvin found another doctor and they took me to my first appointment with her. She did not care what was wrong with me nor did she try to find out and prescribed anti-psychotic medications to help me sleep. She had obviously conferred with the doctor we had fired. We argued but she insisted I take them. She did, however, gave us a referral for physical therapy after seeing how weak I was.

When my physical therapist finally saw me, I was able to stand and walk a few awkward steps and he was very concerned. He saw how I had declined since I had last seen him. He ordered a walker with four wheels, brakes and a seat because of how unstable I was. I was to begin to learn to walk again and begin seeing him three times a week again.

Upon taking the new medications, I got weaker and began to

have more seizure-like episodes. I was unstable, and shaky and had no endurance. The ataxia had returned. We finally decided that the medications were creating part of these symptoms, so I stopped taking them. Almost immediately, I began to do better. Calvin's sister was able to go home, and I was learning to walk again.

Calvin took me to the park every day and I would walk a little farther with my walker each day. However, I have never completely returned to the quality of life (which was not good to begin with) I had before the seizure-like episode. It was actually an episode of Periodic Paralysis made worse by the saline in the IV, the glucose and the Ativan at the hospital, and the other medications prescribed by the doctors who thought I was mentally ill.

I stopped seeing the second PCP and we began to look for another PCP. We could not find a doctor who would take me, so I began to see another nurse practitioner as my new PCP.

Chapter Ten

Periods of Paralysis and a Diagnosis

I began to see the nurse practitioner as my new PCP. She seemed to be a very caring provider. Just after my first visit I had an episode of feeling very strange. Calvin decided to test my bloods sugar level. As it turned out it was very high. We called my PCP, and she checked the blood work I had just completed. It indicated that I had type 2 diabetes. This was quite a shock. She prescribed metformin, a commonly used medication for diabetes.

Not long after that I began to have tremors as well as the episodes of heart racing, muscle weakness with the inability to walk, move, speak or open my eyes. They did not last very long but were very scary. We assumed they were heart related. We taped a few of them hoping to show the doctors.

Due to the rapid heart rate, the PCP ordered a 24-hour EKG. I wore what is called a Holter monitor overnight at home. PVCs, PACs, PJCs, abnormal T-waves, aberrants, ST segment abnormalities, and SVPB/PBCs were diagnosed. In the meantime, I saw a neurologist who was sure I was not having seizures. He did however refer me to a neurosurgeon due to the degenerative disk disease in my cervical spine.

When the neurosurgeon saw me, I was having a problem with ataxia, tremors and partial paralysis and could barely stand or walk. He told me he did not want to operate on my spine for fear it would paralyze me. He also was so concerned with my condition that he told us we should not see any more of the neurologists in Southern Oregon. He said I needed to be seen at a medical clinic in Portland. He wrote a referral to be seen in the neurology department.

I began to get sicker and sicker. My PCP saw me in that condition and was very concerned. We decided to stop the metformin. Almost immediately the tremors stopped. She told us that she thought I had Parkinson's Disease, Amyotrophic Lateral Sclerosis (ALS), or Friedreich's Ataxia.

She followed through on the referral to a Portland clinic attempting to get permission from my insurance. We believe the referral process was being delayed due to the expenses being incurred by my insurance company. Calvin soon discovered the reasons for the delays, which eventually led us to making a change in my supplemental insurance company. My insurer was owned and operated by a group of medical doctors in our town and their profits depended upon keeping expensive medical treatments and procedures at a minimum. Further investigation revealed they had been investigated by the state for making false declarations about tangible assets.

Once again, I was sent to physical therapy with the hope of strengthening my muscles and improving my balance. It became obvious that I was experiencing exercise intolerance. As I was practicing a few leg exercises or working on getting in and out of a chair, standing and walking a few steps, I would get weak and have to sit down or stop altogether. Once I suddenly went into an episode of total body paralysis, though we did not know what it was at the time.

The therapist was so concerned about my body-wide muscle weakness, my balance, the ataxia and the sudden episodes of paralysis that he told us it was time for me to use a power wheelchair. He was afraid I would fall and break a bone due to my severe osteoporosis (bone crush stage). We were able to use one that had belonged to my mother.

One evening I had an episode that was very serious. Calvin called an ambulance, and I was rushed to the hospital. The records from that visit indicated worsening ataxia, generalized weakness, troubled speech and shaking. The doctors and nurses saw these symptoms. Testing was done and nothing obvious showed up in the lab work. The doctor in charge, having read my previous records, diagnosed me with pseudo seizures.

Calvin and I were shocked. He argued with the doctor as I continued to go in and out of the paralysis. Of course, part of this was due to the IV, but we did not know it at the time. They decided to keep me overnight.

After Calvin left, they gave me ativan although Calvin told them not to give it to me. I passed out and did not wake up until the morning. Once I woke up, I was in and out of the paralysis and felt very heavily drugged and felt like I was hallucinating. When Calvin arrived and saw my condition, he did not wait for a discharge. He simply got a wheelchair and wheeled me out of the hospital and took me home. From that day until now, we will not return to that hospital. (We have obtained copies of the hospital records of each visit. It is unbelievable the lies that were written about my condition and me.)

Not long after this incident I was seen at the Portland clinic. I went through more testing and after three, five-hundred-mile trips, I knew no more than I did before my first visit. After having been seen by their top doctors and after having a muscle biopsy, all neuromuscular and mitochondrial diseases had been ruled out. The doctors there told me they did not know what I had, but that maybe it had not been named yet and would be "funny" if they named it after me. I left there in frustration and in tears again, after explaining the strange episodes of paralysis.

During this time with all the medications out of my system, the seizures had now become periods of total paralysis. I was having several each day. Some lasted a few minutes and some several hours. I could not speak, move or open my eyes, during these episodes. They lasted from several minutes to several hours. Sometimes I would choke. I had trouble breathing and my heart would race and help palpitate. I realized I was having them during the night in my sleep. I was waking up paralyzed.

I had one of these while at the Portland clinic while the doctors were giving me a muscle biopsy. They were not paying attention, and I was not hooked up to any machines, so they did not know what was happening. But we know now it was the effects of the lidocaine, they were using.

When I drove the two hundred fifty miles back to Portland to get the results of all the testing, I was told they could find nothing wrong with me that was either neuromuscular or mitochondrial. However, testing indicated changes in the shape and size of my muscle fibers and that I had lactic acidosis. I was dismissed by the doctor and told to just go have fun while I was in Portland. I started to cry and said, "If I could have fun, I would not be here in your office". I asked what I should do now, and he said, "I'm just referring you back to your doctor". I later found out that this doctor is the head doctor of the Muscular Dystrophy Association for Periodic Paralysis! They are supposed to be specialists in Periodic Paralysis.

My periods of paralysis continued. They were getting longer with more heart problems. I gradually got weaker and sicker and began to have trouble breathing even when not in episodes. It was about this time when I got on the Internet and started searching for what could this possibly be that was plaguing me so.

One morning, I typed in the words "periods of paralysis." Suddenly on the screen of my computer with the words, "Do You Have Periodic Paralysis?" As I began to read, I started crying realizing I had found the answer I had been looking for, for years. I found there were boards where people with this disease discussed it with each other. I joined the boards and read everything I could about it.

Through the reading and research of Periodic Paralysis, we discovered that potassium shifting into muscles triggered by many different triggers caused the paralysis. Two types included Hypokalemic Periodic Paralysis if the potassium was low and Hyperkalemic Periodic Paralysis if the potassium was high. We believed I must have the form with low potassium based on the symptoms I was experiencing.

However, to know for sure, we ordered a cardy meter. It is a little device used to measure potassium levels in the soil or other substances. It is not a medical device and therefore our insurance would not pay for it. It cost us almost $250.00.

Calvin began to take readings and record them. We discovered that sometimes my potassium levels during paralysis were too high, too low or even within normal ranges. We purchased potassium citrate in powder form. I began to take it dissolved in a small amount of water when my levels were low, and I began to have symptoms. Within a short time, I began to feel better. Sometimes I took too much and went into hyperkalemia. After experimenting, we began to know how much I could take. I need very little to feel the results.

One day, I discussed my symptoms with someone else with Periodic Paralysis and she told me to check Andersen-Tawil Syndrome. It is the most rare form of Periodic Paralysis. I was shocked when I saw the symptoms and characteristics of the syndrome. Diagnosis was based on full body paralysis from low, high or normal levels of potassium, long QT interval heartbeats and ventricular arrhythmia, and many abnormalities including, but not limited to, webbed toes and curved small fingers and toes and being born with missing teeth. I realized that the other members of my family, who had similar problems, and I must have Andersen Tawil-Syndrome.

I copied as much information as I could about Periodic Paralysis and Andersen-Tawil Syndrome and gave it to my PCP. It was obvious that as much as she wanted to help me, she was very skeptical about this diagnosis. She did however refer me to another neurologist. He was supposed to be a specialist in Periodic Paralysis and was the head neurologist for the MDA in our area.

He started the conversation by telling me I was too old to be asking if I had Periodic Paralysis, He told me he would not diagnose me unless my potassium levels were below 3.5 during an episode. He did not look through my records nor did he view the video we had made to show him of me during an episode full body muscle paralysis.

We left and within an hour I went into an episode, but his office was an hour drive from home. By the time we reached the lab it was 30 minutes too late. My blood lab showed a problem with my creatinine levels and my potassium was at 3.8. He did not bother to call for eight days, though he knew the results within two hours. Someone in his office called and said results were "unremarkable". We had tried to explain that potassium did not have to shift below normal to prove Periodic Paralysis. His lack of knowledge of the latest information on Periodic Paralysis was unbelievable. After being treated so poorly, I decided not to return to him

During a routine mole removal in my PCPs office, I was given lidocaine after telling her I could not have it. She had forgotten. It caused an episode of paralysis during the procedure, but I was treated as if I were a naughty child behaving badly. I was left alone in the room in paralysis until it passed. I was humiliated and did not want to return to her. It just happened to be the one time that Calvin did not accompany me into the PCPs office. In the very beginning, Calvin began to attend my office visits with me to help us avoid some of the misunderstandings that were occurring between myself the doctors. More than one time the doctors would say one thing during an office visit and then at a later time while reviewing my written records, I would find something written that was totally different than what was being said. We also began to hand-carry my medical files. This prevented misinformation about my medical history from tainting the opinions of other providers.

In late October of 2010, I developed a bladder infection and was given a sulpha-based antibiotic. I was the sickest I had been since I began having the episodes. I was in and out of consciousness, having trouble breathing and my heart was beating out of my chest. I had a fever. Calvin called the PCP on a Sunday morning and she agreed to see me the next morning in her office after changing my prescription. I began to take the new antibiotic and got worse.

When I arrived, I could not hold my head up and I begged her to help me. She placed a Holter Monitor on me and told me to come back the next morning after wearing it for 24 hours and then she sent me to the lab. I asked he if I should go to the hospital and she told me "No.". I went home and suffered through another day. It felt like I was dying. I stopped taking the medication and slowly got better by treating the bladder infection with other methods.

The results of the heart monitor revealed I was having long QT interval heartbeats. These arrhythmias can cause fainting and sudden death and are markers for Andersen-Tawil Syndrome. Of special surprise was that there were also periods of bradycardia, an extremely low heart rate, at time throughout the night. We had also recorded the periods of time I was in and out of paralysis. The long QT interval heartbeats and arrhythmias, including bradycardia and tachycardia, occurred at the same times as the paralysis.

The lab work indicated I was in metabolic acidosis (a form of lactic acidosis) a life-threatening condition in which there is too much acid in the body. Both of these things indicated I probably had Period Paralysis: Andersen-Tawil Syndrome. However, my PCP was hesitant to diagnose me. During one office visit she told me that there was not anything remarkable about my heart monitor results. We asked her to look at the written record and after looking closely at the chart, her facial color turned to gray, and she was speechless. She had not read the results and was now looking directly at the readings showing long QT interval heartbeats. This was a blatant example of the incompetence we had experienced for a very long time by many medical providers.

During this time, I continued to decline as I had more and more severe total paralytic episodes. I had tachycardia and palpitations of my heart and I was having difficulty breathing. Sometimes my breathing would actually stop for a few seconds at a time. It felt like an elephant sitting on my chest. It was very frightening. Soon the difficulty of taking breaths in and out began to happen when I was not in paralysis. I found it more and more difficult to breathe. Every time I stood up, ate a meal or exerted myself in anyway, the breathing got worse, and my heart would speed up until it was beating 130 to 140 beats per minute, even while I was eating.

My husband became so concerned with the lack of caring being displayed by my PCP and our insurance company, that in desperation he walked into a medical supply company and told them what was happening and asked if they could help me to get oxygen because I could not breath. After speaking with him for a few minutes, the manager told my husband that she would give all the information he had carried in with him, to one of the technicians and that they would see what they could do for us. She told my husband that they find it is best to get all the information together and then, "Hit them (doctors) between the eyes with the facts".

The technician came to our home and hooked me up with a recording oximeter. I wore it overnight and when he came to pick it up the next morning, I was actually in paralysis. He was able to see the level drop as I was experiencing it happen. It was discovered that my oxygen saturation levels were dropping dangerously low during my episodes of paralysis, and it was apparent that they were low every time I exerted myself in any way. The technician took the information to my PCP, and she had no choice but to sign a referral for me to get oxygen. At that point, we began to look for another PCP and decided to change insurance companies to avoid the need for referrals.

The oxygen therapy helped a great deal. Almost immediately I began to have less episodes of paralysis and the severe tachycardia and high blood pressure eased. Breathing became much easier. We did not know how this helped at the time, but we now understand.

The years of potassium shifting and the depletion from the organs in the body, as it occurs in Periodic Paralysis, affects all the muscles of the body including the heart muscle and the respiratory (breathing) muscles. The muscles can become permanently weakened causing less oxygen to be produced. This weakness of the heart muscle and breathing muscles can be fatal in Periodic Paralysis. If the organs are deprived of oxygen, the heart and the rest of the body are working harder to stay alive. The heart rate and blood pressure automatically increase to dangerous levels.

In my case, apparently, my breathing has become too shallow, and my lungs cannot expel the buildup of carbon dioxide. The effects of metabolic acidosis caused an increase in the carbon dioxide levels my lungs were trying to expel. Damage has been done to most of the organs in my body due to the buildup, including my heart, my breathing muscles and my brain. The oxygen eases the excess work of the heart and other organs, and aides in expelling carbon dioxide.

A month or two before this point, I was in despair over trying to find a doctor who knew about Periodic Paralysis. Then on the evening news, I saw their weekly feature of offering direct calls to doctors with any medical question. I quickly picked up the phone. After a wait of only a few minutes, I was speaking with one of the physicians. I asked her if she had heard of PP or knew of any doctors who might know about it. As luck would have it, she herself had a patient with it. She gave me the name of the neurologist the patient sees.

I went to my PCP with this information and talked her into giving me yet another referral. The neurologist eventually diagnosed me with "probable" Periodic Paralysis. He wrote a letter telling my PCP that I needed to see an electrocardiologist right away. It was several months before I got the referral once again due to the delays of the PCP and insurance company. He described my heart condition, by that point as serious with no treatment, but insisted I needed to have a heart monitor implanted. He also set up a renal specialist to help diagnose what he believed was Andersen-Tawil Syndrome based on all the information being presented to him by my PCP, the neurologist and me.

I did get the diagnosis while in the hospital for the implant. The renal specialist diagnosed "Periodic Paralysis with long QT. Probably a type of Andersen-Tawil Syndrome". (No other type of Periodic Paralysis has long QT except Andersen-Tawil Syndrome.) This was after seeing me in an episode for over 40 minutes with tachycardia sustained above 140 and with long QT arrhythmias and with my past history, all else ruled out and a family history of all the above and my own characteristics and that of my family. Giving me a saline drip and lidocaine during the procedure, by mistake, probably caused the paralytic episode.

Chapter Eleven

Reality and Hope

It has been just over two years since I received my diagnosis. There have been many changes since that day.

After receiving the diagnosis of Periodic Paralysis: Andersen-Tawil Syndrome (ATS) on February 7, 2011, I thought my life would take a turn for the better, but I was wrong. Things got worse in many ways before improving somewhat. The first thing that happened was the doctor who diagnosed me decided he could do no more for me because I could not take diamox to treat the symptoms. I talked with my neurologist who told me that he too did not know what to do for me. And then in May my cardiologist told my husband and me that he could do no more for me either. This was due to the fact that my heart arrhythmias, tachycardia and bradycardia, did not fall into the "extreme" ranges on the heart loop monitor readings (above 180 bpm or below 30 bpm…mine fall into a range of 160 bpm to 41 bpm depending on whether I am hypokalemic or hyperkalemic). Therefore, I am not a candidate for a pacemaker or a defibrillator. Though my condition is serious, there is nothing any doctor can do because I cannot take any kind of medication either.

During that appointment in May, I told the doctor about my frustration and how my symptoms seemed to be getting worse and asked what I should do about my decline. He then decided to refer me to a clinic that specializes in ATS somewhere in the United States. He asked me to find it and then he would write a referral for me. To make a long and complicated story short and simple, I will explain that it was not until October 17, 2011, that I was actually able to see a specialist in another state about one thousand miles away.

During those interim months, I received a letter from the genetic specialist in Germany. It stated that a genetic code had not been found for any of the known forms of Periodic Paralysis or Andersen-Tawil Syndrome in the studies of my blood. The doctor explained that the findings did not mean that I did not have a form of PP or ATS; it just meant I had a type that had not yet been found and named. (30 to 40% of all people with PP or ATS do not have a genetic code found.) It is my assumption that the team in Germany continues to work on finding these unknown codes for the others without known codes and me. Those with ATS symptoms and without a known code are considered to have ATS Type 2. The symptoms are indistinguishable from those with the known codes.

The appointment in another state lasted about 2 hours consisting of a medical assistant going over my medical records and medical history with me and then doing a physical exam. She left and conferred with the neurologist. He came in and reviewed some of the issues with me and also physically examined me.

He believed that since I had other things going on, I did not have ATS Type 2, but rather a type of Periodic Paralysis that was ATS-like and unique to my family. He joked as the other doctors I had seen previously that it would probably be named after my family and me.

He was very kind and very willing to work with my doctors on a consulting basis. However, he did not have any real ideas that would help me, because I am unable to take medications. He suggested a change in the amount of the potassium that I take and a change in the schedule of when I take it. He also told me that he was concerned with my lack of physical activity. He felt I should push myself a little more. Then we left feeling good about what we had discovered and the fact that we had a doctor who was willing to work with us.

As we traveled home, we tried a change in the amount and timing of my potassium. It did not help, and I had more episodes than before. So, I went back to taking it as I felt the need. I also tried pushing myself and ended up in a cycle of total weakness and in and out of paralysis for about two weeks. We had to call in-home healthcare. I have since stopped pushing myself and understand that although exercise is a good thing, it is impossible for me.

I thought about his words, that because I had other things going on, that I did not have ATS Type 2. I did not fit the criteria for his study because of my other conditions. In my family many of us have at least ten other diagnoses also and some have more than ten. These include fibromyalgia, osteoarthritis, degenerative disk disease, heart problems, osteoporosis, pain disorders, blood pressure problems, sleep disorders, constipation (hemorrhoids), exercise intolerance, restless leg syndrome, and female organ dysfunctions.

In order to no longer be confused with Andersen-Tawil Syndrome I have now named the type of Periodic Paralysis affecting my family members and me as "Periodic Paralysis Plus 10 Syndrome" (PP Plus10 Syndrome).

After returning from the trip to the specialist, I finally located a primary care physician who actually wanted to work with me. This was exciting since I had been through three of them in just a few months. We had to leave the first one due to her lack of appropriate care and the other two doctors left town due to being overloaded with patients.

The doctor we found is in another town about forty miles away near my specialists and two better hospitals. She had a background in genetics and was young and energetic. She practiced in a clinic, with eighty-one other doctors, which is open seven days a week. They had their own lab and radiology departments and are open in the evenings as well.

That afforded me the option of getting urgent care when I needed it without going to the ER and easier access to a doctor when I needed one.

While still seeing my previous PCP it was decided necessary that I get a power wheelchair. I could no longer use the power scooter. It had not been designed for me and was not functional for me due to my inability to use my arms and the inability to be able to sit with my back straight for any length of time and a weak and painful neck. We had reverted to Calvin pushing me in my lightweight wheelchair. This was quite a problem because Calvin had fibromyalgia and his back was in constant pain from three separate conditions involving his spine. Pushing me made it worse.

The following is the outline we used to demonstrate my need for a power wheelchair to the insurance company.

Reasons Why I Need a Power Wheelchair:

- ❖ Health Conditions
  - ▪ Periodic Paralysis
    - ➢ Progressive and incurable
    - ➢ Unable to take medications that could help
    - ➢ Partial Paralysis
    - ➢ Total Paralysis
    - ➢ Abortive episodes
    - ➢ Body-wide muscles weakness (myopathy)
      - ▪ Including breathing muscles
      - ▪ Heart
    - ➢ Breathing difficulties
      - ▪ On oxygen therapy
        - ◆ Oxygen levels drop to 81 during paralytic episodes and during sleep
        - ◆ Oxygen levels drop upon exertion
  - ▪ Fibromyalgia
  - ▪ Degenerative disk disease
  - ▪ Arthritis of the spine
  - ▪ Osteoporosis of the spine (bone crush stage) and hips

- Exercise intolerance
  - ➢ Heart works too hard upon any exertion
    - Speeds up
    - Out of breath
    - Weak
  - ➢ Blood pressure increases or drops
- Heart problems
  - ➢ Heart Loop Monitor implanted in my chest
    - Angina
    - Long QT interval heartbeat
    - Tachycardia (147)
    - Bradycardia (44)
    - Arrhythmias
      - ♦ PVCs, PACs, PJCs, Abnormal T-waves, Aberrants, ST segment abnormalities, SVPB/PBC
- ➢ I am unable to do almost anything but sit in a recliner
  - Everything is affected by the above

- ➢ I need to be able to get around on my own
  - My husband is disabled and cannot lift me or push me around
  - Losing/lost my independence

- ➢ My cane is not enough help
  - I don't have enough strength
  - Not enough support
  - I have a problem with balance
  - Problem for falling
    - Osteoporosis
    - Not enough strength to get up
- ➢ My walker is not good enough because I can only walk a few steps
  - I do not have enough strength
  - Not enough support
  - I have a problem with balance and unsteadiness

After a six-month wait, on Christmas Eve, I received a special power wheelchair. It includes a seat that can recline at different angles to help when I go into paralysis and to alleviate the problem, I have with sitting up straight in a chair. It is very taxing on me and can cause paralysis. It has special cushions to help alleviate the pain I feel constantly. Being in the chair aids Calvin when he has to help me during an episode of total or partial paralysis. It also gives me some independence that I did not have previously.

Home healthcare became an option as part of my management plan. I have had to use them two times last year and was able to call on them as needed for blood draws and other necessary medical needs that arise. I have "abortive attacks". These are extended periods of weakness which can last for days or even weeks. During them I am in and out of paralysis and between the episodes my muscles are so weak that I cannot sit up or hold my head up. I am unable to eat, and I am unable to do anything for myself. I sleep most of the time. During these times, Calvin may need assistance to take care of me.

My condition remains untreatable with medication, surgery, heart defibrillators or pacemakers, therefore my heart condition and muscle weakness including my breathing muscles will continue to progress. However, the good news is that it is manageable at this time.

Calvin and I, through necessity and research, have discovered how to improve the quality of my life and lessen the number and severity of my episodes of paralysis. I have gone from having five or more total body paralytic episodes a day to only one or two each month. The abortive attacks are growing shorter and coming less often. We use all natural methods.

We call it "walking a tightrope". These activities include but are not limited to a proper pH balance diet, supplements, potassium, oxygen therapy 24/7, avoiding the triggers that start the paralysis, avoiding all exertion and stress and by monitoring my vitals to include potassium levels, blood sugar levels, oxygen levels, body temperature and blood pressure.

We share these ideas and every aspect of Periodic Paralysis throughout this book in a series of articles. (However, the use of any medications or pharmaceuticals will not be discussed in this book except for the adverse effect it may have on many of us.) These are written in a series of open and heartfelt articles penned over the past several years by Calvin and me. I have written mine from the point of view of a person living with, disabled from and dying of the effects from undiagnosed and mistreated Periodic Paralysis. Calvin has written his articles from the point of view of my caregiver as he watches me living with, disabled from and dying of Periodic Paralysis before his eyes.

As we have put this book together and worked on the editing, it was my intention to edit each of our articles to update them. We have instead decided to publish some of the articles as they were originally written. We believe they will have more impact when read in their original form.

They relate the facts and our emotions in the rawest forms of frustration, anger, despair, fear, distrust, sadness, concern, pain, shock and caring, love, sharing, courage, unselfishness, faith, tenacity and hope. They relate the lies, and a lack of ethics and knowledge displayed by the uncaring, unprofessional doctors and medical professionals. They relate the mistakes made by the unknowing and caring doctors. Names have been changed or abbreviated to protect the innocent and the guilty. They describe the unbelievable and uncaring treatment by family members and friends.

Most importantly, the articles will guide the reader through finding a doctor and getting a diagnosis, to discovering the triggers that cause the paralysis and to managing the symptoms of Periodic Paralysis in all natural ways by "walking a tightrope" and hopefully, achieve a better quality of life for everyone with Periodic Paralysis.

Part II
Understanding Periodic Paralysis

Chapter Twelve
What is Periodic Paralysis?

Introduction

Part One details my medical history, an account of my characteristics, my symptoms and my progressive weakness from birth to the present, which led to my final diagnosis of Periodic Paralysis. In retrospect, it is clear that I have suffered with the disease my entire life, though it was misdiagnosed and mistreated. The lack of a correct diagnosis and proper treatment has led to total and permanent disability. The type I have is obviously inherited and the genetic code has yet to be discovered. Hopefully, this information can and will be used by physicians and other medical professionals as a tool for diagnosing others with Periodic Paralysis in a timelier manner, despite the existence of other diseases and conditions.

Part Two covers many aspects of Periodic Paralysis including, what it is, what causes it, the different forms of it, the aspects of the attacks or episodes of paralysis and the triggers that set them into motion. Each chapter presents the facts and references information based on the research and experiences of Calvin, my husband and caregiver and me, the patient living with the disorder. Each chapter will also include our personal experiences and feelings written in narrative and essay form as we progressed through the process to a diagnosis and management of this disease.

Part One begins with the "end" of my story, before the beginning, to emphasize our desire that others with Periodic Paralysis will not find themselves as totally disabled as I have become. In much the same manner, Part Two must begin with what Periodic Paralysis is "not" before we discuss what it is. This is to emphasize the complexity and misunderstood truths of Periodic Paralysis by both patients with the disorder and medical professionals who diagnose and treat them.

Periodic Paralysis is Not Our Friend

Not long after realizing I had Periodic Paralysis, I heard it referenced on the discussion boards that a few people argue that Periodic Paralysis is our "friend". This idea has been written in medical magazine articles as well and is known throughout the Periodic Paralysis community.

This idea angers me, so I decided to tell the world the truth about Periodic Paralysis in my life and the lives of others who suffer with Periodic Paralysis. In many cases, it is a cruel, devastating disease for which there is no cure, and it destroys the lives of most people who have it. I believe the "friendship" argument is doing a disservice and marginalizes those of us who have severe and totally debilitating forms of Periodic Paralysis.

If someone has a disease that they call their "friend", why would anyone want to donate money for research and treatment or to fund an organization for a disease, which is a "friend"? After all, a friend is a person whom one knows, likes, and trusts. A friend is a supporter, an ally and someone who wishes you well. A friend is a person you know well and regard with affection and trust. That being said, I must disagree with this ideation.

I believe Periodic Paralysis is not our "friend". After all, a friend does not leave you totally paralyzed. A friend does not leave you unable to walk. A friend does not leave you unable to talk. A friend does not leave you in fear. A friend does not take away your quality of life. A friend does not leave you disabled. A friend does not keep away your friends and family. A friend does not keep you from doing your favorite things. A friend does not change the relationship between you and your spouse. A friend does not make you appear to be mentally ill. A friend does not treat you poorly by the very people you most need to help you. A friend does not take away your hope, dreams and desires. So, I must disagree with this ideation that Periodic Paralysis is our "friend". Periodic Paralysis is not my "friend". Periodic Paralysis is not your "friend".

We cannot, we must not treat it as our friend. We cannot "embrace" it as some may argue. We must treat Periodic Paralysis as an enemy that we must battle diligently; daily; minute-by-minute; second by second. Only by doing so, is it possible to keep our "foe" regulated and managed in order to decrease the number and severity of paralytic episodes and the amount of possible permanent damage. We must walk a constant "tightrope" of sorts.

Periodic Paralysis is a very rare disease that in some cases steals one's life away. It is not our "friend", but rather an enemy that must be battled every second of our waking hours and sometimes while we sleep. Many people who suffer from it live in fear and despair as they seek help from doctor after doctor. Some will die before they get the help they desperately need.

Periodic Paralysis is a Disease Unlike Any Other

One of the neurologists, who diagnosed me, recently said to me that Periodic Paralysis is a disease not like any other. It is not a neuromuscular, mitochondrial or autoimmune disease nor is it a muscular dystrophy. It is in a category all its own and needs to be treated in non-conventional ways. He further stated that doctors should keep an open mind and think in unconventional ways when it comes to diagnosing and treating Periodic Paralysis.

The Basic Facts

The following is an overview of the condition gleaned from years of research and my own experience.

What is Periodic Paralysis?

Periodic Paralysis (PP) is an extremely rare, hereditary disease characterized by episodes of muscular weakness or paralysis, a total lack of muscle tone without the loss of sensation while remaining consciousness. It is passed from either the mother or the father to any of the children, male or female. [1]

Ion Channelopathies

Periodic Paralysis was one of the first Ion Channelopathies recognized. An ion channelopathy is a dysfunction of an ion channel, a microscopic tunnel in the cells of muscles called muscle fibers. Particles of potassium, sodium, chloride or calcium, which are electrically charged, known as ions, flow in and out of the cells. They regulate the contraction and relaxation of the muscle. A problem with the flow can cause paralysis.[2] Channelopathies are considered metabolic disorders. [3]

The Three Most Common Forms of Periodic Paralysis

Hypokalemic Periodic Paralysis (HypoKPP)

Paralysis results from potassium moving from the blood into muscle cells in an abnormal way. It is associated with low levels of potassium (hypokalemia) during paralytic episodes. [5]

Hyperkalemic Periodic Paralysis (HyperKPP)

Paralysis results from problems with the way the body controls sodium and potassium levels in cells. It is associated with high levels of potassium (hyperkalemia) during paralytic episodes. [6]

Andersen-Tawil Syndrome (ATS)

Paralysis results when the channel does not open properly; potassium cannot leave the cell. This disrupts the flow of potassium ions in skeletal and cardiac muscle. During paralytic episodes, ATS can be associated with low potassium, high potassium or shifts in the normal (normokalemia) ranges of potassium. Andersen-Tawil Syndrome is discussed in more detail later in this section. [7]

A large percentage of the above known types of Periodic Paralysis have identified genetic markers. This means they can be diagnosed by DNA testing.

Criteria for Making a Genetic Diagnosis

Hypokalemic Periodic Paralysis is caused by a problem in the SCN4A *or CACNA1S* genes. Hyperkalemic Periodic Paralysis is caused by problems in the *SCN4A* gene. Andersen-Tawil Syndrome is caused by a problem in the *KCNJ2* gene. Diagnosis based on genes is referred to as a genetic diagnosis. [5, 6, 7]

Some patients are diagnosed by the symptoms and characteristics. This is called a clinical diagnosis. Those who are diagnosed clinically have symptoms and characteristics identical to others who have known genetic codes. One who is diagnosed with ATS clinically is said to have ATS Type 2 to differentiate. [7]

Symptoms

Although HypoKPP, HyperKPP and ATS are forms of periodic paralysis the mechanism, which creates the muscle weakness and paralysis, is different as described above and the symptoms before and accompanying the paralysis vary. Symptoms can range from simple weakness to total body paralysis with life-threatening heart arrhythmias and tachycardia, breathing problems and choking. Death can occur in some rare cases. The episodes may last from a few minutes to several hours or for many days. The speed with which the potassium shifts may cause symptoms to occur suddenly and without warning or there may be a gradual progression into the weakness or paralysis. [8]

Abortive attacks may also affect some individuals. Occasionally, the common symptoms may begin but the full attack or paralysis may not occur. The person is left with extreme weakness and other symptoms such as extreme fatigue. This may last for hours, days, weeks or even months. In some cases the abortive attack is totally debilitating and actually worse than the episodes of paralysis. [8]

The following symptoms may accompany the paralytic attacks. These are based on my own experiences and the experiences of others I have talked with. Some may cross over. (It is best to use a cardy meter, discussed later in the book, to measure the amounts of potassium before treating, especially if one has ATS or an ATS-like condition.)

Hypokalemic Periodic Paralysis

One who suffers with Hypokalemic Periodic Paralysis may experience a variety of symptoms in relationship to their hypokalemic paralytic attacks including but not limited to the following: varying degrees of muscle paralysis, varying degrees of muscle weakness and stiffness, muscle aches, cramps, odd sensations, rapid and irregular pulse, breathing difficulties, irritation, unusual thirst, stomach and abdominal irregularity, excessive perspiration, unusual tiredness and bladder dumping.

What is Periodic Paralysis?

Hyperkalemic Periodic Paralysis

Someone who suffers with Hyperkalemic Periodic Paralysis may experience a variety of symptoms in relationship to their paralytic attacks including but not limited to the following: varying degrees of muscle paralysis, varying degrees of muscle weakness and cramps, muscle aches, cramps, muscle twitching, tightness in leg muscles, odd leg sensations, rapid and irregular pulse, heart palpitations and irregular heartbeat, breathing difficulties, irritation, unusual thirst, stomach and abdominal irregularity, excessive perspiration, unusual tiredness and bladder dumping, sleepiness and word slurring.

Andersen-Tawil Syndrome

One who suffers with Andersen-Tawil Syndrome may experience a variety of symptoms in relationship to their ATS paralytic episodes including but not limited to any of the symptoms from above depending on whether the attack is hypokalemic, hyperkalemic or normokalemic. They also have long QT interval heartbeats, a life-threatening arrhythmia, which is a marker for ATS. Ventricular arrhythmias are common as is fainting. [7] (More detailed information in Chapter Thirteen).

Triggers

The periodic muscle weakness or paralysis is triggered by a wide variety of activities such as exercise or sleep; foods such as carbohydrates or meat; conditions such as heat or cold; medications such as antibiotics or muscle relaxers; compounds such as caffeine or salt or simply resting after exercise. Many of the triggers are the same for most people but some of the triggers can be unique to each person or the type of Periodic Paralysis. [4]

Treatment

Most individuals with Hypokalemic Periodic Paralysis are able to control the symptoms and paralytic attacks with one or two forms of potassium and avoiding the things that trigger them. Individuals with Hyperkalemic Periodic Paralysis symptoms and paralytic attacks can control their symptoms and paralytic attacks with a diet high in carbohydrates and sugar and by avoiding the triggers. [4, 8]

Controlling the symptoms and paralytic attacks in people with Andersen-Tawil Syndrome is much more difficult. This is due to the fact that these individuals suffer from paralysis due to potassium levels that can be low, high or in normal ranges. Taking potassium may make the symptoms worse. Also, individuals with ATS are usually unable to take any forms of medication. Managing the heart issues by surgery is also a problem because anesthesia can trigger paralysis and deadly arrythmia. For these individuals, natural methods are the best way to manage the symptoms.

Prognosis

For most people with Periodic Paralysis the weakness and paralysis are intermittent. There is a beginning and end and between the episodes the individual is normal. However, for some individuals the weakness can linger or become permanent. Some people will become disabled and require the use of a power wheelchair. In some cases, ATS can cause death. [8]

More information on each of the above issues is discussed in great detail throughout the following chapters.

Chapter Thirteen
Andersen-Tawil Syndrome

Introduction

In Chapter Twelve Periodic Paralysis is discussed in terms of what it is and what it is not. It has been determined that it is certainly not our "friend" as some would argue. Nor is it a neuromuscular (though that is how it is usually categorized), mitochondrial or autoimmune disease nor is it a muscular dystrophy. It is in a category all its own. It is an Ion Channelopathy, a type of metabolic disorder, a dysfunction of an ion channel, which opens and closes in response to specific signals. Potassium is allowed through the channels in error. The potassium enters the muscles causing paralysis. There are several types, Hyperkalemic Periodic Paralysis, high potassium: Hypokalemic Periodic Paralysis, low potassium and Normokalemic Periodic Paralysis, with normal potassium levels. The symptoms, triggers and characteristics were discussed as well as the types of treatment and management.

Andersen-Tawil Syndrome (ATS) will be discussed in great detail in this chapter. This is due to the fact that I have a form of Periodic Paralysis, which is much like Andersen-Tawil Syndrome, as do other members of my family. Most of the over forty members of our discussion board and their families also believe they have Andersen-Tawil Syndrome or a variant of it.

What is important to note here is that specialists in the field, of which there a very few worldwide, argue that only one hundred cases exist on the entire planet. Of those, only about sixty are diagnosed genetically based on their DNA and known as ATS1 and about forty are diagnosed clinically; that is, based on their symptoms and known as ATS2. ATS1 and ATS2 are indistinguishable, impossible to tell apart. [7, 14]

Based on our experience we have concluded that there are many, many more individuals and families who have a variant of Andersen-Tawil Syndrome which has yet to be named or discovered genetically. These people are overlooked and not included in the count, because they have other diseases and conditions, coexisting with the ATS. The "specialists" in the field normally do not see patients. They are involved in research and probably get their funding for only the "pure" form of ATS. As far as I know, they do not study, diagnose or treat anyone who has any variation or added conditions.

This leaves hundreds, maybe even thousands, of people who are being overlooked, undiagnosed and untreated by the medical profession. Many are treated with scorn and labeled as having conversion disorder. All of them are suffering just like others with Periodic Paralysis who have a known genetic code and are diagnosed. In fact, they are suffering more due to the stress of not being diagnosed and not being believed.

I was diagnosed with Andersen-Tawil Syndrome after first being diagnosed as having Periodic Paralysis by a neurologist. I was not diagnosed by a specialist but by a renal specialist who saw me in paralysis, studied my medical records, my symptoms and characteristics, studied the information about ATS I provided for him, and with everything else being ruled out, he had no other choice but to diagnose me with a "form" of Andersen-Tawil Syndrome, as he called it.

Upon traveling a thousand miles to another state (the entire time in and out of paralysis); hoping to get some help with my severe symptoms; to see a "specialist", I was told that he did not believe I had ATS. He said I had other symptoms that did not fit the ATS description and the characteristics I had were "subtle". Although he discussed the possibility of it being a variant unique to my family and me and it would probably be named after us, he did not add that information to the letter he sent to the referring doctor, nor did he suggest any way for that to happen. It also was never discussed that I could very well have more than one disease existing with ATS. So, for my family, the others and me with ATS-like symptoms, it will be discussed in detail. Someday, the genetic code will be found, probably too late for some if us.

The Facts

Andersen-Tawil Syndrome (ATS) named after Ellen Andersen and Dr. Al-Rabi Tawil is a serious form of Periodic Paralysis. It has the potential for being fatal due to serious arrhythmias of the heart, which can accompany the attacks of paralysis. The underlying cause is only partially understood, and no treatments exist. [9] Andersen-Tawil Syndrome was given a name in 1971. One parent usually passes it, and it is an uncommon cause of periodic paralysis (accounting for approximately 10% of all periodic paralysis cases). It is characterized by three particular elements: periods of paralysis, distinctive face, skull and skeletal abnormalities, and prolonged QT interval heartbeat and abnormal cardiac rhythms usually ventricular in origin. However, individuals affected may display only one or two of the three components. [7, 72]

Some of these components and symptoms were found in my mother, possibly through her father, and many of her descendants, specifically, two of her three sons and me, her only daughter. Many of her grandchildren and great grandchildren also have varying degrees of the characteristics and symptoms.

Some of the manifestations of this condition are serious and life threatening. Each family member of someone diagnosed with ATS should be well educated about this syndrome, in particular, regarding the episodes of paralysis (full body or partial), the heart complications, the strange effects of most medications and the serious complications of anesthesia.

The following information describes the scope of Periodic Paralysis in the several forms in which it is manifested. Andersen-Tawil Syndrome is a hypokalemic (low potassium) form, though it can also be seen with high potassium or normal potassium levels.

An individual is born with Andersen-Tawil Syndrome and symptoms may begin in early childhood or not until later in life. Members of the same family can have varying degrees of it or some of the characteristics without actually having it.

During an attack, brought on by many triggers to include carbohydrates, sugar, medications, exercise, heat, cold, periods of sitting too long, stress (good or bad), etc.; potassium leaves the organs it belongs in and goes into the muscles where it does not belong and paralyzes the muscles (totally or partially). The depletion of the potassium in the other organs can cause symptoms such as irregular heartbeat, weakness, fainting, numbness, tingling, breathing issues, choking/swallowing problems, and exercise intolerance. After many years the body can become permanently weakened.

It is important to get a diagnosis for proper treatment to avoid the permanent disabilities. It is also important so one can avoid the triggers and hopefully control the episodes as much as possible. Most over-the-counter medication, as well as those prescribed by physicians, such as antibiotics and painkillers can cause serious consequences. Many medications can cause an opposite effect such as sleeping aids can keep you awake and agitated.

Executive Functioning (EF) Disorder can accompany ATS. There are three primary layers of executive functions: self-regulation, organization and high order reasoning skills. It is associated with many disabilities: attention deficit hyperactivity disorder (AD/HD), learning disabilities (LD), tourette syndrome (TS), obsessive compulsive disorder (OCD), autism, depression, bipolar, etc. It is important to have these conditions diagnosed as early as possible for proper treatment, training, and education.

Distinctive Face, Skull and Skeletal Abnormalities of ATS

- ❖ Widely spaced eyes.
- ❖ Short stature.
- ❖ Scoliosis.
- ❖ Webbed toes or fingers (partial or total between second and third toes).
- ❖ Unusual short fingers.
- ❖ Low set ears.
- ❖ Broad forehead.
- ❖ Small jaw.
- ❖ Protruding jaw.
- ❖ Broad nasal root.

Other Characteristics of ATS

- ❖ Ventricular arrhythmia.
- ❖ Abnormal heart rhythm.
- ❖ Long QT interval heartbeat.
- ❖ Irregular heartbeat.
- ❖ Discomfort.
- ❖ Fainting caused by irregular heartbeat.
- ❖ Dental abnormalities (born with missing teeth & late or non-loss of baby teeth).
- ❖ Low-set ears.
- ❖ Widely spaced eyes.
- ❖ Abnormal curving of fingers (little fingers curve inward).
- ❖ Abnormal curving of toes.
- ❖ Short stature.

A Few Other Lesser-Known Anomalies

❖ Clubbed thumbs.
❖ Short opening for the eyes between the eyelids.
❖ Abnormal smallness of the head.
❖ Slowed degree of maturation of child's bones.
❖ Looseness of the muscles and soft tissue surrounding a joint.
❖ Small cheekbones.
❖ An abnormally low position (drooping) of the upper eyelid.
❖ Cleft palate.
❖ High arched palate.

The above characteristics and abnormalities can be quite subtle, only partially present or seen in members of the family without periods of paralysis. [7, 14, 72]

Criteria for Making a Genetic Diagnosis

❖ Testing of DNA will show mutations on chromosome 17q23 in KCNJ2. [73]

Criteria for Making a Clinical Diagnosis

❖ A clinically definite diagnosis requires two of the following three features:
  ➢ Periods of Paralysis.
  ➢ Long QT interval heartbeats or ventricular arrhythmias (identified on ECG or Holter Monitor).
  ➢ Characteristics typical of ATS including:
    ◆ Ears that are low set,
    ◆ Wide eyes,
    ◆ Small jaw,
    ◆ Curved fifth finger,

♦ Webbed fingers or toes (the second and third
♦ Toes)

❖ A diagnosis can be made also with one of the three characteristics listed above and a diagnosed family member having two of the three. [72]

(I should note here that I was diagnosed based on all three features. Other family members of mine should be able to be diagnosed with ATS, or at the very least Periodic Paralysis, using my diagnosis. However, no other doctor will diagnose my other family members, including a brother and a daughter, who have periods of paralysis, ventricular arrhythmias and characteristics listed above).

Conditions That Can Accompany Andersen-Tawil Syndrome

Malignant Hyperthermia

Malignant Hyperthermia is a rare, hereditary, life-threatening muscle disease that causes serious muscle contractions and high fever with the use of some general anesthesia. [10, 11]

Neuroleptic Malignant Hyperthermia

Neuroleptic Malignant Hyperthermia is a rare, neurological, life-threatening disorder that causes rigid muscles, a raise in body temperature, delirium, cognitive problems and autonomic nervous system issues from taking anti-psychotic drugs. [12]

Serotonin Syndrome

Serotonin Syndrome is a rare life-threatening reaction to certain drugs that causes too much serotonin to be produced. The increase produces symptoms in just minutes to hours.

Symptoms include agitation, diarrhea, rapid heart rate, hallucinations, fever, coordination loss, vomiting, nausea and sudden blood pressure changes. [13]

Prognosis

For most people with Periodic Paralysis the weakness and paralysis are intermittent. There is a beginning and end and between the episodes the individual is normal. However, this is not the case for most individuals with Andersen-Tawil Syndrome, a very serious, form of Periodic Paralysis. It is a life-threatening condition due to the heart arrhythmias, especially the long QT interval heartbeat, that accompany the periodic paralysis attacks. Most medications and anesthetics can be lethal, due to the paradoxal effects. There is no treatment due to the problem with shifting potassium levels in low, high and normal ranges. Surgery for heart issues is not usually preformed due to problems with the anesthesia. The episodes of paralysis are usually more serious involving breathing and choking issues. Without being able to use medications, or surgery, the disease becomes progressive. Muscles continue to weaken, including the breathing muscles. Heart issues progress. The most common cause of death is cardiac arrest due to heart arrhythmia or respiratory failure due to weakened breathing muscles. [8, 27]

Period Paralysis Plus 10 Syndrome A Form of ATS?

We know there are three types of Periodic Paralysis: Hypokalemic Periodic Paralysis with symptoms from low potassium, Hyperkalemic Periodic Paralysis with symptoms from high potassium and Andersen-Tawil Syndrome with symptoms from low, high and normal ranges of potassium. A large percentage of these forms of Periodic Paralysis have known genetic DNA codes and a smaller amount have unknown genetic DNA codes at this time. Researchers continue to search for the as yet undiscovered markers.

In the meantime, some individuals with unknown genetic DNA codes are lucky enough to find a doctor who is willing to give them a diagnosis for Periodic Paralysis based on their symptoms, but most doctors refuse to give a diagnosis. This is usually based on the lack of a true understanding of the disease and shortage of the most recent information on the part of the physician.

It is difficult to believe that a doctor who sees a patient who is having periods of partial or total paralysis, with fluctuating blood pressure and heart rate among the other common symptoms of the syndrome, everything else ruled out, would not give the patient a diagnosis of Periodic Paralysis. What could be the reason for not wanting to help someone who is suffering?

Calvin and I created a website to help others with Periodic Paralysis (Periodic Paralysis Network), especially those who cannot get help from their doctors or who cannot take the traditional medications. We have a discussion board on the website. We currently have over forty members. Most of them have Anderson-Tawil Syndrome ATS-like symptoms and characteristics, as do other members of their families. Very few of them can get a diagnosis for Periodic Paralysis let alone ATS.

Most of them have been looking for answers for many years and have been to a plethora of doctors and specialists. Nearly all of them have been humiliated by being diagnosed with conversion disorder or have been called hypochondriacs in their medical records.

The interesting thing about these individuals and their other family members is that they all have more than one condition co-existing with their periods of paralysis or muscle weakness, problems with potassium shifting and heart issues. As in my case, the other conditions were masking the real disease, or the medications were creating symptoms that looked like something else.

As we discussed these issues among ourselves over time, it became clear that there were too many similarities for this to be a coincidence. I decided to take a survey of our members to discover the other diagnosed diseases or conditions plaguing them. I wanted to know how many of them were the same for each of us. The following are the results:

First, although none of us has a known genetic code that has been discovered yet, we all have symptoms of periods of paralysis, total and/or partial, which involve the shifting of potassium, either, up, down or in normal ranges.

Next, we all have symptoms of blood pressure changes during them, which can be up or down or fluctuating. We all also have heart arrhythmias (some long QT) and tachycardia or bradycardia or both during the attacks. Most have problems breathing and some with choking. (These fit the ATS description. It is certainly ATS-like.)

Third, we have at least ten other identified and diagnosed conditions, which are the same. The conditions, which appeared over and over again in each one of us are:

❖ Fibromyalgia/Chronic Fatigue.
❖ Osteoarthritis.
❖ Degenerative disk disease.
❖ Heart problems, tachycardia, bradycardia, arrhythmia,
❖ long QT).
❖ Pain disorders.
❖ Blood pressure problems, (high or low).
❖ Sleep disorders, (insomnia, sleep apnea).

* ❖ Constipation (hemorrhoids).
* ❖ Exercise intolerance,
* ❖ Female organ dysfunctions.

It is certainly ATS-like. Almost everyone that contacts me believes they have ATS due to their symptoms and characteristics. However, no ATS specialists will see us, and those that do get seen are told it is not ATS because of the other things accompanying it. These specialists appear to be "purists" studying only the pure and clear-cut cases.

I have chosen to no longer include "ATS" in my medical description. I do not want to be linked to the "purists" in any way because they appear to discount us, and our conditions. It is unfortunate for them because they will not be able to get the credit for discovering yet another form of Periodic Paralysis.

It is overwhelming what we individually and as a group are enduring every day. None of us have less than ten diagnosed conditions.

The following is the list of the other symptoms, diseases and conditions that were listed in the survey.

Cyclic vomiting syndrome, high cholesterol, diabetes type 2, peripheral polyneuropathy, arachnoids cysts in the brain, loss of peripheral vision, poly cystic ovarian disease, migraines, osteoporosis (bone crush stage in spine and hips), spina bifida oculta, crooked little fingers, small brain ischemia, intolerance to most medications, paradoxal effect to most medications, hypoglycemia, intolerance to anesthesia, cataracts, costochondritis, gluten intolerance, fibrocystic disease, esophageal reflux, esophageal hernia, diverticulitis, hearing loss, lactic acidosis, metabolic acidosis, hypoxemia, (low blood oxygen), restless leg syndrome, stress fracture of the foot, neuromas (nerve tumor) in both feet, painful and tight calf muscles, fibroid tumor (uterus), ovarian cysts, chronic bladder infections, born without eye teeth or wisdom teeth, small jaw, 2-3 toe partial webbing, totally webbed second-third toes, crooked little finger, extremely dry skin, gerd, weak eye muscles, fasciculations, temporomandibular disorders, reflex sympathetic dystrophy, cervical and uterine cancer, uterine and ovarian cysts, vertigo, high clotting, blood clots, asthma, low set ears, hypermobile joints, gastritis, syncope, muscle spasms, depression, obsessive compulsive disorder, memory loss (short term), chronic fatigue, edema, unnamed lumps in breasts, herpes simplex A (lips-cold sores), gastroparesis, myalgia, myositis, osteoarthritis, myoclonic jerks, teeth problems (still have baby teeth as an adult, impacted teeth, crowded teeth), dysphagia (trouble swallowing), lumbar spinal stenosis, many cysts, fatty tumors, hyperthyroid, clotting disorder, memory deficit, compressed pituitary, kidney cyst, allergies, goiter, hardening of the arteries in legs, trouble climbing stairs, low platelet count, mastectomy and hysterectomy, straight spine, vertigo, tinnitus, atrial septal defect, complete heart block, scoliosis, pitting edema, thyroid hormone resistance disease, seizures, cluster headaches, severe sleep apnea, rectocele, pulmonary hypertension, candida, acute pancreatitis, chronic pancreatitis, Barret's esophagus, heart attack, gall bladder issues, carpal tunnel, exercise intolerance, and kidney stones.

At this point it is difficult to know if the other symptoms, diseases and conditions are at all related to the Periodic Paralysis in each of us, but it would seem somewhat likely. New research indicates many of the above conditions are also ion channelopathies, forms of metabolic disorder. They include fibromyalgia, malignant hyperthermia, chronic fatigue, long QT syndrome, seizures, congenital hypoglycemia, inherited cardiac arrythmias, migraines, involuntary movement, epilepsy, some autoimmune diseases and hypertension. [14, 9]

Also, many of the symptoms and conditions listed, which are coexisting with Period Paralysis, can certainly be related to the basic shifting of potassium, and other ions at the same time, in and out of our muscles and other organs, damage is obviously done creating conditions like osteoporosis and degenerative disk disease.

It is obvious that many of the issues are definitely Andersen-Tawil Syndrome-like: intolerance to anesthesia, exercise intolerance, crooked little fingers, born without eye teeth or wisdom teeth, small jaw, 2-3 toe partial webbing, totally webbed second-third toes, syncope (fainting), teeth problems (still have baby teeth as an adult, impacted teeth, crowded teeth), dysphagia (trouble swallowing), intolerance to most medications, paradoxal effect to most medications, low set ears, heart problems, tachycardia, bradycardia, arrhythmia, (long QT), blood pressure problems, (high or low).

New ion channelopathy connections are being discovered every day, but not fast enough to help people with, as yet unknown variants of, Periodic Paralysis, according to a physiologist who recently contacted me. He told me thousands of connections have been made to date, thus leading to possible cures or treatments for those conditions. My own research indicated that pharmaceutical companies are working on new drugs aimed at treating the ion channelopathies.

It has been suggested that some very expensive DNA testing may be able to pinpoint the mutation causing our Periodic Paralysis Plus 10 Syndrome and it would be best to use as many family members in the study as possible. At this point there is no funding available nor any institutions or organizations willing to work with us in this endeavor. So, for now, it is my hope that someday the information I provide in this chapter and in this book can and will be used to locate the genetic mutation and give it a name, thus hopefully finding a cure or proper treatment.

Update

As we are editing and getting ready for publishing, there has been a new development regarding DNA testing. My family and I have been accepted into a genetic study. This particular study is designed for individuals who have been clinically diagnosed (based on symptoms) with Andersen-Tawil Syndrome and later DNA testing ruled out any of the known mutations.

A blood sample was drawn from me has been sent to be studied. It is the plan of the genetic specialists to do exome sequencing to rule out known genes. I was told there are seven of them. I have had only the three main ones ruled out, but there are more rare genes they want to rule out before enrolling more of my family members. They believe there is a new or undiagnosed form of Andersen-Tawil Syndrome yet to be discovered. A few other families are also in the study. Apparently, each of the families has ATS-like symptoms with many more medical issues, just as I have described above. (See more about genetic testing in Chapter Thirty-One.) It is their plan to do "exome sequencing" to rule out the "known genes". I was told there are "7 of them". I have had only the "main 3 ruled out", but there are "more rare genes" they want to rule out before enrolling more of my family members in the study (see Appendix for photographs of subtle ATS characteristics).

Chapter Fourteen
What is an Ion Channelopathy?

Introduction

Part One details my medical history, that is, my life with Periodic Paralysis and Part Two details the aspects of Periodic Paralysis. So far, we know the basic facts about the three forms, Hypokalemic Periodic Paralysis, Hyperkalemic Periodic Paralysis and Normokalemic Periodic Paralysis as well as Andersen-Tawil Syndrome. This includes symptoms, triggers, treatment and prognosis. Chapter Twelve begins with what Periodic Paralysis is not, as well as what it is. This chapter will continue the discussion of just what Periodic Paralysis is not as well as what it is, an ion channelopathy, which is a complicated and complex system. We have decided to not go into great detail about ion channelopathies but will discuss the basic facts in as easy to understand terms as possible.

Ion Channelopathies are Metabolic Disorders

As discussed previously, Periodic Paralysis is not a neuromuscular, mitochondrial or autoimmune disease nor is it a muscular dystrophy. It is a rare condition like no other, called an ion channelopathy. Ion channelopathies were first recognized in 1971 and Periodic Paralysis was one of the first to be discovered. An ion channelopathy is a dysfunction of an ion channel. [2,15]

Ion channels are like a microscopic tunnel in the cells of muscles. The tunnels are called muscle fibers. Ions, which are molecules or atoms, flow in and out of the muscle cells through membranes or gates. Each of the gates is shaped exactly for the correct ion or molecule to enter. The ions are made up of what we call minerals, electrolytes or proteins. Some of the common ions are potassium, sodium, magnesium, chloride and calcium. They are electrically charged, and each has its own size or shape, so to speak. If the gates or membranes are faulty in size or shape, an inefficient or improper flow through the membranes can and does cause muscle weakness and paralysis because they regulate contraction and relaxation of the muscle.

Through research, I have discovered that channelopathies are classified as a class four metabolic disorder. Disorders of metabolism are usually inherited and are involved in chemical and physical processing, which use and make energy in the body. These processes include breathing, circulation of blood, food and nutrient digestion, elimination of waste through bowel and bladder and temperature regulation.

Unfortunately, ion channelopathies are not usually categorized nor listed in medical writing or studies as metabolic disorders. This poses a problem for recognition, diagnosis and treatment by physicians and other medical professionals. I have found and heard Periodic Paralysis, which is a channelopathy, referred to as, a neuromuscular disease (affecting muscles and/or nerves also known as myoneural), a muscular dystrophy (wasting of muscle and eventual early death), and a disease of the nervous system (nothing to do with the nervous system), therefore, none of these is correct. Periodic Paralysis is a metabolic disorder, a condition which is based in the faulty cellular level of how energy is produced in our bodies. [16]

To clarify, even further, Periodic Paralysis is a channelopathy which is a mineral metabolic disorder. Metabolism disorders involving minerals are conditions in which there is either not enough or an overabundance of minerals in an indivdual's blood. Minerals have many functions in metabolism and the functions of the human body. They are important in bone and muscle building and growth. Organs, cells and tissues need minerals in order to function properly. So, a dysfunction of minerals in the body affects many processes and functions.

What is an Ion Channelopathy?

Potassium, the main mineral involved in Periodic Paralysis, is involved in making proteins from the amino acids and plays a role in carbohydrate metabolism, so a dysfunction involving it, can affect more than just muscles. [2, 15]

The doctors we see for this condition are almost always neurologists. This is a problem when seeking a diagnosis and treatment because Periodic Paralysis is not neuromuscular disease and although it affects the muscles, the treatments involved should not be those used for neuromuscular diseases. Some confusion about this may come from the fact that the Muscular Dystrophy Association (MDA) lists it as one of the diseases they research and treat (more information on this to be discussed later). They are known for diagnosing and treating muscle wasting diseases. Periodic Paralysis is not a muscle wasting disease though on rare occasion there can be muscle wasting.

The probable reason we all end up with a neurologist, or a number of them, is because the symptoms look like a neurological disease. Neurologists, however, can be good for ruling out a neuromuscular disease, but at the point it is ruled out, then an individual should be referred to a doctor specializing in metabolic disorders. However, this is the point when conversion disorder or hypochondria becomes the diagnosis instead.

This clarification in the medical field could help us to get better treatment and quicker diagnoses, by seeing the correct physicians. That being said, an endocrinologist should be the correct doctor to see. However, I find that many of them are not aware of Periodic Paralysis. The last one I saw, knew nothing about it and refused to help me. He could not get me out of his office fast enough. He told me I needed to find a specialist somewhere in the country specifically researching Periodic Paralysis and ion channelopathies. I told him, "Long story short, been there, done that" and exited the examination room. He kept my co-pay and billed my insurance for an office call.

Last summer, the Andersen-Tawil Syndrome specialist I saw in another state, was a neurologist and referred in his findings letter to my referring physician, that I was on oxygen. He believed this to be problematic because "oxygen does not typically help patients with neuromuscular diseases". Surprise!!! Surprise!!! Periodic Paralysis is not a neuromuscular disease!!! It is a channelopathy, a fourth-class metabolic disorder, which is a mineral metabolic disorder! (The use of oxygen is discussed later in another chapter.)

When we as patients see a doctor, we are assigned a diagnosis, disease or reasons for that visit. Each patient has a form, usually in triplicate, attached to their chart. The form has a large number of possible diseases or diagnoses listed with a number assigned to each. The diseases are categorized. These names and numbers are universal, used worldwide. They are the method for assigning a diagnosis and for billing insurance companies. By the end of the visit, several of the diseases may have been checked. This system is called the ICD-10 Codes Registry, (International Classification of Diseases). [17]

Periodic Paralysis has been assigned the number: G723 (G72.3) and is categorized as a disease of the nervous system and further sub-categorized as a disease of the myoneural junction (also known as neuromuscular) and muscle. Although it is an ion channelopathy, a mineral metabolic disorder, it is listed as a nervous system disorder, the type being a myoneural junction and muscle disorder. A myoneural junction is where nerves and muscles connect. The muscles and nerves respond to the neurotransmitter acetylcholine and cause the muscle to contract. A myoneural junction disease is characterized as a condition in which strength in the muscle fluctuates due to use of the muscle, so

What is an Ion Channelopathy?

Periodic Paralysis is not a myoneural junction disorder.

Often in medical literature, Periodic Paralysis is listed as a muscle myopathy. This simply means a muscle disease. It is listed as such because it is a condition, which affects the muscles and ICD-10 Codes Registry, and HIPAA Compliance Validation Services has chosen to categorize it in that way. Muscle myopathies are either inherited or acquired. Periodic Paralysis is categorized as an inherited muscle myopathy. These are further broken down into more categories including: inflammatory, infectious, endocrine, toxic, metabolic etc. [18]

Since it is a channelopathy, which is a mineral metabolic disorder affecting muscles, it is a metabolic myopathy or a metabolic muscle disease. Therefore, it has been classified as a muscle myopathy, not to be confused with neuromuscular diseases, muscular dystrophies or diseases of the nervous system.

In review Period Paralysis is an ion channelopathy, a fourth-class metabolic disorder, which is a mineral metabolic disorder. It affects muscles and it is therefore categorized as a muscle myopathy which means it is a disease of the muscles. However, it is a disease in and of itself and very different from the other muscle myopathies, such as the muscular dystrophies, the nervous system diseases and the neuromuscular diseases. It therefore needs to be recognized, diagnosed and treated in much different ways than the other myopathies.

This creates a problem for finding a doctor who can and will treat Periodic Paralysis. This is discussed in detail in another chapter, but due to the unique issues relating to it, in my opinion, it is best to search until you can find a Primary Care Physician who is willing to learn and research the disease with and for you. Also, be sure to let your doctor know the number ICD-10 G72.3 is the one he or she needs to check off on your HIPAA Compliance Validation form for your diagnosis of Periodic Paralysis.

Metabolic Disorder

Fourth Class = Mineral Metabolic Disorder (potassium, sodium, calcium)

Ion Channelopathy = C23.550.177

Affects Muscles

Muscle Myopathy = G72.3[2]

Muscle = Affected by Potassium (Mineral)

Metabolic Muscle Myopathy. [19, 20]

In conclusion, if you have access to a computer connected to the Internet there is a wealth of information available to read about ion channelopathies. The study of ion channelopathies has been around for several decades and there are a number of diseases attributed to the malfunction of ion channels. In very simplistic terms each cell has an outer membrane. Every substance inside our body has chemical and electrical properties. The cell membrane regulates the passage of chemical substances and electrical charges. Approximately 95% of the body's potassium is contained within the cells. The other 5% is contained in the blood stream. The kidneys help regulate serum blood potassium levels in the body. Diseased kidneys will alter serum blood supply of potassium and can cause muscle paralysis especially in someone who also suffers with an ion channelopathy induced mutation or chronic disease. Causes of potassium induced muscle paralysis are difficult to diagnose.

Chapter Fifteen
Description of Paralytic Attacks

Introduction

We know what Periodic Paralysis is and is not. It is not our "friend" nor is it a neuromuscular, mitochondrial, or an autoimmune disease. It is in a category of its own. It is an ion channelopathy, a dysfunction of an ion channel, a form of metabolic disorder. There are several types including Hyperkalemic Periodic Paralysis, Hypokalemic Periodic Paralysis, and Normokalemic Periodic Paralysis. There are periods of paralysis involved with each type. Symptoms, triggers and characteristics were discussed, and types of treatment and management were addressed. Andersen-Tawil Syndrome was discussed at length as well as the possibility of a new form of Periodic Paralysis we call Periodic Paralysis Plus 10 Syndrome.

This chapter will discuss at length the various ways in which the paralytic episodes can manifest themselves. Depending on the potassium levels; high, low or in normal ranges found in the blood serum levels, (to be discussed later), and the speed with which the potassium shifts, the episodes or attacks can be markedly different. Episodes may be as simple as dizziness, numbness or tingling, passing out, sudden dropping or falling to the ground or partial paralysis. They may be as serious as full body paralysis including heart arrhythmia, choking, the cessation of breathing and cardiac arrest. Attacks may happen as often as several a day or one or two in a lifetime. They may last from just a few minutes to hours at a time. Some individuals with known genetic markers for Periodic Paralysis may never go into paralysis.

I wrote the following to present to my doctors to describe what was happening to me periodically, before I knew about Periodic Paralysis.

My Symptoms During Episodes

"Usually, I wake up in the morning and I am paralyzed. I find I can't move. I cannot open my eyes. My mouth is open. I cannot breathe through my nose. I have urges to swallow but cannot so there is a choking sound in my throat every few minutes. Sometimes my heart will race or beat irregularly, though usually, there is no problem with my heart. My mouth is very dry. I cannot speak

As I begin to come out of it, my mouth will start to get saliva, my eyes will open but I can only see what is in front of me, since I cannot move my head. Sometimes my eyes will jerk around when I first open them, usually jerking up. My body will sometimes jerk a little. Sometimes there is a big breath my body will take.

Sometimes, I will go back into it. My eyes close, I feel very hot, and all the symptoms return. Sometimes there will be a few jerks as I go back into it.

During all of this I am awake and am aware of everything going on around me. Sometimes I begin to cry, due to the frustration, and fear. I can feel the tears running down my cheeks.

If I have these at times other than upon waking, the symptoms are the same. I get a strange sensation of heat body wide, usually beginning in my back. My eyes will close and then my body goes limp. I may have a few jerks as I am going limp. My mouth will open, and I am in it... unable to move, speak or open my eyes.

Sometimes, I do not go too deep. It is all the same, but I am able to open my eyes and can speak a little with a tight tongue and tight lips. My mouth is still open, however. I cannot move my body.

Once one of these begins, it may last up to 45 minutes to an hour, or can be as short as about ten minutes, if it is a second or third one in a row.

It takes about fifteen to thirty minutes to come out of it all the way. I am always left with lingering weakness for many hours that can linger into days. Speaking is difficult. Walking is difficult. My arms and hands come back sooner than my legs. I begin to get feeling back in my body. I can move my lips. I begin to breathe thru my nose again. It is difficult to speak or move but it gradually comes back. Speech is very difficult; my lips do not want to move. My tongue is difficult to move. I will suddenly have an urgency to urinate. If, at this point, I get help to the bathroom, I am like a rag doll, especially my legs. My arms flail, like a child just learning to stand and walk, balancing herself.

For many hours, I remain too weak to do much of anything but sit up in bed or sit in a recliner. I must use my walker or a wheelchair.

It is difficult to know what brings these episodes on. I know that sleep has something to do with some of them, but not all of them. I know that sometimes, when I wake up during the night with an urgency to urinate, I am coming out of one, because I have all the symptoms previously discussed. My arms and hands and legs are numb, and feeling is just coming back. My mouth is tight and dry. Walking is difficult." (May 28, 2010)

Symptoms That Accompany the Paralytic Attacks

The symptoms that follow are based on my own experiences and the experiences of others I have talked with and from research. Some may over-lap, so it is best to use a cardy meter (discussed later in the book), to measure the levels of potassium before treating, especially if one has ATS or an ATS-like condition before treating based on the symptoms.

Hypokalemic Periodic Paralysis Symptoms

When potassium shifts into lower ranges in normal individuals, hypokalemia, low potassium levels in the blood, will occur for anyone and a myriad of symptoms can be experienced. Potassium regulates contractions of smooth muscles so when potassium is low muscle twitches, muscle spasms, charley horses and restless leg syndrome can occur. It plays a part in arranging the energy sources in the body so low levels of potassium can cause one to feel tired, fatigued and achy. It can also cause one to feel anxious, irritable and depressed. Potassium stops the destruction of bone, so when levels are low, osteoporosis can develop. Very low levels of potassium in the body can be dangerous, even deadly.

If an individual has Hypokalemic Periodic Paralysis and potassium shifts into lower ranges, he or she can and will experience a combination of the same myriad of symptoms as well as paralysis and it can be equally as dangerous and deadly.

When potassium levels are low which is usually between 2.5 to 3.5 mEq/L, the following symptoms can occur: tiredness, pain in the muscles, cramping, upset stomach, constipation, lightheadedness, depression, mood swings.

Potassium levels below 2.5 mEq/L affect many functions of the body including the muscles, digestion, kidneys, electrolyte balance, the liver and the heart.

Muscles: fatigue, pain in the joints, muscle weakness, muscle weakness after exercise, muscle stiffness, muscle aches, muscle cramps, muscle contractions, muscle spasms, muscle tenderness, pins and needles sensation, eyelid myotonia (cannot open eyelid after opening and then closing them).

Digestion: Upset stomach, loss of appetite, vomiting, constipation, diarrhea, bloating of the stomach and full feeling in the stomach, blockage in the intestines called paralytic ileus.

Heart: Anxiousness, irregular and rapid heartbeat, angina, prominent U waves, inverted or flattened T waves, ST depression, elongated PR interval.

Kidneys: Severe thirst, increased urination, difficulty breathing, too slow or shallow breathing, lack of oxygen in the blood, sweating, increased blood pressure, metabolic acidosis.

Liver: The brain function becomes affected: Irritability, decrease in concentration, lack of clear thinking, confusion, slurring of speech, seizures.

Paralysis: Episodic muscle weakness, episodic partial paralysis, episodic total paralysis episodic flaccid paralysis (limp muscles, without tone).

Laboratory blood changes: Increased number of neutrophils in blood, increased number of white blood cells in the blood, reduced number of eosinophils in blood, increased number of lymphocytes in blood, low blood sodium, low blood potassium, elevated Serum CPK (creatine).

Laboratory urine changes: excess protein in urine, excess sugar in the urine, excessive acetone in urine, and presence of renal casts in urine. [5,6, 22,37, 68]

A Description of My Hypokalemic Periodic Paralysis Episodes

My potassium levels shift into low levels at times depending on the trigger (to be discussed later) that sets it into motion. When that happens, my symptoms are much as described in the narrative at the beginning of this chapter. I suddenly get a strange sensation of heat body wide, usually beginning in my back then it spreads to the rest of my body. Nausea may accompany this. I begin to feel very heavy and weak. My heart begins to beat faster, and I start to breath faster. My blood pressure increases, and my oxygen levels drop. My lips feel numb and swollen. I feel as though I am being pushed back into my recliner. My eyelids become very heavy, and my eyes will close and then my body goes limp. I may have a few jerks as I am going limp. My mouth will open, and I can only breathe through my mouth. When I reach this point, I unable to move or speak or open my eyes. I am, however, able to hear and am aware of everything going on around me. I may stay like this for a few minutes to a several hours. During that time, my heart rate, breathing and blood pressure fluctuate between normal and increased levels. My oxygen levels fluctuate between normal and low. Sometimes my breathing will stop for several seconds, a very frightening experience. My body will try to swallow but is unable to so there is a choking sensation and odd sounds are emitted from my throat. At times my heart will beat erratically causing me much stress.

Once an episode begins, it can be as short as ten minutes or last several hours. Sometimes I begin to come out of it and can open my eyes but then I go back into it. This can happen several times over several hours. Coming out of it is as described above.

Hyperkalemic Periodic Paralysis Symptoms

When potassium shifts into higher ranges in normal individuals, hyperkalemia, high potassium levels in the blood, will occur for anyone and a myriad of symptoms can be experienced and can be dangerous, even deadly. If an individual has Hyperkalemic Periodic Paralysis and potassium shifts into higher ranges, he or she can and will experience a combination of the same myriad of symptoms as well as paralysis and can be equally as dangerous and deadly.

When potassium levels are at a slightly elevated level there may be no symptoms. At a moderately higher level, which is usually between 5.5 and 6.5 mEq/L, there may be some symptoms involving muscles, digestion, kidneys, electrolyte balance, the liver and the heart.

Potassium levels above 6.5 mEq/L are very serious and usually require medical attention.

Muscles: Fatigue, weakness, pins and needles, tingling or numbness in the extremities, muscle contraction, muscle rigidity, muscle cramps, muscles stiffness, muscle twitching, muscle cramping, reduced reflexes, muscle contraction involving tongue, tightness in legs, strange feeling in legs.

Digestion: Discomfort, nausea, vomiting, stomach cramps, diarrhea, vomiting.

Heart: Palpitations, chest pain, irregular heartbeat, slow heartbeat, weak pulse, absent pulse, heart stoppage, small P waves, tall T waves, QRS abnormality, P wave abnormality, QT lengthening, fast heartbeat.

Kidneys: Breathing problems, wheezing, shortness of breath, fast breathing, feeling hot, low blood pressure.

Liver: The brain function becomes affected: Irritability, sleepiness, confusion, seizures, loss of consciousness.

Paralysis: Episodic muscle weakness, episodic partial paralysis, episodic total paralysis.

Laboratory blood changes: Elevated blood potassium, serum sodium level elevated, Serum CPK (creatine).

Laboratory urine changes: Elevated urine pH level. [6, 23, 39, 41, 45]

A Description of My Hyperkalemic Periodic Paralysis Episodes

My potassium levels also shift into higher levels at times depending on the trigger (to be discussed later) that sets it into motion. When that happens, my symptoms are different in some ways than described above when I have an episode from low potassium.

I begin to have a severe weakness and feel very tired. I begin to have difficulty with my speech. I slur my words, stutter and sometimes strange sounds will come of my mouth like "ah" or "aaahhh" or a "sushing" sound. I have difficulty with coherent thought and speech. I get frustrated and cry easily. I am able to hear and am aware of everything going on around me. During this time, I get weaker and shaky, feel tingly and eventually slip into paralysis. Once in the paralysis, my muscles tighten and I begin to have one part of my body start to jerk every ten to twenty seconds, usually one of my legs. I feel strange, itchy sensations and then the muscles will contract and jerk violently with each contraction. An "uh" sound may be emitted from my mouth with each contraction. It is very painful. This cycle may last for several minutes to several hours. I may also have pain and burning in other parts of my body, especially my buttocks and thighs. I also have shortness of breath and a decrease in blood pressure and heart arrythmias including long QT interval heartbeats and drops in oxygen levels. My breathing will stop at times. I will eventually fall asleep but wake up suddenly with more jerking and hyperventilation. The longest episode I had like this was seven hours long.

Normokalemic Periodic Paralysis Symptoms

For some individuals, periodic episodes of paralysis may occur when potassium shifts within normal ranges. This is called Normokalemic Periodic Paralysis. Some studies indicate that it is actually a variant of Hyperkalemic Periodic Paralysis. It should also be noted here that paralyzed muscles swell and fill with potassium. When the swelling begins to subside the level of potassium may return to normal levels. This may happen quickly and by the time the blood sample is taken the level of potassium may have already returned to the normal ranges, thus appearing to be Normokalemia.

If someone has this condition or appears to have it, when this happens, he or she can and will experience a combination of the same myriad of symptoms either Hypokalemic Periodic Paralysis or Hyperkalemic Periodic Paralysis. Normokalemic Periodic Paralysis can be seen in individuals with Andersen-Tawil Syndrome.

A Description of My Normokalemic Periodic Paralysis Episodes

I have had periods of paralysis as described in both Hypokalemic Periodic Paralysis and Hyperkalemic Periodic Paralysis when my blood potassium levels were in the normal ranges according to a cardy meter and lab testing.

Andersen-Tawil Syndrome

An individual with Andersen-Tawil Syndrome may experience the symptoms described previously depending on whether the potassium shifts into high or low ranges. The symptoms will be based on the triggers and will coincide with hypokalemia, hyperkalemia or normokalemia as described previously. They also experience long QT interval heartbeats, a life-threatening arrhythmia in which the heart takes longer than it should to recharge, and they have ventricular arrhythmias. That is a problem originating in the lower chambers of the heart. They include premature ventricular contractions known as PVCs; bigeminy, trigeminy, and quadrigeminy beats in which PVCs occur every second, third or fourth beat; ventricular tachycardia in which there are at least three PVCs in a row and ventricular fibrillation a beat without any organized contraction which is life threatening. [7, 14, 72]

A Description of My Andersen-Tawil Syndrome-like Periodic Paralysis Episodes

My episodes of periodic paralysis include the three types as described above; Hypokalemic Periodic Paralysis, Hyperkalemic Periodic Paralysis and Normokalemic Periodic Paralysis as well as the description of those that accompany Andersen-Tawil Syndrome. I experience, PVCs, bigeminy and trigeminy, ventricular tachycardia Long QT interval heartbeats and other types of arrhythmias as recorded on Holter monitors and ECG's.

Abortive Attacks

Abortive attacks are periods of extended time anywhere from hours, days, weeks or months in which some individuals are totally debilitated by extreme muscle weakness without going into full paralysis. The previously described common symptoms may begin but the full attack or total paralysis may not occur. The person is left with severe weakness and other symptoms such as extreme fatigue. It is difficult to do anything physically and it also can affect cognition abilities, such as memory, thought processing and speech and some become very fragile emotionally. The individual may want to sleep and may have no appetite. In my own case the abortive attacks are totally debilitating and actually worse than the episodes of paralysis. When I am in them, I wish I could slip into paralysis and get it "over with". I have experienced no worse feelings of weakness and helplessness in my life other than being in a full body state of paralysis.

Other Types of Periodic Paralysis Episodes

Although distinct episodes of total, full body paralysis are a clear sign of Periodic Paralysis, it must be noted here that not every paralytic episode is full body or total paralysis. An individual may be only partially paralyzed. Only his or her legs may be paralyzed, or they may only be weak. Episodes may occur as sudden falls or dropping to the floor. Feet or legs or arms may go numb and tingly. Muscles in the calves may become very tight and painful. An episode may include overall weakness with arrhythmias and fluctuating blood pressure. Walking may suddenly become difficult due to a weak foot.

Each of these attacks or episodes has a clear beginning and a clear end. Each episode is intermittent. They come and go. Most people will be normal between them, or their muscle strength will improve between them. However, some individuals over time may develop permanent muscle weakness.

Making a Diagnosis

The misconception of only full body, total paralytic attacks for diagnosing Periodic Paralysis is misleading and a very real problem for individuals who need a diagnosis. If someone has periods of muscle weakness with a clear beginning and end, is normal between the episodes or their muscle strength improves between episodes or attacks and everything else being ruled out, Periodic Paralysis should be included in the options for a diagnosis.

The first full-body, total paralytic attack that I recognized happened to me when I was sixty-one years old. However, for decades I had been experiencing episodes or attacks of partial paralysis and muscle weakness, numbness and tingling, tight and painful calves, strange sensations in my legs, a totally numb arm for two months, dropping to the floor when my leg gave way under me, overall weakness with arrhythmias and fluctuating blood pressure, inability to walk due a suddenly weak foot. All were attacks of Periodic Paralysis as the results of potassium shifting, yet not total, full body paralysis (see appendix for photographs of paralytic episodes).

Chapter Sixteen
Potassium

Introduction

We know that Periodic Paralysis is an ion channelopathy, a dysfunction of an ion channel, and a form of mineral metabolic disorder. This is because potassium, which is a mineral, is directly related to the paralysis of the muscles. We know that many things cause the potassium to shift, which in turn triggers episodes or attacks of partial or full body paralysis or muscle weakness. Many symptoms can accompany the episodes. In this chapter, potassium and potassium shifting and how it relates Periodic Paralysis is discussed by Calvin Hunter.

Potassium and Potassium Shifting

It is an established fact that too much potassium in the blood stream will have an impact on muscle function especially if there are complications with body organs and especially the kidneys. The inverse is also true with too little potassium in the blood stream having an impact on muscle function. In a few individuals, potassium levels in the blood stream fluctuate outside of normal ranges and this condition results in muscle paralysis. The term Periodic Paralysis is used to describe unusual effects of potassium on muscle function. There are three conditions that are used to describe various levels of potassium in the blood stream: hyperkalemia, hypokalemia, and normokalemia (high, low, and normal potassium blood concentrations). Research scientists have identified several specific causes of abnormal potassium shifting in the blood stream. Periodic Paralysis can be caused by genetic mutation of cell membrane, illness and disease and environmental factors. Ion channelopathies and metabolic acidosis are two well-known causes of potassium induced muscle paralysis.

Potassium Levels

So, who or what determines high, low and normal potassium blood concentrations? We must rely on science to provide the answers. Just about everyone has undergone a blood draw. A nurse or professional phlebotomist in a laboratory setting with the use of needle extracts a sample of blood from a vein. Several vials of blood are drawn and sent to a medical laboratory for analysis. Medical labs perform a variety of tests usually ordered by a doctor to get an idea of the levels of various substances in the body. There are many minerals present in our bodies, which work together to support normal life and metabolic functions. The main minerals are sodium, potassium, magnesium, and calcium. There are numerous other elements that make up our bodies also including vitamins, antibodies, enzymes, other minerals and metals, living organisms, and a host of other organic and inorganic materials. In a perfect world, they all work together to keep us healthy and alive. The body works to maintain certain levels of each substance in order to maintain optimal efficiency. If we get too much or too little of any one of these life-supporting substances, our bodies do not work as well and in some instances, it can be life threatening. The body has a remarkable ability to manage all these substances and keep us functional and alive.

In order to determine what constitutes a high, low or normal level of any substance samples have to be taken from a large number of people in the general population and over an extended period of time. The samples are compared, and numbers are assigned which establish normal ranges through statistical analysis. Once the normal ranges have been established then our individual blood sample can be analyzed and compared to the larger population.

The typical normal blood serum potassium level falls within 3.5 to 5.0 range. If a sample falls within this range than it is considered to be normal potassium reading. This holds true for the majority of people. In the case of someone suffering with a chronic illness or disease, their samples might fall well above, well below or even within a normal range as compared to the general population. For anyone suffering with Periodic Paralysis the parameters governing normalcy are different due to the way in which potassium and other minerals are metabolized. A person with Periodic Paralysis cannot depend on someone else to determine normalcy. Potassium readings need to be taken in a frequent and consistent manner to uncover patterns and associations with other daily events and activities.

A person with Periodic Paralysis experiencing a state of full body muscle paralysis might have a blood concentration level of potassium measured at 3.75. Within a short period of time the same person might be free of any symptoms and still register a blood potassium level of 3.75. For another person with the same reading, they might not have any noticeable symptoms until potassium levels rise above 4.5 or drop below 3. Each person with the disease is unique in how their body reacts to potassium concentrations and shifting. In order to gain some level of understanding, predictability and control over this disease, each person must understand their individual metabolic chemistry and their individual states of normalcy. These are some of the mysteries surrounding the disease, which lead to so much misunderstanding, misdiagnosis and mistreatment. Understanding these concepts requires a stretch of conventional understanding of bodily processes and functions that is something most medical providers are incapable or unwilling to do.

To further complicate matters, when someone is experiencing full body muscle paralysis it is nearly impossible to get a blood sample taken. Rushing someone in a state of muscle paralysis to a medical lab is impractical. It is dangerous to move someone while they are in a state of muscle paralysis due to the muscle and joint damage that can occur. It is an absolute waste of time and resources and nothing of importance about the patient or the disease will be revealed. Periods of muscle paralysis fluctuate as does the level of serum potassium. Attempting to get a blood draw during an episode of muscle paralysis is one of those things misinformed doctors do in a misguided attempt to diagnose the disease. Even the top specialists employed by specialized treatment facilities that we visited did not understand the role of potassium shifting and muscle paralysis in individuals with Periodic Paralysis.

Potassium shifting does not happen in isolation. Other elements such as sodium, calcium, and magnesium have an effect on potassium levels inside and outside of the cells. These elements work together keeping cells performing at their very best levels and changes in one chemical concentration effects concentration levels of other chemicals. Sodium plays a key role in potassium moving through cell walls. The process involves both negative and positive charges and cell membrane channels, which allow the flow of substances from inside and outside of the cells.

Another reason why Periodic Paralysis is so difficult to diagnosis is due to the speed with which potassium shifts from the cells into the blood stream and back into the cells. The kidneys work hard to maintain certain potassium levels throughout the body and catching a spike or decline of potassium in the blood stream is difficult. Taking a sample reading is similar to taking a photograph of a moving object. Multiple readings over an extended period of time need to be analyzed to get an accurate picture of how potassium is behaving inside the body. Potassium and other mineral levels shift very rapidly depending on a multitude of variables and once again we are faced with the difficulty of getting the blood draw during an episode of full body muscle paralysis.

The use of a cardy meter at home partially rectifies this situation. However, the Food and Drug Administration do not approve the device for use on humans. The manufacturer of the cardy meter also does not recommend the use of the device to measure serum potassium levels in humans. We have used the device over several years and it has been a vital part of our at-home medical kit we have used to understand and manage Susan's episodes of muscle paralysis. It is a personal decision and one that has served us well.

One of the greatest challenges individuals with Periodic Paralysis face is the difficulty they encounter when convincing medical professionals to consider abnormal potassium shifting as a cause of their symptoms. This is especially true when getting them to consider metabolic acidosis as a cause of potassium shifting. Metabolic acidosis has serious consequences on the body including the respiratory and cardiovascular systems. [21]

Approximately ninety five percent of all potassium in the body is contained within the cells and the remaining five percent is what is used for measurement purposes. There are not any tests available that measure potassium concentrations inside of cells. So, when we talk about potassium shifting, periods of paralysis or Periodic Paralysis, we are looking at the potassium levels in the blood stream.

Value of Potassium Readings

Once Susan and I figured out that taking an occasional blood potassium reading was useless in making a diagnosis and getting Susan to a lab during an episode of full body muscle paralysis was dangerous, we began researching other methods of measuring potassium levels in the blood. The value of the readings taken over a period of time with the use of a cardy meter provided us with valuable information about

Susan's blood potassium levels during periods of muscle paralysis. In the beginning, Susan was in a state of paralysis most of time. We began taking vital readings and recording those readings on a homemade chart. With our backgrounds in teaching and science, we were familiar with the use of charts and graphs and set about to customize our own unique forms. With the aid of these tools, we began to identify patterns and trends. We established cause and effect relationships and expanded to sampling urine, saliva, blood pressure, and oxygen levels, respiration, temperature and also kept notes about what Susan was eating and drinking.

Over a period of several years, we were able to determine individualized normal ranges for Susan and from that point we were able to begin interventions. The cardy meter proved invaluable not necessarily to get a specific reading but rather to identify trends specific to Susan. At times when Susan was in full body muscle paralysis, her serum potassium levels were at the range of 4. At these times Susan was experiencing symptoms related to Hyperkalemia. At times when Susan was in full body muscle paralysis her serum potassium levels were around the range of 3. Her symptoms were related to Hypokalemia. The same held true when her readings were around 3.5 and still experiencing muscle paralysis.

With these readings and other information gathered over an extended period of time, we knew Susan probably suffered with a genetic mutation of muscle cells or ion channelopathy and also from metabolic acidosis being aggravated by pharmaceutical medications and imbalances in her body pH. We discovered the importance of maintaining a balance between alkaline and acid levels through diet and natural supplements. During this same period of discovery, we were both busy researching everything we could find over the Internet that might be related to the role of potassium in the body.

Chapter Seventeen
Triggers

Introduction

The last chapter discussed several aspects of potassium including potassium levels and potassium shifting. Each type of Periodic Paralysis has a separate set of symptoms depending on whether the serum potassium levels are low, high or normal. The shifting in the levels of potassium creates a different set of symptoms that may accompany the paralysis.

This chapter will discuss the triggers that cause serum potassium levels to shift thereby causing episodes of Periodic Paralysis. There are some common triggers among those with the different forms of Periodic Paralysis and there are some triggers, which are unique for each individual. Triggers can be certain medications, foods, activities, stress and even sleep. It is important to know one's triggers in order to avoid having episodes of paralysis, which can lead to permanent damage to major body organs.

What are the Triggers of Periodic Paralysis?

There are many triggers that set into motion partial and total paralysis and other symptoms. It is important to discover these triggers because we need to stop the episodes or attacks, if possible, in order to regain the quality of our lives and to prevent the damage being done to our organs as the potassium shifts and concentrations fluctuate. Potassium shifting can cause a myriad of conditions including permanent tightness of the calf muscles, muscle wasting of arm and leg muscles, restless leg syndrome or even osteoporosis. The muscles that assist in breathing and swallowing can weaken over time and be affected during attacks. This can seriously affect the intake of oxygen and expelling of carbon dioxide. Excessive carbon dioxide in the blood stream can be deadly. Dangerous arrhythmias of the heart can also occur when an individual is in an episode or attack.

Between attacks, the muscles usually return to normal or strengthen, but over time with repeated episodes of paralysis, progressive and permanent weakness of the muscles is possible. This includes the heart and breathing muscles. This can lead to heart failure and respiratory failure, thus eventual death.

Other complications can include respiratory arrest and aspiration pneumonia which can lead to death. Though rare, these can occur with Hypokalemic Periodic Paralysis. Complications of Hyperkalemic Periodic Paralysis include bi-directional heart arrhythmias and permanent weakness of the muscles, which also can be deadly.

As discussed previously, in the case of those with Andersen-Tawil Syndrome, the paralysis leads to tachycardia and serious arrhythmias, including long QT intervals, which can lead to cardiac arrest or sudden death. Avoiding paralysis is absolutely necessary, due to these life-threatening effects. [24]

There is no doubt that avoiding or stopping the paralytic attacks or episodes is essential. It is imperative that a person with Periodic Paralysis be fully aware of the activities, foods, medications and elements that can trigger Periodic Paralysis. [4]

The Common Triggers of Hypokalemic Periodic Paralysis

Some triggers typically responsible for causing potassium to shift in Hypokalemic Periodic Paralysis include excessive carbohydrates, alcoholic beverages, sodium and exercise. [22]

The Common Triggers of Hyperkalemic Periodic Paralysis

Some triggers typically responsible for causing potassium to shift in Hyperkalemic Periodic Paralysis include excessive carbohydrates, exercise, cold temperatures, excessive potassium rich foods or medications, stress, rest after exercise, fatigue and fasting. [23]

Other Triggers for Periodic Paralysis

Other triggers can include simple carbohydrates (processed sugar, processed flour), complex carbohydrates (some grains, wheat, rye), red meats, sodium, caffeine, MSG, alcoholic beverages and large meal portions.

All aspects of sleep have set my episodes into motion including falling asleep (during and after waking), stress, dehydration, fasting, sitting too long in one position, climate changes, fatigue, heat and cold.

For me, exercise acts as a trigger for paralysis. Some people with Periodic Paralysis are able to exercise without triggering an episode of muscle paralysis but more often the condition referred to as "exercise intolerance" is more common. Episodes of paralysis can occur during periods of exertion, immediately after exertion or can be delayed for hours or days. Typically, a period of rest after exercise will act as a trigger for muscle paralysis.

Some people have reported feeling the effects of electromagnetic force (EMFs). There are also times when I cannot explain why the muscle paralysis occurred. I try to follow all the rules established to avoid or lessen paralytic attacks and they still occur for reasons unknown to me at this time.

Over-the-counter Medications:

Most over-the-counter medications can set muscle weakness or paralysis into motion for people with Periodic Paralysis. The following is a list of some medications compiled from a list of my own known offenders, some which others have told me about, and some I found in my research.

❖ Cough Syrup
❖ Eye Drops
❖ Glycerin Enemas
❖ NSAIDs

If the following ingredients are contained within any of the products you use, they are also known to trigger symptoms:

❖ Sodium Hydroxide
❖ Edetate Disodium
❖ Stearic Acid

These ingredients may be in any of the following:

❖ Lotions
❖ Oils
❖ Hair Dyes
❖ Suppositories
❖ Soaps
❖ Shampoos
❖ Deodorants
❖ Beauty Products
❖ Skincare Products
❖ Emollients
❖ Ointments
❖ Creams
❖ Colognes
❖ Powders
❖ Hair Gels

Triggers

- ❖ Mousse
- ❖ Enemas
- ❖ Toothpastes
- ❖ Mousse
- ❖ Perfumes
- ❖ Antiperspirants
- ❖ Shaving Creams
- ❖ Cosmetic Products
- ❖ Hair Sprays Tonics
- ❖ Bath Salts
- ❖ Pharmaceutical Medications

Most prescription drugs set muscle weakness or paralysis into motion for people with Periodic Paralysis. The following is a list compiled from my own known offenders, some which others have mentioned to me and some I found in my research. If one must take a drug, it is better to begin with one quarter of a normal dose to make sure it will work for you.

- ❖ Saline Drips
- ❖ Glucose Infusion
- ❖ Oral Corticosteroids
- ❖ Beta Blockers
- ❖ Tranquilizers
- ❖ Analgesics
- ❖ Puffers for Asthma
- ❖ Antibiotics
- ❖ Cough Syrups
- ❖ Lidocaine
- ❖ Anesthetics
- ❖ Epinephrine
- ❖ Antihistamines
- ❖ Contrast Dye for MRIs
- ❖ Muscle Relaxers
- ❖ Intravenous Corticosteroids
- ❖ Pain Killers

- ❖ Eye Drop Dilator
- ❖ Adrenaline [4]

If an IV is needed, mannitol can be used (or diluted solutions in extreme cases).

Drugs Affecting Long QT Interval Heartbeats

For those who have Andersen-Tawil Syndrome there are special medication precautions due to the long QT interval issue and the possible risk of torsades de pointes, an uncommon and deadly form of ventricular tachycardia.

There are extensive lists of drugs and medications that can cause long QT interval heartbeats. The list is extensive, so we recommend the reader use any one of many search engines found on the Internet to view additional information.

We also would ask the reader to utilize Internet search engine capabilities to research drugs and medications known to cause torsades de pointes heartbeats.

Now that most of the offending elements and experiences, which can trigger attacks of Periodic Paralysis, have been listed and discussed, a chapter will follow later in the book on how to discover which of these things are triggers for each person.

Chapter Eighteen
Prognosis

Introduction

In review, it is now known that certain medications, foods, activities, stress or even sleep can cause potassium to shift, which sets an attack into motion. These are called triggers. Knowing one's triggers is essential in order to avoid the attacks or episodes because they can cause permanent damage to organs in the body as well as lead to permanent muscle weakness. This leads us to want to know just what to expect so this chapter will discuss the prognosis or what is going to happen to someone who has this disease.

How Bad Will It Get? The Truth

When I realized that I had Periodic Paralysis, I wanted to know what to expect. How long will I live? How bad will I get? Can this disease be reversed if I get proper treatment? Will I lose my ability to walk? Will I ever drive again? Will I need to be in an assisted living program? Is there medication to stop the total paralytic episodes? What are my chances of dying from the long QT interval heartbeat? Will my breathing continue to get more difficult until I can no longer breathe on my own? Is there any medication I can take if I get another bladder infection? What happens if I need an operation and cannot use anesthetics? What can I do to stop the pain in my shoulder and back since I cannot take any pain medications? When I go into cardiac arrest, is it worth trying to save me? Will I end up on dialysis due to kidney failure? Can I travel? What will happen if I end up in the Emergency Room again and they cannot help me with any medications?

My research to answer these questions, led me to an inadequate amount of information; both in the number of articles and the amount written. I found only a few short blurbs. These passages were and are copied over and over on the different websites related to the condition. Most are simply written by professional people who have no form of Periodic Paralysis and no real understanding of the disease. As well as being short and lacking information, I find the content to be simply misleading such as indicating that muscle damage can be reversed and that most people do well on medication. The specialists in the field write little more of what to expect in the studies of and articles about Periodic Paralysis. It seems strange that a disease as serious and as complex as Periodic Paralysis has only two or three short and misleading sentences written about what to expect for the rest of our lives!

I now know, there are no doctors who can tell me. My renal specialist told me that he is unable do anymore for me since the diamox did not work. My neurologist tells me that he does not know what to do for me. My cardiologist says my heart condition, due to the Periodic Paralysis, is "not treatable" for me. I am, "not a candidate for a pacemaker ", "possibly a defibrillator later". My Primary Care Physicians (PCP) will not treat anything that has to do with my disease. Even the Muscular Dystrophy Association (MDA) doctors I saw did not recognize Periodic Paralysis nor did they know how to diagnose it correctly. I was told by one of the MDA Healthcare Coordinators, that they need me to educate the MDA doctors so they will know how to treat me. This is not at all comforting. No one can tell me how to treat my symptoms or what to expect.

The following is what I do know about myself, and my own answers to the previous questions:

I am sixty-four years old and was diagnosed with Periodic Paralysis (PP) on February 7, 2011, at the age of sixty-two. The type I have is like Andersen-Tawil Syndrome Type 2 but is yet unnamed. I have had episodes of partial and total paralysis for many years. During the episodes, my potassium shifts are low, high and within the normal ranges. Due to several misdiagnoses and a lack of proper diagnosis and treatment for over fifty years, I have become totally and permanently disabled with weak muscles throughout my body including those involved with my vision, digestion, breathing and my heart. I must be on oxygen constantly and cannot exert myself in any way. The electrical workings of my heart are defective. I have had a heart loop monitor inserted in my chest to monitor the tachycardia and arrhythmias, which include long QT interval beats. I now spend my days in a recliner, often unable to walk farther than across a room. I must use a motorized wheelchair for anything farther. If I did not have the help of my husband, I would have to live in an assisted living program. I was misdiagnosed for many years. The medications given to me medical professionals made me worse.

Through the past years of my physical decline, I have had to give up my career as a special education teacher, my hobbies to include hiking, walking, swimming, exercising, fishing, camping, traveling, shopping, cooking and baking. I had to sell, and move away from, a beautiful home in the mountains of Utah. I can no longer drive. I have lost many friends, because I could not keep up with them or entertain any longer. I have lost contact with family members who did not understand or did not want to watch my decline or who thought I was a hypochondriac. I have lost the connection I once had with my grandchildren because I can no longer keep up with them or continue a meaningful relationship with them. The relationship with my husband has changed from husband and wife to caregiver and patient. Many of the over thirty-seven doctors I have seen in the past eight years have treated me poorly and as if I was mentally ill.

I have spent the past several years working diligently to get a diagnosis and treatment for the ailment that cruelly stole the quality of my life. The most difficult part of this, for me is knowing that I may not have become this seriously ill if just one of more than thirty-seven medical providers I saw before my diagnosis would have taken me seriously.

According to many people that I am in contact with from different parts of the world, my situation is not that unusual for someone with Periodic Paralysis. In our quest to understand PP and receive an appropriate diagnosis and treatment, many medical professionals do not take us seriously. Some facts about Periodic Paralysis that we have in common include the following and need to be asserted by every person with PP.

Muscle weakness, which is permanent, can develop. Breathing and heart problems can develop and cause death. Many individuals cannot tolerate the medications. Recurring episodes of paralysis can make future episodes worse and develop continuous muscle weakness. There are complications of the heart, kidneys, speech, swallowing, breathing and permanent damage to the muscles. Power wheelchairs may be needed. Oxygen saved my life. One may not be able to be employed.

In my opinion, the majority of people with this disease end up in a situation similar to mine; very, very ill; but they are misdiagnosed, underdiagnosed, called mentally ill, or hypochondriacs. They are diagnosed as suffering from conversion disorder or having pseudo seizures. They are laughed at and scoffed at by many medical providers who do not understand Periodic Paralysis. I have been told that I am too old to have Periodic Paralysis and another person I know was told their skin color ruled out the possibility they suffered with the disease. Most of the medications we are given to treat PP come with side effects and cause symptoms to worsen. I have been dismissed by doctors and experienced open ridicule. My medical records are filled with misinformation and derogatory remarks.

Prognosis

Treatments in the form of medications are withheld. Many people with Periodic Paralysis are listed as dying of things such as, unknown muscle wasting disease, accidental drowning in a swimming pool or bathtub, sudden early cardiac arrest, strokes, or failure to thrive. I believe many people who are misdiagnosed and undiagnosed end up taking their own lives. The death certificate reflects the cause of death as suicide without mention of the reason why the suicide occurred. Many people give up the daily struggles and die alone.

One of our main reasons for creating our website, the Periodic Paralysis Network, and writing this book, is for these people. They need to be diagnosed and get the proper medications and treatment before it is too late. We are hopeful that the medical professionals who see our website and read this book will become more aware of this disease and gain enough information to begin appropriately diagnosing their patients with Periodic Paralysis before it is too late.

In conclusion, many people with Periodic Paralysis will live normal life spans and their disease will be minor with occasional weakness. Some may actually not even have episodes of muscle paralysis. Others will have moderate disability and receive proper medical treatment and medication. They will respond well and may even reverse some of their weakness. But other people with Periodic Paralysis will have mild, moderate or severe disability and they will not receive proper diagnoses or treatment. They will become more disabled as the symptoms progressively worsen. They will suffer needlessly and may die due to complications. So, for some individuals, Periodic Paralysis is a terminal condition.

Terminal?

Last year I became extremely ill. We had to call our local home health care. We were hoping they could come to the house and evaluate me by doing some lab work to see if I was in metabolic acidosis (to be discussed in the next chapter) or had some other infection of some type. I was hoping they could help Calvin take care of my needs. He is disabled too and cannot lift me. I could do nothing for myself. I could not eat. I slept most of the time and I was in and out of total body paralysis for weeks.

A nurse and physical therapist came to our home. Upon evaluation it was decided that I did not qualify for their services due to some technicalities with my insurance and Medicare, mostly due to the fact that my symptoms were intermittent. We did get a visit from the nurse a few times over the following weeks but never got blood drawn. With each visit we discussed the ways we could get some services from them, as I needed them. They personally thought we deserved and needed the help from them.

It was decided that I might qualify for services under the hospice wing of their organization. Hospice is care and support to individuals with life-limiting conditions or illness and their families during later stages of the disease. Hospice is chosen and begins when comfort and management is chosen rather than attempting to reverse or cure the condition or disease. This was and is absolutely the case for me.

I have a disease with no known cure. There is no treatment I am able to use. I am getting progressively weaker, and my breathing gets more difficult. I could die at any minute from arrhythmias. Because I cannot tolerate antibiotics, a simple infection can kill me.

Prognosis

We had to discuss this with my Primary Care Physician. After recovering from the severity of the illness and regaining some strength, I researched the issues and wrote a paper arguing the possibility of receiving services through hospice. On my next visit, we discussed these issues and presented her with a letter.

The doctor decided that hospice was an option for me. I did indeed fit the definition of being "terminal". I am in an advanced stage of a disease called Periodic Paralysis, it has an unfavorable prognosis because of lack of treatment and medications, and it has no cure. It was decided that when I felt it necessary, I could begin the hospice services. In the meantime, a standing order for blood work was set up and the home health care could draw it when needed. The doctor also agreed, at my request, to sign a "Do Not Resuscitate Document (DNR)". This means that if my heart stops or I stop breathing, there is to be no CPR, or any other type of life-saving measures used. This document is displayed in plain view when and if an ambulance is called and recorded at the nearby hospitals.

And so, we now know that Periodic Paralysis can be a terminal condition for some individuals. It is in fact killing me. I cannot at this time tell anyone else what to expect or how bad it will get. The next chapter will discuss the serious complications, which can accompany Periodic Paralysis and make it terminal.

Chapter Nineteen
Complications

Introduction

In Chapter Eighteen the prognosis or what to expect if one has Periodic Paralysis was discussed. For many people with Periodic Paralysis (PP) their life span will be normal with very mild symptoms, but for others there may be severe complications and their life may be shortened. This chapter will discuss in detail some of these major complications including exercise intolerance, progressive muscle weakness, heart issues, the need for oxygen, lactic and metabolic acidosis and kidney issues.

Progressive Muscle Weakness

Muscle weakness is a decrease in the strength of muscle and the need for extra effort in order to move the affected muscles in the body. It can involve the function and movement of one or more muscle groups. It can be very mild for some and totally debilitating for others. It can be the inability to do specific things like walking upstairs or reaching above one's head. Muscle weakness is the result of a number of diseases of the skeletal muscles. These include the muscle dystrophies, the inflammatory muscle diseases, the neuromuscular diseases and the muscle myopathy diseases. The cause of the muscle weakness will determine which muscle or muscle groups will be affected. A generalized muscle weakness is one that involves the entire body. [27, 28, 29, 30]

In Periodic Paralysis, which is a mineral metabolic myopathy, also known as an inherited myopathy, there is generalized weakness, because the muscles of the entire body are involved. There is no loss of sensation or feeling, however. The weakness is usually most noticeable in what are called the proximal muscles, those closest to the trunk, and the largest of the muscle groups. The weakness is equal on both sides of the body. And, although the weakness and paralysis are intermittent and have a beginning and an end in most cases, for some the weakness becomes chronic, or occurring over a long span of time or it returns often. The chronic weakness can become slowly progressive and fixed or permanent. Once it becomes chronic it can cause muscle wasting and fat or lipid can replace the muscle as we have seen in a previous chapter. At the point the muscle weakness becomes permanent, it will not go away and at this point it is progressive meaning it will steadily continue to worsen. [25, 26]

Symptoms

The symptoms of progressive muscle weakness begin with general muscle weakness. The weakness gradually increases as endurance decreases and muscle wasting can be seen. The progressing weakness can cause an imbalance of the joints causing restricted movement. This in turn can lead to deformities as well as stiffness. This begins in the thighs, shoulders and upper arms and the muscles closest to the trunk. Then as it advances it spreads to the muscles of the feet and hands. [25, 31]

In Periodic Paralysis the large muscle groups are obviously affected, those attached to bone and also the muscles for breathing, talking and eating, the muscles of the throat and the eyes and of course, the heart being a muscle, it can be affected also. This means that as it progresses some of the functions of the body that can be affected are, but not limited to, standing, walking (gait, coordination and reflexes), sitting, rising from a chair, using arms (reaching above the head), and hands (writing, typing and feeding oneself), talking, eating, chewing, swallowing, digestion, elimination (bladder and bowels), breathing, vision and heart rate and rhythm. Once it begins to affect the muscles of the chest, the breathing or respiratory muscles, Periodic Paralysis becomes terminal. [25, 32]

Complications

My own symptoms of muscle weakness came on very gradually as would be expected, though as a child I experienced weakness for as long as I can remember. I first noticed a problem with walking up inclines and then stairs.

Diagnosing

Tests can be performed to confirm the muscle wasting. Of course, a physical examination would be first, then laboratory studies including a study of muscle enzymes would be in order, as well as, electromyography (study of electrical activity of muscles), which can confirm the myopathy and types of radiology (MRIs, x-rays) may be used. The most invasive of the tests is a muscle biopsy. A surgical procedure, using anesthesia, is performed to remove a piece of muscle to study in a laboratory. [25]

If a muscle biopsy is performed few abnormalities will appear for an individual with Periodic Paralysis unless permanent damage to the muscles has occurred. Changes in size and shape of muscle fibers may be found as well as lipids. There may also be changes in the vacuoles, an increase in fibers with internal nuclei and the formation of excess connective tissue. [33]

Care should be given if a muscle biopsy is to be used. Lidocaine is a serious trigger for paralysis and arrhythmias in Periodic Paralysis. I had a muscle biopsy performed, before my diagnosis, to rule out mitochondrial disease. I had some complications with the lidocaine. The test results did indicate, however, the existence of mild muscle myopathy. It was discovered that I had changes in size and shape of some muscle fibers. Also noted was the existence of fatty tissue.

My Experience with a Muscle Biopsy

I had been seen at a neurological clinic in a large medical center in the Pacific Northwest in 2009, two hundred fifty miles away from my home. After an examination and weakened muscles were discovered, it was decided a muscle biopsy was in order to test for mitochondrial disease as other conditions had already been ruled out. During the procedure they used lidocaine and I went into a paralytic attack. They ignored what was happening to me. The two physicians were too busy discussing one of the doctor's upcoming trips to Japan to do some lecturing. He was discussing taking his son on the trip with him.

I was choking and my heart was in tachycardia and arrhythmia and my chest was tight and in pain and I could not move, speak or open my eyes. I was not hooked up to any devices for monitoring, but when they heard me, they asked what was wrong. I could not answer, and then one doctor hollered, "Are you asleep?" I was finally able to barely answer that I was having one of those episodes (paralysis) and that my chest hurt, and my heart was pounding. No one did anything to help! They just went back to their conversation. I continued through the attack as the procedure continued and then slowly recovered. My husband and a nurse had to leave me on the table for a while afterward and then finally help me off and into a wheelchair due to my weakness. I was very weak the remainder of the day and night.

When I returned a month later (had to drive two hundred fifty miles each way) to get the results of the previous exam and muscle biopsy, I was told that nothing showed up on the biopsy and their conclusion was that I had nothing neuromuscular nor mitochondrial and had no diagnosis for me.

Complications

Calvin and I asked about the periods of paralysis that I was having. I told him I had one while I was having the muscle biopsy and asked him if he remembered hollering at me and me telling him about it? He denied even being in the room!! Then he dismissed me and said, "Go have a good time while you are here in our city". I told him that, "If I could have a good time, I would not be sitting in this consult room with you". I had episodes all the way there in the car and had them all the way home. We asked him what to do and he said he was referring me back to my Primary Care Physician and dismissed us.

It is interesting the results of the biopsy indicated I had myopathy, changes in size and shape of fibers, indicative of Periodic Paralysis but I did not know this until I got the records just a few months ago, three years after the fact! Also in the records were the results of a lab test indicating that I was in lactic acidosis the day of the original exam. On that day, a young neurologist examined me. Unfortunately, he left the facility before the biopsy was performed and before I could see him again. He had written in his notes that he believed I had Periodic Paralysis. The other two neurologists, who took over after he left, obviously ignored the lab report and the previous doctor's conclusions.

Due to the doctors' lack of concern and negligence, my diagnosis and treatment were set back almost a year. If I could have been diagnosed a year sooner, I may not have become as seriously ill as I now am. I have recently spoken with the young neurologist after finding and reading his notes. He apologized for having to leave before he could see me again, and for the actions, and non-actions, of his colleagues. He also told me he was not surprised when he heard my account of their behavior.

The most disturbing thing about this is that I discovered these doctors were the Periodic Paralysis specialists for my region! How could I have been treated so poorly and how could these doctors have missed diagnosing me?

(*Begin Report*)

The Muscle Biopsy Result:

SURGICAL PATHOLOGY

SOURCE OF SPECIMEN: A Muscle Biopsy, Myopathy

Final Pathologic Diagnosis:
Skeletal muscle left quadriceps, biopsy:

- Mild type 2 fiber atrophy
- Mild variation in type 1 fiber size
- Mild increase in lipid

The patient is a 61-year-old woman with a long history of weakness and
difficulty walking. She describes episodes of weakness and separate episodes of ataxia. EMG and nerve conduction studies were normal.

Myofiber size: Variable:
Most fibers are between 50 and 80 microns in diameter. There are rare
fibers up to 100 microns and scattered fibers less than 40 microns.
No increase in internalized nuclei
Angular atrophic myofibers
Comment(s): Mild
Round atrophic myofibers
Comment(s): Mild
Hypertrophic fibers
Comment(s): Rare
Atrophy of both type 1 and type 2 fibers
Comment(s): Many of the type 2 fibers are mildly angular and the type
2's are generally smaller than the type 1's (25-70 versus 40-100 microns).

The type 1 fibers are all polygonal, but vary in size.
Comment(s): Lipid is increased in both fiber types, more in 1's than

Complications

2's.
*Comment(s): There is a single angular, darkly staining fiber.
There is variation in fiber size and increased lipid similar to that
seen
in the frozen sections.*

(End Report)

Treatment for Progressive Muscle Weakness

As written in the chapter on prognosis, if one has Periodic Paralysis, we know there is no cure or treatment for permanent progressive muscle weakness. There is no way to strengthen the muscles involved in breathing once they are permanently weakened. Although the literature regarding permanent muscle weakness indicates that physical therapy can be helpful for all individuals with muscle weakness, this is not true for those with Periodic Paralysis. It can actually be more harmful to exercise due to exercise intolerance, which will be discussed later. [34]

Exercise Intolerance

We know that there are two types of involvement of muscles in individuals with Periodic Paralysis. There are attacks of paralysis of the muscles, which are intermittent, and there is a myopathy or a progressive, permanent muscle weakness, which can occur. Some individuals experience one or the other and some experience both conditions, though it is less common to have both, and it is very rare to have only the progressive, permanent muscle weakness. If an individual develops the progressive, permanent form of periodic paralysis, it begins as exercise intolerance, usually in the legs and feet, which progressively spreads to the rest of the muscles in the body.

In exercise intolerance the individual is not able to do

physical exercise or exertion that would be expected from someone of his or her age and overall health level nor for the amount of time expected. He or she lacks stamina. The individual may also experience extreme pain and fatigue after exercising or exertion and other symptoms such as a feeling of heaviness in the muscle groups. Exercise intolerance is a symptom rather than a condition or disease. It is a common symptom found in several diseases including metabolic disorders. Periodic Paralysis is a mineral metabolic myopathy.

Food and oxygen are normally converted into energy and delivered to the muscles, but this cycle is disrupted in individuals with exercise intolerance. The muscles are unable to use the nutrients and oxygen and therefore, enough energy may not be generated to the muscles and he or she is left with little or no energy. The degrees of low energy can be mild or extreme and the symptoms may occur during exercise or exertion, or they can occur later, even the next day.
Symptoms

Symptoms

Symptoms of exercise intolerance include fatigue, muscle cramps, insufficient heart rate, depression, changes in blood pressure and cyanosis. Fatigue may show within minutes of beginning to exercise with shortness of breath or dizziness. This is a sign that sufficient oxygen is not being processed. For individuals with severe exercise intolerance this can happen after doing simple tasks such as eating, sitting up in a chair or writing. Muscle cramping and stiffness also will appear within a few minutes of beginning to exercise. This can linger for days after the exercising. There may also be a delayed reaction of hours and the pain may begin while one is sleeping causing one to awaken. The heart rate does not increase enough to meet the needs of the muscles during the activity. Depression is often seen in individuals with exercise intolerance. Not being able to do the things a person wants to

Complications

do or should be able to do can create anxiety, irritability, bewilderment and hopelessness leading to depression. Standing up or walking across a room may be all that is necessary for an individual's blood pressure to rise significantly. Cyanosis is a serious condition that indicates there is not enough oxygen in the blood. The individual may appear to look blue in the face and hands and needs immediate medical attention.

Exercise intolerance can be seen in the small muscle groups as well as the large muscle groups. Writing or other fine motor skills can be affected causing cramping, fatigue and spasms. Tachycardia (fast heart beats) can occur from increased breathing rate during exercise or exertion and this rapid breathing increases from fatigue of the diaphragm and chest wall. Vision may become blurry due to fatigue of the eye muscles. The oral muscles, those involving the mouth, may be affected making speech difficult and making chewing of harder or tougher foods a problem. [27, 28, 30, 31, 32]

Diagnosing

Diagnosis would be based on the symptoms above and the diagnosis of the root cause, which in this case is Periodic Paralysis.

Treatment

For most individuals with Periodic Paralysis who have exercise intolerance, it is best to avoid physical activity and exertion because it can lead to muscle cell damage (muscle wasting), exhaustion and a condition called lactic acidosis, a form of metabolic acidosis (also discussed in this book). It also can be a trigger for attacks of paralysis. [35, 36]

My Experience with Exercise Intolerance

My own symptoms of exercise intolerance began as having a

problem keeping up with others in exercise classes, walking up inclines and stairs and later during and after physical therapy. I would get fatigued, out of breath and dizzy after only a few short minutes. I would develop terrible pain in my legs during the exercising or activity and would have to stop. The pain and fatigue would be worse the following day. This continued to gradually worsen until now it takes less and less activity to create the symptoms.

Now, I cannot walk more than a few steps at a time. I cannot sit up straight in a chair for very long to do a puzzle, sew or talk with friends. I can no longer wheel myself in a wheelchair. I cannot talk on the phone for very long. Fine motor skills, like writing or sewing by hand, cause my hands and fingers to cramp. Any exertion or exercise causes my blood pressure to rise; I get short of breath, fatigued and will later go into an attack of paralysis.

A muscle biopsy revealed signs of muscle cell change or damage and replacement with fat or lipids. I have been diagnosed with metabolic acidosis and lactic acidosis, all related to the exercise intolerance from the progressive and permanent muscle weakness I experience due to the continued and unchecked (over the years before my diagnosis) shifting of potassium from Periodic Paralysis, which is a mineral metabolic myopathy.

Heart Issues

Abnormal heart rhythms are serious and life-threatening complications for individuals with Periodic Paralysis. Each of the three forms, Hypokalemic Periodic Paralysis, Hyperkalemic Periodic Paralysis and Anderson-Tawil Syndrome, has a specific pattern of irregular heartbeats, which makes it easy to identify on an electrical study of the heart called an electrocardiogram (EKG). It is not necessary to explain or understand each irregular heartbeat or pattern.

Complications

They are however, referenced in the following sections for recognition and for diagnosis by physicians and patients.

Hypokalemic Periodic Paralysis

When an individual with Periodic Paralysis begins to experience a decrease in potassium, there is a decrease in the "T" wave. The next step is an "ST- segment depression" and then the "T" waves become inverted or "flip". At the same time the "PR" interval becomes prolonged, and the "P" wave enlarges. A "U" wave appears after the "T" wave and can be seen on the mid-precordial leads. When the "U" wave becomes larger than the "T" wave develops on the EKG, the potassium level in less than 3 (<3). As the potassium levels decrease further, the "T' and "U" wave combine into a prominent "U" wave on the EKG. This makes the "T" waves visible.

At this point, in severe hypokalemia, a person might also develop ventricular tachycardia (fast heartbeat) and/or ventricular fibrillation. The fibers of the ventricle of the heart contract in an uncontrolled and random manner. When this happens, without immediate medical help, the individual will die because the heart can stop beating suddenly and unexpectedly from cardiac arrest. Occasionally atrioventricular block, which is a sudden pause, or bradycardia, which is a slow heartbeat (under 60 beats per minute) can occur. So, in episodes of hypokalemia in individuals with Periodic Paralysis, there may be either a fast heartbeat or a slow heartbeat along with the specific arrhythmias. [41, 42]

Hyperkalemic Periodic Paralysis

If an individual has mild to moderately high potassium levels in his or her blood, "P" wave becomes smaller in size and a peaked "T" wave develops on an electrocardiogram (EKG). In more dangerous higher levels of potassium, it affects the electrical conduction of the heart in the sinoatrial (SA) of the heart. The SA is the "pacemaker" of the heart and responsible for the contraction of a heartbeat.

On an EKG the "P" wave disappears, and the ventricular contraction lengthens. This appears on an EKG as a "QRS complex". The overall pumping of the heart decreases to below 60 beats per minute and this is called bradycardia. The pulse becomes weak and heart block may occur. There may also be an increase in the heart rate called ventricular tachycardia. Arrhythmias in the form of ventricular fibrillation may also occur. So, in episodes of hyperkalemia in individuals with Periodic Paralysis, there may be either a fast heartbeat or a slow heartbeat along with the specific arrhythmia. [38, 39, 40, 41]

Andersen-Tawil Syndrome:

In an individual with Andersen-Tawil Syndrome, the heart complications are very distinctive, extremely serious and some of the arrhythmias are life threatening. They can include prominent two-phased "U" waves, down sloped terminal "T" waves which are prolonged, wide "TU" waves, premature ventricular complexes (PVCs), ventricular arrhythmias, including ventricular tachycardia, ventricular tachycardia which is bidirectional (BVT), supraventricular tachycardia, ventricular fibrillation, long QT interval heartbeat (a ventricular tachycardia) and torsades de pointes.

He or she may have no symptoms although they are experiencing arrhythmias, or they may have minor symptoms despite experiencing a serious number of arrhythmias and tachycardia or they may be very symptomatic. Regardless of the symptoms, a person is at high-risk for sudden death from an arrhythmia, namely the long QT heartbeat (LQT), the torsades de pointes and the ventricular fibrillation.

The changes, which are most common and affect the heart most often in Andersen-Tawil Syndrome, are the ventricular arrhythmias. This is a disruption in the lower chambers of the heart. In the long QT heart beat the heart muscle takes longer than normal between beats to recharge. When this condition is not treated it leads to uncomfortable feelings, syncope, (fainting) or cardiac arrest. The long QT interval heartbeat is one of the distinguishing features used to identify and diagnose Andersen-Tawil Syndrome.

There may be no actual, underlying cardiac disease in individuals with Andersen-Tawil Syndrome, but rather they are born with the predisposition to develop, under certain circumstances (triggers), the ventricular tachycardia and arrhythmias identified here. However, cardiomyopathy, a disease of the heart muscle, often develops in persons with Anderson-Tawil Syndrome. The heart becomes thickened and/or enlarged and weakens. This leads to heart failure. [7, 24, 38, 40, 43, 66, 72]

Diagnosing

Diagnosing Hypokalemic Periodic Paralysis, Hyperkalemic Periodic Paralysis or Andersen-Tawil Syndrome, based on the patterns on an EKG or a twenty-four-hour Holter Monitor, should be very straightforward based on the previous outlined information, when combined with the other symptoms unique to Periodic Paralysis, especially the intermittent paralysis or muscle weakening occurring as the EKG is being recorded. However, in many cases, this is not being used as part of the diagnosis and is often overlooked, misread or ignored.

My Own Heart Issues

I wore my first Holter Monitor for twenty-four hours many,

many years ago. I was experiencing heart palpitations and angina (chest pain). The reading indicated I was experiencing PVCs (premature ventricular complexes, an extra beat from the ventricle) and PACs (premature atrial complexes, an extra beat from the atrial). These are usually considered benign, or harmless in most cases and that is just what I was told. I was told to, "Go home and do not worry about it". However, with the passing out episodes since I was eleven, the other symptoms I was experiencing and my family history, the PVCs and PACs were an indication of potassium shifting.

After many EKGs and more Holter Monitor readings over more recent years, more heart abnormalities were recorded. They are as follows: PVCs (an indication of ATS), PACs, PJCs (premature junctional contraction, an abnormal beat between regular beats and shows on an EKG as an inverted "P" wave and becomes a QRS complex...indicating hyperkalemia), SVPB/PVC (supraventricular premature beat that originates in the atria/premature ventricular complex, an indication of ATS), errants (rapid irregular heartbeats, indicative of ATS), ST segment abnormalities (a sign of hypokalemia), non-conducted PACs (skipped beat), abnormal T waves (signs of hypokalemia, hyperkalemia and ATS), supraventricular fibrillation (an indication of ATS), tachycardia (heartbeats over 100 per minute) (mine was 147 per minute) (signs of hypokalemia, hyperkalemia and ATS), bradycardia (heartbeats less than 60 per minute) (mine was 44 per minute) (indication of hypokalemia and hyperkalemia). I experienced angina and was diagnosed with mild mitral valve prolapse. I was told my heart was small; especially the left side and that occasionally it would work hard and cause the above symptoms. It was not until the long QT interval heartbeat (a marker for ATS) was discovered that I finally got taken seriously and was later diagnosed with Andersen-Tawil Syndrome. We know now that I have a variant of Periodic Paralysis that is much like ATS, as yet unnamed. [42, 43]

It should be noted here that my mother was also diagnosed with much of the same heart conditions. She developed cardiomyopathy, which caused congestive heart failure. This is what eventually caused her death.

The Need for Oxygen

My Experience with Oxygen

Some people who have Periodic Paralysis may need oxygen therapy. I am one of them. I first noticed a breathing problem during total paralytic episodes. I was unable to move in any way, speak, or open my eyes. I had tachycardia and palpitations of my heart and I was having difficulty breathing. It would actually stop for a few seconds at a time. It felt like an elephant sitting on my chest. It was very frightening. Soon the difficulty of taking breaths in and out began to happen when I was not in paralysis. I found it more and more difficult to breathe. Every time I stood up, ate a meal or exerted myself in anyway, the breathing got worse, and my heart would speed up until it was beating 130 to 140 beats per minute, even while I was eating.

Finally, I was tested, and it was discovered that my oxygen levels recorded on an oximeter were dipping into seriously low levels during total paralytic attacks and upon any type of exertion. I was put on oxygen therapy for the periods of time I was in paralysis and during the night when I had my most serious episodes. It was not long before I realized I needed it twenty-four hours a day.

I am doing much better now that I am on oxygen therapy. I am having fewer episodes of the paralysis and the severe tachycardia has eased. I am breathing much easier. Understanding why I needed the oxygen and how it helps is discussed in this section. [18, 25, 26, 35]

Symptoms

The potassium shifting and depletion that occurs in Periodic Paralysis (PP) can affect all the muscles of the body including the heart muscle and the respiratory (breathing) muscles. The muscles can become permanently weakened and this includes the heart and breathing muscles. This weakness of the heart muscle and breathing muscles can be fatal in Periodic Paralysis. The diaphragm is the primary breathing muscle. The intercostal muscles are secondary breathing muscles. Breathing involves all the muscles from mouth to lower abdomen. Paralysis of the diaphragm can cause respiratory arrest or the sudden stoppage of breathing. [44]

If the organs are deprived of oxygen, the heart and the rest of the body are working harder to stay alive. This can cause an individual with PP to develop hypoventilation. This is a condition in which one is barely breathing due to weak breathing muscles which prompts him or her to breath less and less over time. Eventually one will get accustomed to getting by on less oxygen while excess carbon dioxide is stored in his muscles and organs. This can cause long-term problems including damage to most of the organs and muscles in the body, but the heart and brain are particularly vulnerable. Oxygen therapy may be necessary at this point. [47] Based on the above information, it is important to understand that when someone with Periodic Paralysis begins to hyperventilate during an episode with tachycardia, this is due to the body trying to compensate by expelling the excess carbon dioxide. This is a good thing, though he or she may be trying to stop the process, because it may be scary. A caregiver should allow the person to hyperventilate without resorting to such things as using a paper bag. [45]

And so, if an individual, who may or not be on oxygen

therapy, begins to have difficulty breathing during an episode of partial or total paralysis or at any time; he or she may get some relief if they breathe in through their nose and breathe out as hard as they can through the mouth to expel the carbon dioxide. It is good to do this until the breathing becomes easier and oxygen levels rise. The use of a portable finger oximeter is helpful in self-monitoring oxygen levels at home.

One can develop a serious condition of metabolic acidosis if the carbon dioxide levels are allowed to rise and remain in the body. Metabolic acidosis affects the cardiovascular and respiratory systems. It can cause potassium to shift out of the cells creating hyperkalemia. Hyperkalemia, which is high levels of potassium, and metabolic acidosis, a pH imbalance in which the body has accumulated too much acid and does not have enough bicarbonate to effectively neutralize the effects of the acid, can be life threatening. [21, 46]

Some individuals with Periodic Paralysis and Andersen-Tawil Syndrome must be careful with exercise if they begin to have trouble breathing while exerting themselves. It is best not to make your body work too hard because it can be due to exercise intolerance and it can cause the adrenalin to run thus causing potassium shifting, and the cycle can begin anew; weakening the muscles and organs which can cause tachycardia and arrhythmias including the long QT interval heartbeat which can lead cardiac arrest. Or it may be that one's breathing organs and cardiac muscles are weakening, and oxygen therapy may be indicated to ease the excess work of the heart and other organs.

Diagnosing

If an individual with Period Paralysis begins to have breathing problems, it would be best to have it checked out with you Primary Care Physician. The doctor can refer you to a pulmonologist or have your oxygen levels tested using an oximeter with a recorder overnight or for twenty-four hours.

Conclusion

I now understand why I need to use oxygen. Over the years of potassium depletion and shifting, my cardiac and breathing muscles have become weak and cannot do the job they need to do. My heart is working overtime. Hypoventilation has developed. My breathing has become too shallow, and my lungs cannot expel the buildup of carbon dioxide. Damage has been done to most of the organs in my body due to the buildup, including my heart, my breathing muscles and my brain. The oxygen eases the excess work of the heart and other organs, and aides in expelling carbon dioxide.

However, due to the body-wide organ damage, I am unable to do anything that requires any exertion. I get worn out very easily and the tachycardia begins quickly. This is also due to the exercise intolerance I experience due to Periodic Paralysis.

Kidney Issues

Kidney function can be affected in individuals with Periodic Paralysis. We know that when potassium shifts, calcium carbonate from the bone is released. This increase of calcium carbonate can lead to the formation of kidney stones. We also know if one has chronic metabolic acidosis, as a result of Periodic Paralysis, his or her kidneys can be affected because metabolic acidosis also causes an increase or shifting of potassium into the body fluids causing an increase of calcium carbonate. The use of the commonly used diuretic for patients with Periodic Paralysis, acetazolamide, also known as diamox, can cause kidney stones. [5]

Osteoporosis

When potassium shifts in the body, as it does in Periodic Paralysis, calcium carbonate from the bone is released. This causes a loss of the bone crystals in the bones leading to osteoporosis. Chronic metabolic acidosis, as a result of Periodic Paralysis, also causes the potassium to shift, thus creating bone loss or osteoporosis. [48, 21]

My Experience with Osteoporosis

In 2005 as we were preparing to move, my left foot suddenly began to hurt when I walked. It gradually got worse during the move, so I had x-rays taken at the hospital in the new town shortly after arriving. However, the radiologist did not find anything wrong. It did not improve so, finally after quite some time, I got a referral to a podiatrist who did another set of x-rays and was able to diagnose a stress fracture and also discovered I had an extra bone in the same foot which was causing some of the pain. I was put in a walking boot cast and wore it for about a year.

In 2008 I was shocked to discover I had severe osteoporosis considered to be at the "bone crush stage" in my spine and hips. Several years earlier I had been diagnosed with osteopenia, which is a less serious degree of osteoporosis. It had progressed very quickly. I could not understand this because I had taken a calcium tablet each day with my multi-vitamin since I was in my early thirties. I knew that my mother also had osteoporosis considered "off of the chart", but a bigger surprise was that two of my brothers in their fifties also had osteoporosis severe enough to require daily medication.

Due to the fact I had already had a fractured foot, I was sent to an endocrinologist for treatment for the osteoporosis. I was told that my condition was severe, and I needed to treat it very aggressively. I was put on a new medication called "forteo". I had to inject it into my thigh every night for at least a year. I dutifully did this painful chore for nearly a year until the day I ended up in the seizure-like episode and ended up in the hospital. I believe this medication, or the combination of it and the other medications I was on, was the cause.

I know now through research there is a connection between Periodic Paralysis and the osteoporosis. Some individuals with Periodic Paralysis can develop early bone loss due to the potassium shifting out of the bones and other organs as it shifts into the muscles. During the shifting, there is a loss of the bone crystals causing bone-loss or osteoporosis.

Metabolic Acidosis/Lactic Acidosis

Metabolic acidosis and lactic acidosis are complex conditions, which can be difficult to understand, but fairly easy to diagnose based on symptoms and lab results. However, in individuals with Periodic Paralysis, they are often overlooked, missed on the lab reports and testing for them is often not requested as a possibility for obvious symptoms. Because Periodic Paralysis is a mineral metabolic disorder and it affects the breathing muscles, individuals with it appear to be susceptible for developing these conditions. Episodes of paralysis are triggered by metabolic and lactic acidosis.

This section, just as the section on heart issues, will be as simplified as possible but some terms will be included which, will be specifically used for recognition and diagnosis by physicians and patients. (More technical information about metabolic acidosis can be found at the end of this chapter.)

Complications

Metabolic Acidosis

As we have previously learned, metabolic acidosis is a pH imbalance (the balance between the acid and alkaline), in which the body accumulates an excess of acid in the body fluids and does not have enough bicarbonate to neutralize the effects of the acid effectively. An individual can develop metabolic acidosis, if the carbon dioxide levels are allowed to rise and remain in the body.

We know that metabolic acidosis affects the heart and breathing. It results in potassium shifting out of the cells and into the bloodstream creating hyperkalemia, too much potassium. The combination of metabolic acidosis and hyperkalemia is a serious condition and can be life threatening leading to shock and death.

Symptoms of Metabolic Acidosis

Some of the more common symptoms of metabolic acidosis are muscle weakness, bone and muscle pain, headache, chest pain, tachycardia, heart palpitations, abdominal pain, rapid breathing, shortness of breath, confusion, drowsiness, a lack of energy and paralysis for persons with Periodic Paralysis. If metabolic acidosis becomes severe it can lead to shock (a lack of an appropriate flow of blood in the body) or death. However, the symptoms of metabolic acidosis are sometimes not very obvious or specific, depending on the cause. It should be noted that in some individual's metabolic acidosis could be mild and ongoing (chronic).

In chronic metabolic acidosis an individual's bones and kidneys are affected. When potassium shifts in the body, calcium carbonate from the bone is released. This causes a loss of the bone crystals leading to osteoporosis. When the kidneys are affected, and this can be seen by the formation of kidney stones.

Diagnosing Metabolic Acidosis

There are several methods that can be used to diagnose metabolic acidosis; usually more than one will be utilized. The arterial blood gas test is the most important and decisive one used.

The most widely used methods are listed below:

* ❖ Arterial blood gas: If the pH balance is low (below 7.75) and bicarbonate levels are low, then metabolic acidosis is present.
* ❖ Anion gap: subtracting chloride and bicarbonate levels from sodium. If elevated (>16 mmol/l) it can indicate metabolic acidosis and lactic acidosis
* ❖ Serum electrolyte levels (high potassium)
* ❖ Urine pH: acidity levels
* ❖ Glucose/sugar levels
* ❖ Kidney function
* ❖ Full blood count
* ❖ An EKG: This will show heart complications such as arrhythmias

Treatment and Management for Metabolic Acidosis

The best way to treat and manage metabolic acidosis for individuals with Periodic Paralysis is to avoid the causes. It may develop due to an unbalanced diet, exercise or exertion, medications (it should be noted here that diamox or acetazolamide may cause it.), illness, infections or too much potassium, or it may be chronic. Eliminating the medication, avoiding exercise or exertion, eating a balanced pH diet, lowering the level of potassium or treating the infection or illness, will manage the acidosis. Using bicarbonate or increasing alkaline will neutralize the acids. In severe cases, dialysis may be needed. Mechanical assistance or ventilation for breathing may be necessary. [48, 49]

Lactic Acidosis

Lactic acidosis is a form of metabolic acidosis that occurs when blood pH levels in the blood and lactic acid become unbalanced. This is the result of oxygen levels dropping. It forms if the carbohydrates get broken down and are used for energy from the low oxygen levels. The lactic acid increases in the bloodstream more quickly than it can be expelled. Too much lactic acid in the body creates an increase of pyruvic acid. Too much pyruvic acid in the body creates metabolic acid in the body. It can cause mental confusion and lead to a coma. It affects the function of the liver and can develop into multiple organ failure, which can lead to death.

Lactic acidosis can develop in individuals with metabolic disorders, especially ones that do not supply enough oxygen to tissues in the body. This kind is known as Type A lactic acidosis. Because Periodic Paralysis is a disorder in which hypoventilation (slow and shallow breathing) can occur when the breathing muscles weaken, individuals with it, can and do develop metabolic and lactic acidosis.

Symptoms of Lactic Acidosis

Some of the more common symptoms of lactic acidosis are frequent urination or absence of urine output, anemia, low blood pressure, abdominal pain, an enlarged liver, weight loss, breathing problems, hyperventilation, muscle pain, weakness, tiredness, irregular heartbeat, lightheadedness, dizziness, profuse sweating, loss of appetite, nausea, vomiting, headaches, sensitivity to light, moist skin, clammy and cold skin, chills and dry eyes, nose, mouth and throat. As it progresses the hands and feet turn blue, blood pressure drops, heart rate slows, a person feels disoriented and confused and unconsciousness and paralysis set in for someone with Periodic Paralysis.

Diagnosing Lactic Acidosis

A lactate test is used to determine the amount of lactic acidosis in the blood. The normal values are between 0.5 and 2.2 mmol/L. Above 2.2 (>2.2 mmol/L) would indicate an individual has lactic acidosis. It is best not to use a tourniquet when testing for lactic acidosis because it can cause the results to be falsely elevated.

Treatment and Management for Lactic Acidosis

The best way to treat lactic acidosis is to treat the underlying cause as in metabolic acidosis. In the case of Periodic Paralysis, it is best to avoid the causes. It may develop due to an unbalanced diet, exercise or exertion, medications, illness, infections, too much potassium or it may be chronic. Eliminating the medication, avoiding exercise or exertion, eating a balanced pH diet, lowering the level of potassium or treating the infection or illness will manage the acidosis. In severe cases, dialysis may be needed. Mechanical assistance or ventilation for breathing may be necessary. Lactic acidosis may be difficult to avoid in individuals with Periodic Paralysis due to the chronic low oxygen levels from the weak breathing muscles. Oxygen therapy may be necessary.[50, 51]

My Experience with Metabolic and Lactic Acidosis

Some of my laboratory tests over the years indicate I have been in metabolic acidosis. At those times I have been deathly ill, and the doctors ignored my condition. I have proof of this in my past laboratory results. I was able to obtain them after requesting my records from previous doctors and from the hospital. We discovered that they were caused by the medications I was prescribed including acetazolamide and some antibiotics, which caused high levels of acidity in my body and low oxygen levels.

I also have been in lactic acidosis and discovered this nearly two years after the fact. A year ago, one year after I had been diagnosed, I received a copy of my medical records on disk from my last two primary care doctors. I had each of them for only a few months. Both of them left town due to being overloaded with patients by the management of their medical group.

The disk had no record from either doctor but a few records from other doctors including the report from a Neurology Clinic at the major medical center in Portland, Oregon. I had been seen there in April of 2010 and the results of a lab test that were done there.

The young doctor I saw there was wonderful but left the medical center after my initial visit. However, he wrote in his report that he thought I had Periodic Paralysis and that I should be put on diamox to see if it would help, if the muscle biopsy I was to have done showed no mitochondrial disease. The two doctors, who took over, obviously ignored his report. They did the muscle biopsy (which showed no mitochondrial disease, but it did indicate atrophy of the muscle fibers, and variation in the size and shape of both type 1 and type 2 muscle fibers as well as an increase in lipid, all an indication of muscle wasting) and ignored the results of the Amino Acid Plasma Quantitative Test which came back abnormal indicating that I was in lactic acidosis.

These results could have helped to diagnose the Periodic Paralysis much earlier. It had been recommended in the Amino Acid Test report that I have more tests done and be followed up for the condition. However, not one word was ever said to me about this by any of the three doctors at the neurology clinic or by my primary care physician at the time, nor the two doctors who later became my PCPs, or by the specialist in another state.

The following is the results of the Amino Acid Plasma Quantitative Test (The original report is found in the appendix):

Aspartic Acid (<2, 0-6) and 3 Methylhistidine (<;6, 0-64) were low and Proline Plasma (501, 110-360), Alanine Plasma (744, 230-510), Valine (331, 150-310) Plasma, Tyrosine Plasma (107, 45-74), Homcysteine Plasma (11.9, 4.0-12.0), and Pyruvic Acid (0.146, 0.030-0.107) were all high. Lactic Acid was high also (1.8, .5-1.6)

"The high Alanine Plasma indicates: Primary or Secondary Lactic Acidosis or Hyperammonemic Syndrome. Clinical findings may be episodic. Further workup may be warranted."

"Hyperprolinemia is consistent with Mitochondrial Dysfunction or may indicate Type 1 or Type 2 Hyperprolinemia. Further analysis may be warranted."

"Recommend measurement of blood lactate and repeat of the Plasma Amino Acid Analysis."

When I returned to the neurology clinic for the results, I was told everything came back "normal", I was told to go have fun while in Portland. The doctors had either not read this lab work or had ignored it. Once again, my condition worsened due to the absolute incompetence of another group of medical specialists.

Here is the timeline:
- ❖ 4/20/10 Saw Dr E
- ❖ 4/20/10 Lab work was done
- ❖ 4/22/10 Specimens arrived in NC for testing
- ❖ 4/22/10 Testing done
- ❖ 4/26/10 Entry of results into computer

Complications

- ❖ 5/11/10 Received by Dr C
- ❖ 6/04/10 Muscle biopsy by Dr C and Dr L (Dr E gone)
- ❖ 7/14/10 Visit with Dr L for results of testing...told all was "normal"
- ❖ 7/14/10 Case closed by Dr L
- ❖ 7/14/10 The results faxed to my PCP
- ❖ 1/07/11 Diagnosed with Andersen-Tawil Syndrome

The results ruling out mitochondrial disease, but not ruling out a metabolic disorder, of which Periodic Paralysis is, and then with the recommendation of Dr. E, I should have been considered for a diagnosis of Periodic Paralysis and been given a trial of diamox in July of 2010.

That was six months before I got my diagnosis. The diagnosis came after changing my insurance company, getting three specialists on my own and firing my PCP. I could have been treated much sooner and not been labeled once again as a hypochondriac by several more medical professionals, when I was in metabolic acidosis and lactic acidosis and needed oxygen. I probably could have avoided the heart loop monitor implantation from which I nearly died and maybe could have had the lactic acidosis treated appropriately, which to this day I have not found a doctor who has addressed it.

Several months ago, I was able to speak with Dr. E, the young doctor who ordered the Amino Acid Plasma Quantitative Test. He explained that it was a rare test seldom used. He said that the test did indicate that I had lactic acidosis and that it looks like it can actually be used to diagnose Periodic Paralysis since it indicated I had a metabolic disorder (Periodic Paralysis) and lactic acidosis. He was happy to know that he had chosen Periodic Paralysis as his top choice for my diagnosis. He apologized for how I was treated at the Neurology Clinic and for leaving me at that critical time. He also told me that he was not surprised at all to know how Dr. L and Dr. C treated me.

He told me that he was going to research locating a specialist in ion channelopathies who may want to help my family and me. He said that Periodic Paralysis is an ion channelopathy (which we already know), a disease not like any other. It is not neuromuscular or a mitochondrial disease. It is in a category all its own and needs to be treated in non-conventional ways.

He told me that of the few patients he has had with Periodic Paralysis, they were all diagnosed with conversion disorder before they got their diagnosis. He explained that Periodic Paralysis is so different that it looks "fake" to doctors. He believes all doctors need to be educated (one reason why we are writing this book). He advised the best thing we could do is to find a doctor with an open mind and who will think "outside of the box" when it comes to diagnosing and treating people like us.

Knowing I have chronic or recurring metabolic acidosis and lactic acidosis saved my life. Calvin researched it and discovered that a pH balanced diet, supplements, oxygen and potassium bicarbonate all help the conditions. He set out to get these things for me. One at a time we tried them. Immediately, I began to improve. My lab work showed improvements and my heart tests were all in normal ranges. Although there are some things going still going on, my breathing was better, and I began to have fewer episodes of paralysis.

Before making the changes, I was experiencing long QT interval heartbeats and other arrhythmias and my blood pressure was very high. I was having more and more difficulty breathing and was dying and it was happening very quickly.

Complications

That is why I now eat a pH balanced diet, do not do anything to exert myself in any way, take potassium bicarbonate as needed, and am on oxygen twenty-four hours a day. If I stray from this plan my symptoms will quickly return. So, each day I manage my metabolic acidosis and lactic acidosis and stay balanced by doing what I refer to as "walking a tightrope". This is further discussed in Section Three.

Acidosis

Due to the seriousness of acidosis, Calvin has written a more technical article to better explain it and understand how it is diagnosed.

Calvin writes: There are many causes of abnormal potassium shifting. Genetic mutations and acidosis are two identifiable causes. Variations of the first type include Andersen-Tawil, which can be identified through locating genetic markers. Variations of the second type can be identified through measurement of bodily fluids acidity or pH. Periodic Paralysis is a disease characterized by varying degrees of muscle paralysis. From the perspective of this layman, Periodic Paralysis thus muscle paralysis is attributable to abnormal potassium levels inside and outside of cells. The terms Hyperkalemia and Hypokalemic are used to describe high and low levels of serum blood potassium. Both the speed and degree of the potassium shifting produce physiological symptoms.

The pH or acidity levels of the blood stream play a key role in potassium shifting. Metabolic acidosis is a medical condition that happens when the body produces too much acid. It can also occur when vital organs such as the kidneys do not perform properly. A primary function of the kidneys is to regulate the acidity or pH level of the body. The body maintains a continuous level of 7.35. Any changes in this optimal level of body pH or acidity can have serious and even fatal consequences.

The acidity or alkalinity of any substance is measured on a scale of 1 through 14. Pure water has a pH level measure very close to 7. Anything with a pH level below 7 is considered acidic. Anything with a pH level above 7 is considered alkalinic. pH is a measure of hydrogen concentration and activity. One of the tests performed during a standard blood draw is the measurement of Anion Gap. According to Wikipedia:

> *"The anion gap is the difference in the measured cations and the measured anions in serum, plasma, or urine. The magnitude of this difference (i.e., "gap") in the serum is often calculated in medicine when attempting to identify the cause of metabolic acidosis. If the gap is greater than normal, then high anion gap metabolic acidosis is diagnosed."*

A high anion gap number should warrant any medical professional to inquire deeper into the causes of increased acidity especially in cases of patients suffering with unexplained muscle paralysis. This is what led Susan and I to a deeper understanding of the disease. It also led us to treatment options outside the realm of medical professionals. A high anion gap number indicates the serum blood is highly acidic and the body is out of pH balance. It is a red flag that gets missed because most medical professionals do not understand the importance of pH levels in the body and how acidity affects potassium shifting and muscle function. For someone prone to abnormal cellular functions due to genetic mutations, high acidity can cause full body muscle paralysis, which is typical of Periodic Paralysis. Most medical professionals are incapable of connecting the dots even with verifiable science right in front of their eyes.

According to the Wikipedia:

"Acidosis is an increased acidity in the blood and other body tissue (i.e., an increased hydrogen ion concentration). If not further qualified, it usually refers to acidity of the blood plasma.

Acidosis is said to occur when arterial pH falls below 7.35 (except in the fetus- see below), while its counterpart (alkalosis) occurs at a pH over 7.45. Arterial blood gas analysis and other tests are required to separate the main causes". [52]

Determining a condition of metabolic acidosis is all about the accurate measurement of acidity within the body. Acids have been determined to play a key role in potassium shifting. The following excerpt was taken from a comprehensive publication regarding metabolic acidosis.

"A metabolic acidosis can cause significant physiological effects, particularly affecting the respiratory and cardiovascular systems." Metabolic acidosis can cause *"Shift of K+ out of cells causing Hyperkalemic".* [22]

Measurement of Anion Gap

After having some conversations with a medical lab technician regarding the science behind the measurement of anion gap, I discovered many alarming issues that are worth sharing. The first issue relates to how a state of metabolic acidosis is determined. As further research on my part has pointed out, there are three types of measurements and several methods used to determine a state of metabolic acidosis. Here is the first response I received from a medical lab in this area regarding the measurement of metabolic acidosis and anion gap.

"Anion gap (AG or AGAP) is a value calculated using the results of an electrolyte panel. It is used to help distinguish between anion-gap and non-anion-gap metabolic acidosis. Acidosis refers to an excess of acid in the body; this can disturb many cell functions and should be recognized as quickly as possible, when present. AG is frequently used in the hospital and/or emergency room setting to help diagnose and monitor acutely ill patients. If anion-gap metabolic acidosis is identified, the AG may be used to help monitor the effectiveness of treatment and the underlying condition.

Specifically, the anion gap evaluates the difference between measured and unmeasured electrical particles (ions or electrolytes) in the fluid portion of the blood. According to the principle of electrical neutrality, the number of positive ions (cations) and negative ions (anions) should be equal. However, not all ions are routinely measured. The calculated AG result represents the unmeasured ions and primarily consists of anions, hence the name "anion gap."

There are two ways to calculate the anion gap with or without the potassium.

Our lab calculates with the potassium and our reference range reflects this.

Anion gap = ([Na+] + [K+]) - ([Cl-] + [HCO3-])

The second method is without the potassium:
Anion gap = ([Na+]) - ([Cl-] + [HCO3-])

And the third method being: "Modern analyzers make use of ion-selective electrodes which give a normal anion gap as <11 mEq/L. Therefore, according to the

> *new classification system, a high anion gap is anything above 11 mEq/L and a normal anion gap is between 3–11 mEq/L.* [8]?

> *All 3 methods are valid calculations, but you have to use the correct reference range for the calculation that you are using, and reference ranges are not interchangeable. Reference ranges are important because reference (normal) ranges are dependent on instrumentation, testing methodology and populations (age, sex, race) served. These ranges are not universal and are determined by the clinical laboratory scientists who performed your testing."*

It took me a very long time to understand what this meant. After doing more research, more questions naturally were conceived. I asked the same lab to look at three separate lab reports. I told them that one report was conducted at our local hospital. I told them that the second report was conducted at a hospital in another town about forty miles away. (I concealed the fact that this report was an identical copy of the lab conducted at our local hospital). The only changes were in the letterhead of the hospital where the lab was reproduced. The third report was from another lab that I was talking with for further clarification about the testing methodology. Here is the second reply that I received from the original lab.

> *"The method used to test the Sodium, Potassium, and Chloride assays is ion-selective electrodes. The Carbon Dioxide is enzymatic and detected by a colorimetric method. The anion gap reference range was determined using literature and confirmed by our actual patient population."*

The second reply answers my original question about the testing methods used to determine acidity. What they are saying is that they use "literature" (of unknown origins) and "actual patient population" to determine the standard by which they determine what is normal and what is outside of normal range. The sample used to determine normal ranges was from their patient populations and not the general population. This would cast doubts on the reliability of their established norms. In the first response they failed to mention a third testing technique but then in the second response stated that they used the third type using "ion-selective electrodes" (after I introduced the information). I caught them in several blatant lies about their testing methods and also was able to determine the norms to be unreliable due to the narrow scope of the sample populations being tested.

The twisting and turning of the facts permeate the entire medical profession. This is just one example. When pressed for answers to questions about the credibility of tests, you will never get the truth until people are pressed into a corner. The only way to get the facts is to take one of them to court and have them testify under oath. For a person with life-threatening muscle paralysis this kind of misinformation equates to a death sentence. And this is only the tip of the iceberg that we have uncovered.

One of the most interesting and telling parts of the above exchange occurred as the lab was asked to examine three separate medical labs and their response not knowing that the second lab was only a copy of the first. On the second lab report, which came from another hospital, the standards had been changed. Let me explain. The first lab was taken at our local hospital. Susan's anion gap number came back as twenty-two, which fell far outside the normal ranges, identified on the lab analysis as any number between three and twelve. When this same lab result was sent to the hospital in the nearby town (a subsidiary or sister hospital to the one in our community) the report got altered. The anion gap number stayed the same but the number describing acceptable normal ranges had changed. The new normal range was displayed as anything between three and twenty-four. The hospital in the nearby town refused to respond to my calls and refused to reply to any email messages. Simply put, the same blood draw and measured potassium level was reported by one lab as normal by both labs, but the normal range was different for each reporting hospital. Depending on which lab reports someone was looking at the interpretation would be different. That difference could mean the difference between life and death for someone with undiagnosed Periodic Paralysis. Periodic Paralysis requires thoughtful scrutiny and interpretation of test results. A business-as-usual attitude is unacceptable, and patients are dying as a result of no one paying close attention to what is going on with modern medicine.

It is a losing battle trying to get laboratories to explain what they are doing and how they are doing it. And to make matters even more confusing, the standards get changed even as copies of identical lab reports are distributed through different outlets. All the labs in question were taken at our local hospital and the acceptable norms were changed for no explainable reason as the labs were transferred from one facility to another. One set of reports showed Susan's anion gap as within normal ranges. Several of Susan's labs changed reflecting that her anion gap was higher than normal and that she was in a state of metabolic acidosis during the times she was in the hospital. No one at our local hospital ever questioned the high acid readings and the hospital has not responded to inquiries. If they had actually taken the time to look closely at Susan's laboratory results (considering the unusualness of her physical condition), her condition would have been identified and proper treatment given. A simple infusion of potassium bicarbonate or oxygen therapy might have reversed the paralytic outcomes of having too high a level of acidity in her body. Something as simple as hyperventilating might have helped her expel the excess carbon dioxide thereby reducing the acidity levels in her body.

Susan's potassium levels taken at the hospital and local lab usually returned as being within normal ranges, so it was important for them to look at her physical symptoms to further identify her condition. She was having heart arrhythmias and trouble breathing due to high acidity. She was in a state of hyperkalemia due to high potassium levels (which were determined to fall within normal ranges by the hospital but actually were in high ranges for her).

The people need to be held accountable for their actions but for most people this is beyond their reach. As we discovered it is nearly impossible to hold incompetent medical professionals accountable in court. It is cost prohibitive for most people and finding a medical doctor who is willing to testify against another medical doctor or hospital is nearly impossible. They have the resources and we do not. Attorneys are expensive and medical insurance companies have unlimited resources to win. My conclusion is that you take your life into your own hands when you walk, crawl or get delivered by ambulance through their doors.

Metabolic Acidosis

I wouldn't go as far as to assume there is some kind of massive conspiracy going on to keep people ill, but as we all know, stranger things have happened and especially when we are dealing with pharmaceutical companies, the Food and Drug Administration and the American Medical Association. They all prosper from the perpetuation of human illness, misery and disease.

Several things are certain at this point in time: medical professionals have very little knowledge of the science behind those numbers we see on laboratory reports and have very few treatment options for serious illness outside of administering pharmaceutical drugs or performing invasive surgeries. For most people this does not mean a lot because they never get seriously ill but for a smaller percentage of the population, suffering with rare forms of illness and disease, it means the difference between life and death. They are left alone to figure out what is causing symptoms that medical professionals are unable to address. We have very few people who are real healers in this country or people who understand the basics of the rudimentary causes of human disease. This opens the doors to quacks and charlatans and very sick people get taken advantage of in their personal quest to find wellness.

My favorite form of quackery involves the use of "positive thoughts" to control disease processes or cure metabolic based illnesses. When people are desperate for answers to mysterious health conditions that medical professionals are unable to diagnose or treat, they will spend everything they own to find a cure. These unfortunate individuals are often pushed into the shadows and left to die alone.

There were several primary resources that I used to help me understand what was causing Susan's muscle paralysis. *Acid-base pHysiology' written by Kerry Brandiss* taught me more about metabolic acidosis than all other books and research articles combined. It describes the fundamentals of metabolic acidosis in great depth and detail. The information contained inside this text saved Susan's life. As it turned out, this topic has been around for quite a while and this subject is taught to medical students at medical schools. Throughout this entire process, I often asked myself "where were the doctors when this subject was being taught to them at medical school?" Another research article of great importance is *Metabolic Acidosis by Joseph C. Charles, MD and Raymond L. Heilman.*

Since most metabolic processes are invisible to the human eye it is necessary to gather information by other means. Samples of blood, urine, and saliva all contain a wealth of information about what is going on inside of our bodies. Using medical devices to measure blood pressure, temperature, pulse rate, breathing rate, and brain and heart functions gives us detailed information about what is happening beneath our layers of skin. Without the medical tests and devices, the practice of medicine is left in the realm of subjective interpretations and baseless speculation, which is something I discovered many medical professionals engage in on a very regular basis. Unfortunately, many medical professionals do not use their tools of the trade and deadly consequences are the result. There are countless tests we can perform on our bodies that help us paint a mosaic about our bodies. When we are ill these tests and observations are particularly useful in forming conclusions about what might be causing our illness and the best way to treat the symptoms. In the case of Periodic Paralysis all these same rules apply but at an even more critical level. But there seems to be one major problem when doctors encounter Periodic Paralysis. Most medical professionals do not understand Periodic Paralysis or believe that such a disease or condition exits. Doctors will go out of their way to avoid a diagnosis of Periodic Paralysis mainly due to their narrow vision.

Every licensed medical doctor in the United States with the American Medical Association (AMA) has engaged in some form of higher education at an approved medical institution. The curriculum at these places of higher learning is standard throughout all these institutions. In other words, all doctors are exposed to the same types of learning opportunities. The texts are the same, the academic demands are the same, the experiential learning opportunities are the same and everyone gets the same basics in physiology, chemistry, statistics, disease and medical practice. The practioners are taught traditional ways of addressing illness and disease. They are taught how to evaluate patients and how to treat identifiable medical conditions. For the most part this system works for the majority of people. People get sick, they go to the doctor and the doctor diagnoses their condition and prescribes a treatment. The treatments are administered, and most people recover. The system works most of the time. When a doctor encounters a patient showing symptoms that cannot be quickly connected to some cause then more medical tests are ordered. The patient is referred to a medical specialist who practices in a particular specialty area. Usually, the specialist will diagnose the cause of the disease or illness and prescribe a treatment. The patient will typically heal and return to normal life. In some cases, the patient will develop limitations and be expected to learn to cope with those limitations with the help of some assistive technologies such as pacemakers, wheelchairs, artificial limbs, and other aides. The system works most of the time for most people.

On rare occasions medical doctors and specialists are unable to diagnose the cause of a particular illness or disease and unable to prescribe an effective treatment. Oftentimes the treatments they prescribe aggravates the patient's symptoms. When medical professionals encounter such cases, they generally believe that the patient is imagining the condition and creating their own symptoms as a result of some form of mental illness. They are referred to medical specialists of the mind commonly known as psychiatrists. Very few doctors will go the extra mile to diagnose difficult cases. They have just so much time scheduled each day and must see a certain number of patients in order to pay the overhead. The cases that are easiest to diagnose and treat turn the highest profits for the doctors. Least amount of time spent equals the greatest profits. But the doctor still bills for an hour of time even though they only spend an actual ten minutes with a patient. The cases that are most difficult to diagnose and treat return the lowest profits. It is difficult for most laypeople to believe this reality. This knowledge makes most people cynical and causes them to give up their search for answers to difficult questions. You are left to your own devices for care and treatment, if you have a disease that is nearly impossible to diagnose and impossible to treat.

Once the patient has entered into the realm of specialized psychiatric treatment, they are administered pharmaceutical drugs, surgeries and other forms of treatment designed to alter their state of consciousness. Psychiatrists attempt to make sad people happy and dysfunctional people functional through the use of drugs, surgeries and therapy. It is all neat and tidy for the medical community but tragic for many people who still suffer with an illness or disease that is very real and not imaginary such as Periodic Paralysis.

People who suffer with Periodic Paralysis have a disease that is typically misdiagnosed as somatic in origins rather than being founded in chemical, electrical and metabolic imbalances, which are brought about by genetic and environmental factors. They are treated with disrespect and basically left alone at home with no hope for a better tomorrow. They are treated with pharmaceutical drugs that increase symptoms rendering the patient totally paralyzed. Most people who suffer with Periodic Paralysis suffer with other debilitating diseases, which complicate normal metabolic processes. More specialists are called in to treat problems with kidneys, heart, and lungs, which often are a result of medication-induced acidosis.

There is not any way to identify how many people die each year from complications caused by acidosis mainly because the cause of death in these individuals is listed as things such as heart failure, kidney disease, liver failure, and respiratory arrest. Very seldom does anyone look at what caused the kidneys to fail, heart to die as a result of uncontrolled tachycardia, or lungs to stop the normal function of taking in oxygen and exhaling carbon dioxide. This all goes unnoticed, and patients die in the darkness of incompetence. The truth about Periodic Paralysis is that it is difficult to identify and difficult to treat. There is no known cure that I am aware of but there are ways to manage the severity of paralytic episodes.

We hear people talk about pH levels all the time and in a variety of contexts. People with fish aquariums are constantly monitoring and adjusting the pH level of the fish tank. Water treatment plants constantly monitor the pH balance of our drinking water. Fortunately, water itself has the correct pH balance needed to support all kinds of life. Water can be the carrier of elements that alter the pH balance of the organisms it enters but also can carry away unwanted amount of harmful chemicals which are capable of causing all types of nasty illnesses and diseases. Our bodies naturally maintain a slightly alkaline pH level, which is measured just above the number seven on a pH scale of one to fourteen. A number of one is the most acidic and a number of fourteen the most alkalinic or less acidic depending on your viewpoint. Our bodies are constantly at work to maintain a specific number around 7.35 and will do anything including taking marrow from bone to maintain an optimum pH balance.

Diet has much to do with how our bodies maintain a proper pH balance. If your diet contains all the vitamins, minerals and other things such as amino acids then it is easier for your body to maintain a proper pH balance. If the pH balance moves one direction or another by only a few degrees for any extended period of time, then you become seriously ill and quite possibly die. In order for us to stay alive and functioning, we must maintain a specific pH level. What we put inside of our bodies in the form of foodstuff, chemicals and things that are either acidic or alkalinic, either aid or take away from the smooth functioning of the body. A condition known as metabolic acidosis occurs when the body becomes more acidic.

Metabolic Acidosis is one of the main causes of potassium shifting. A highly acidic system leads to high levels of acid in the body and causes the organs in charge of riding the body of acid to work extra hard. If this overworking takes place over time, then these organs become diseased and fail. When our internal organs do not work properly then our bodies become contaminated, and all sorts of things begin to happen. When there are high levels of carbon dioxide present in our bodies then our lungs work harder to expel the excess carbon dioxide. When the blood stream contains an abnormal amount of potassium (>5%<) due to acidity then the excess potassium causes the muscles to malfunction.

Diaphragm muscles control breathing function but if these muscles are in a state of paralysis due to an increase in potassium, then a person experiences labored breathing or as some people report having the feeling of an elephant sitting on their chest. While the body is trying to expel excess carbon dioxide and the diaphragm muscles are in paralysis due to abnormalities in serum and cellular potassium levels, the heart works harder, and heart arrhythmias can occur. If breathing is not returned to normal and muscle tissues oxygenated, then serious damage and possible death will follow. People are often placed on mechanical ventilators to force oxygen in and carbon dioxide out when abnormal lung function occurs.

As you can probably see this process heads quickly in a downward spiral and a person is at risk of death on the way to the emergency room (ER). If they make it to the ER, then they are faced with people fumbling around with insurance forms and taking vitals and samples of urine and blood. A catheter is inserted for the convenience of the staff and precious minutes tick away while permanent damage is being done. In many cases even with the test results staring them in the face, the ER staff is not capable of correctly interpreting the results. In many cases they are not capable of reading monitors correctly. It is all very alarming. I have sat by Susan's bedside in an ER many times and watched her nearly die as incompetent doctors and nurses fumbled the ball. When you visit an ER, you are placing your life into the hands of strangers who might not be there for the reasons you would hope.

As we discuss on our Periodic Paralysis Network web site and Face Book page, it is important for everyone to eat a balanced diet, which includes foods that are high in alkaline and low in acid. Vegetables, fruits and grains are generally more alkaline and meats and processed foods (canned and package goods have no nutritional value and don't deserve the food label) are more acidic. The alkalinity or acidity of substances is measured in terms of pH. The human body strictly maintains a pH level of 7.35 in the serum blood level on the alkaline side of the scale. The urine pH has wider fluctuations depending on a number of variables such as time of day, hydration and dehydration, type of foodstuff consumed, and the filtration ability of the kidneys. The pH level reading in saliva also fluctuates throughout the day. As the pH number falls and our bodies become more acidic, we become very ill and at risk of death if the causes are not corrected.

Anyone with potassium shifting that is caused by a genetic mutation of the cell membranes also needs to be aware that metabolic acidosis causes excess potassium to be released from cells into the blood stream. Potassium shifting caused by metabolic acidosis is treatable but the potassium shifting caused by the genetic mutation is more difficult to manage. Both things combined might be part of the reason why people with Periodic Paralysis have such serious and life-threatening episodes of muscle paralysis. Left untreated the combination of these conditions can cause muscle paralysis that can result in death if left untreated. Most doctors do not understand the dynamics involved in this process and patients are left untreated and suffer with major organ damage and failure.

Part Three:
Managing Periodic Paralysis

Chapter Twenty
Treating and Managing Periodic Paralysis

Introduction

Though misdiagnosed and mistreated for sixty-one years, the signs and symptoms of Periodic Paralysis existed from the time I was a small child. I have a form that is obviously inherited but the genetic mutation is unknown. I am now totally and permanently disabled due to lack of a diagnosis and proper treatment in a timely manner. We now know that Periodic Paralysis is an ion channelopathy, a form of metabolic disorder, a rare disease like no other. We know what causes it, the different forms of it, the aspects of the attacks or episodes of paralysis and muscle weakness and the triggers that set them into motion. We understand why we need to be able to stop or prevent the attacks. Now we will learn how to treat and manage the symptoms to gain a better quality of life by what I call 'walking a tightrope'.

Part One starts with the "end" of my medical story, rather than the beginning. Part Two begins by explaining what Periodic Paralysis is "not". Part Three, in the same manner, will begin with the final overall outline of the plan or method we call 'walking a tightrope' and the remainder of this section will go into great detail and expand on each component including how to discover your triggers, how to relieve your symptoms, how to get a diagnosis, how to find a doctor and how to monitor the symptoms.

Our method was created after trial and error in my own quest for relief of symptoms, treatment and management for my form of Periodic Paralysis. How effective it is for all other types will be determined in time as other people adopt this approach. We call it 'walking a tightrope' because every single step or component must be strictly followed and adhered to or it will not work. Each step depends on the one before it and the one following it. One misstep can set everything into motion once again. An individual will become out of balance and paralytic episodes and other symptoms will repeatedly occur. One will fall off the 'tightrope'.

This method or plan can be modified and individualized for each person with Periodic Paralysis. Calvin and I had no doctors assisting us and gleaned as much information as possible over the Internet and in discussion with other people who experience Periodic Paralysis and Andersen-Tawil Syndrome. Each component will be discussed and elaborated on in the following chapters.

The Outline

How To Treat, Control and Manage Periodic Paralysis?

- ❖ Educate Yourself.
  - ➢ Join a Periodic Paralysis Community.
  - ➢ Search the Internet.
  - ➢ Read books.
- ❖ Identify and eliminate all known triggers.
  - ➢ Record symptoms and possible causes.
  - ➢ Monitor symptoms.
  - ➢ Keep a journal.
- ❖ Relieve your symptoms.
  - ➢ Avoid all known triggers.
    - ▪ Avoid all pharmaceutical drugs including over-the-counter medications (consult with the doctor beforehand).
    - ▪ Avoid stress.
    - ▪ Minimize physical activity.
    - ▪ Avoid temperature extremes.
  - ➢ Eat a pH balanced diet consisting of 70% alkaline and 30% acidic foods.
    - ▪ Avoid processed foods (eat from the farm and not from the factory).
    - ▪ Use organic foods.
    - ▪ Drink distilled water.
  - ➢ Use organic natural nutritional supplements.
    - ▪ Vitamins.

- Probiotics.
- Calcium Citrate.
- Magnesium Citrate.
➢ Stay well rested.
➢ Stay well hydrated.
➢ Use a Cardy Meter to measure serum potassium before treating muscle paralysis.
  - Take potassium when needed (if low potassium).
    • Research different types and forms of potassium.
    • Purchase potassium from a reliable natural organic source.
  - Take glucose or carbohydrates as needed (if high potassium).
➢ Use oxygen during periods of muscle paralysis.
  - Breathing problems.
  - Low oxygen levels.
  - Heart problems.
➢ Use meditation and mental imagery.
  - Practice
❖ Monitor your vitals.
➢ Obtain medical equipment.
  - Cardy meter.
  - Oximeter.
  - Stethoscope.
  - Wrist blood pressure device.
  - Ear thermometer.
  - PH monitor.
  - Blood sugar monitor.
❖ Getting a Diagnosis.
➢ The Plan.
  - Process of elimination.
    • Gather the facts.
    • Lab work.
    • Periods of paralysis, documented.
    • EKGs.
    • Oximeter recordings.
    • Genetic testing?
    • Previous medical records.
    • Chart the triggers.
    • Document potassium use.
    • Gather and chart family information.
❖ Getting Proper Treatment.
➢ Assemble a team of doctors (knowledgeable about PP

or willing to learn).
- PCP.
- Neurologist.
- Electrocardiologist.
- Nephrologist.
- Endocrinologist.
- Counselor or therapist.
- Others as needed for symptoms.
- MDA doctors.
➢ Direct the team.
  - Primary Care Doctor.
  - Paramedics.
  - Emergency Rooms.

Making Lifestyle Changes

Calvin writes: It will take a great deal of self-discipline to make healthier lifestyle choices. It has been my experience that people generally do not make personal changes unless they are faced with some painful consequences for the continuation of old habits or ways of behaving. People with chronic addictions have proven that some people will continue to put harmful substances inside their bodies even in the face of death. The majority of people will become very ill before making the connection between ill health and poor diet.

If you are having difficulty ridding yourself of poor lifestyle choices, you are like many millions of other people. This is precisely why we see millions of Americans today classified as obese. Many people need some type of outside intervention and support to make major lifestyle changes especially when it comes to stopping the consumption of poisonous substances such as nicotine, alcohol, caffeine, salt, artificial sweeteners, processed sugar and foods, animal fat and pharmaceutical drugs. Drugs obtained legally and illegally are especially difficult to discontinue.

My personal awareness about the relationship between personal health and proper nutrition and diet was expensive in terms of poor health. I had to become seriously ill before waking up to the fact that I was consuming things that were causing my poor health. For me it was important to go through the pains of withdrawals in order to teach myself lessons that would not be soon forgotten.

Pain is a great teacher. Experiencing the discomfort and pains involved in ridding ourselves of unhealthy chemical substances helps guarantee future success. Making changes takes time and a lot of patience and persistence is required. Caution should be used when attempting to quit any chemical substance especially those substances known to cause physical addiction. Medical advice should be sought before discontinued use of any chemical substance that is known to be addictive. Non-addictive substances are much easier to eliminate. Going 'cold-turkey' could kill you so exercise great caution when eliminating harmful chemical substances from your daily routine.

Difficult but Successful

Susan writes: We understand it is difficult at first to give up so many things like, caffeine, sugar, white flour and fats and then add a great deal of more fresh vegetables to the diet. We understand it will be work to discover all the triggers that set the symptoms in motion. Avoiding them may be even more difficult if they are things you enjoy. Monitoring vitals and recording them constantly may be overwhelming to begin with but needed for baselines. However, when the attacks or paralysis begin to stop and one can regain his or her life, it will be worth the efforts.

Many people who contact us have developed their own plan based on our methods. Like me, they are 'walking a tightrope' every minute of each day and they are enjoying the successes of decreasing the number of paralytic episodes and lessening the severity of the attacks. We hear about how much weight they have lost and how much better they are feeling and how other symptoms have been alleviated. Many of them believed they were close to death when they found our website and decided to implement our program, so they are thankful to be alive, as well.

They tell us about their struggles in the beginning to change and how difficult it is at times to continue each day 'walking the tightrope" but they are grateful to gain control and regain their lives.

After following our plan, one of our friends Tanya wrote us about her success:

> *"For the past few months, I've been feeling better. What I learned on here was about my diet. I eat a VERY low carb diet. At first it caused more symptoms, but my body has gotten used to it and I'm feeling better. This diet is really hard but worth it. I also listen to my body and instead of pushing myself and getting over tired I stop and rest... I also still have lots of pain and weakness in my legs...but I'm still improved, and this is the first relief I've had in over 20 years."*

> *"...trying to make adjustments to the low carb diet. I've been doing the low carb diet and it was doing pretty good. I lost 28 lbs. and only had a few days of episodes when I was sick from a virus. In 6 months, that was really good..."*

We wish all of you success also!! (See appendix for photographs of before, during and after following the plan).

Chapter Twenty-One
Educating Yourself

"DISCUSSION GROUPS, WEBSITES, INTERNET AND BOOKS"

If a person has been diagnosed with a form of Periodic Paralysis, whether it is by the discovery of a DNA mutation, by clinical means (which is based on symptoms) or self-diagnosis, they should learn everything they are able to about every aspect of the disorder. It is also necessary that they educate their family members and friends. Knowing about and understanding the syndrome will ease fears and assist with proper diagnosis, management and treatment. Also, the knowledge that other people obtain will aid the patient during paralytic episodes.

Joining a Periodic Paralysis discussion group or board on the Internet is one of the best methods to discover information about Periodic Paralysis. Being part of a Periodic Paralysis community is vital. You will know that you are not alone. You will receive encouragement, support, empathy and sympathy when needed. You will gain information and knowledge from other people who live with the same enemy on a daily basis. People share information and ask questions. There are several types of groups. Some groups are called listservs, which allow you to post questions and get answers using email. Some groups are Facebook pages. Some groups are specific to the type of Periodic Paralysis, like Familial Hypokalemic Periodic Paralysis. Some are for individuals with all forms, and some are specific to and restricted to only people who have a known genetic mutation. Some have doctors who will answer questions, though they do not always respond or do not respond in a timely manner.

The Periodic Paralysis Network is an online community of people who are affected by Periodic Paralysis. Our focus is on educational resources and self-reliance. Our approach to treatment focuses on the self-monitoring of vitals and the management of pH levels through the elimination of triggers and awareness of proper nutrition and supplementation. This approach evolved from the inability of the medical community to provide appropriate medical diagnosis and treatment.

We have a discussion board, and we also have a Facebook page for discussion and support with over forty members, which is used more frequently. The members prefer it to be a private board for confidentiality reasons. On our Facebook page there is a wide variety of information posted about many aspects of Periodic Paralysis. Membership is open to the public and we interact in real time nearly every day with other members. We occasionally take polls and many members research and post scholarly and non-scholarly articles. We now have web cam discussion groups, and we continue to do research and provide the latest information to our members. Anyone wishing to join our Facebook page discussion group may contact us on our website or they may contact us at: http://www.facebook.com/groups/periodicparalysisnetwork/

In addition to joining a discussion group, everyone should also research Periodic Paralysis on the Internet. There are many Web sites with updated and quality information. Many other Web sites are not so careful about the accuracy of posted information and the reader should exercise caution before forming any conclusions about Periodic Paralysis. Most of the available research is difficult to read and understand. Some is very misleading, especially for those with unknown variants. Very little information exists on how to deal with the symptoms in a natural way, which is necessary for many people who have medication intolerances.

The Periodic Paralysis Network (PPN) is our website which contains a wide range of information. The Periodic Paralysis

Educating Yourself

Network was created to provide a hands-on approach to understanding the disease, getting a proper diagnosis, managing the symptoms, and assisting caregivers and family members. We attempt to discuss issues relating to Periodic Paralysis in practical language. Our hope also is that the medical professionals dealing with individuals with Periodic Paralysis may come to our site and learn more about how to recognize, diagnose and properly treat their patients in a timely manner.

The following are some comments written to us by some of our members"

> *"Thanks Susan...Your advice to me has been the absolute best and most knowledgeable I have found...Also everything you write here about the breathing issues is what I figured out for myself but haven't had a decent doctor to listen to them yet. With regards to blood pressure, your bid was much better than the doctors. I actually thought the same as you. Good for you for all the research you are doing. You are a pioneer whose efforts will benefit many people.*
>
> ~Tammy
>
> *"What you do now will help people now and for many years to come. You will leave a lasting mark in this world. Some people I've seen that are well bodied and have done nothing with their lives. Here you are sick and making a difference!!...Girl...keep going and do your thing. You situation is difficult...but it can be used for the good of many others. Martin Luther King, Mother Teresa, Susan Q Knittle-Hunter"*
>
> ~Tanya

> *"Hello. You have made a huge impact on my life in the best possible way. Thank you from the bottom of my heart, for being there when I have needed you, listening to me and guiding me in the right direction. You are a great and wonderful woman! Also you have forever touched my life in a great and meaningful way. Know that you are loved and appreciated!"*
>
> ~Tamira

The third method for learning about Periodic Paralysis is by reading about it in books. However, only a few books exist with information about Periodic Paralysis and what is available is very specific to certain types or variants. They are also difficult to read and understand. This book, *Living with Periodic Paralysis,* was written in part for that reason and with that in mind. It is a culmination of all aspects of the condition in one book written in an easy-to-read format of narrative style, essays and technical input where necessary. It is also designed so the reader does not need to read from cover-to-cover, although that is a possibility, but rather a particular topic can be searched for and found easily for quick answers.

Another group member wrote the following passage about our book:

> *"Sometimes it is a very lengthy and odd trip we take to a diagnosis for those of us suffering from rare diseases such as the Periodic Paralyses and Andersen Tawil Syndrome, and then there are those of us like Susan and I who still do not have an official genetic diagnosis so the trip continues.*
>
> *For the diagnosed, this book offers the latest information on diet and treatment for these unusual but rarely diagnosed conditions. It will also present the trip that Susan has begun and continues, in order to aid her family*

and my family and possibly your family on the road to better management of your disease.

For the undiagnosed, a roadmap to diagnosis to help make your trip a little easier than ours has been outlined.

For the medical professionals dealing with these conditions, a picture from the patient's point of view as well as a quick source for a tremendous amount of information.

For those that doubt these strange disorders actually exist; that they are all "in our heads" or greatly exaggerated, the proof is provided to change your minds.

For all of those out there dealing with these issues, I just want to say, "Keep on truckin'!"

~ Karen Carr Biehl

Thanks to each one of you for your kind words and support. We learn as much from you every day as you learn from us. We admire your strength and marvel at what you each must overcome daily. It is for you and your families, as well as our own, that we work so hard each day seeking out the answers for understanding, diagnosing, treating, managing and possibly curing Periodic Paralysis. You have all become our friends. It is wonderful communicating and sharing with you and it is a joy to know you.

~Susan and Calvin

Chapter Twenty-Two
Discovering Your Triggers?

"CHART, JOURNAL AND MONITOR"
Introduction

One of the most important things a person with Periodic Paralysis can do, no matter what type we have, is to discover what causes, starts or triggers our episodes of muscle weakness or paralysis. The goal is to regain the quality of our lives and to prevent the damage being done to our organs as the potassium rises, shifts and depletes in our bodies.

In the case of people with Andersen-Tawil Syndrome, the paralysis leads to tachycardia and serious arrhythmias, including long QT intervals, which can lead to cardiac arrest. Avoiding paralysis is absolutely necessary, due to these life-threatening effects.

As we know from previous discussions, certain foods, medications, conditions and activities can trigger many of the paralysis events. To begin with, the easiest way to decide what caused an episode would be to look at anything new or different; a new type of bread, a new antibiotic, a new activity, a new shampoo, stressful event (good or bad), or a chilled or over heated room.

Discovering our triggers requires a little bit of time to follow a simple plan. In a matter of a few days or weeks, it may be possible to draw some useful conclusions about the possible triggers of a paralytic event.

In the fields of medicine and education, it is said, "If you did not write it down, it did not happen". This can be applied to our method for discovering our triggers. The first thing we must do is to write everything down. Creating a journal is a good way to make sure this is done. I have created a chart, which can be added to a journal to make the process easier

Living with Periodic Paralysis

(see a copy below).

Several necessary components are included on this chart:

❖ A 24-hour time frame
❖ A section to write possible triggers
❖ A section to write down symptoms one may be experiencing
❖ A section to record the muscle weakness and paralysis
❖ This section becomes a graph of the periods of weakness or paralysis

Once the information has been gathered for a few weeks, it will be easy to see trends or connections of a particular food, medication or activity to muscle weakness or paralysis.

Next, knowledge of the more common triggers is needed for PP attacks. The following is a partial list I have compiled for convenience in this chapter. You may also refer to Chapter Seventeen:

Symptoms

Understanding and becoming familiar with the symptoms is another important part of completing the chart. As much information that can be added will be helpful. In this section anything may be included from "**feeling well**", or "**none**", to some of the known symptoms for Hyperkalemia and Hypokalemia in the following charts. You may also refer to Chapter Fifteen:

Possible Symptoms for Hypokalemia

❖ Episodic muscle weakness
❖ Episodic partial paralysis
❖ Episodic total paralysis
❖ Episodic flaccid paralysis (limp muscles, without tone)
❖ Muscle weakness after exercise

❖ Muscle weakness
❖ Muscle stiffness
❖ Muscle aches
❖ Muscle cramps
❖ Muscle contractions
❖ Muscle spasms
❖ Muscle tenderness
❖ Pins and needles sensation
❖ Eyelid myotonia (cannot open eyelid after opening and then closing them)
❖ Irritability
❖ Severe thirst
❖ Abdominal bloating
❖ Nausea
❖ Vomiting
❖ Constipation
❖ Excessive urination
❖ Sweating
❖ Tachycardia
❖ Irregular heartbeat
❖ Palpitations
❖ Dizziness
❖ Fainting
❖ Breathing problems (barely breathing)
❖ Hypoventilation
❖ Increase in blood pressure
❖ Irritability

Possible Symptoms for Hyperkalemia

❖ Episodic muscle weakness
❖ Episodic partial paralysis
❖ Episodic total paralysis
❖ Muscle contraction or rigidity during an attack
❖ Muscle weakness
❖ Muscle cramps
❖ Muscle stiffness
❖ Fasciculation (muscle twitching)
❖ Pins and needles sensation
❖ Cramping pain
❖ Reduced reflexes
❖ Muscle contraction involving tongue
❖ Slurring of words
❖ **Tightness in legs**
❖ Strange feeling in legs

- ❖ Tingling sensations
- ❖ Pulse issues (absent, slow, or weak)
- ❖ Irregular heartbeat
- ❖ Heart palpitations
- ❖ Breathing problems (wheezing, shortness of breath, fast breathing)
- ❖ Mild hyperventilation
- ❖ Decrease in blood pressure
- ❖ Nausea
- ❖ Feeling hot
- ❖ Sleepiness

Possible Triggers

Our diet can be one of the biggest contributors to episodes of paralysis.

- ❖ Simple carbohydrates: processed sugar, white flour, etc.
- ❖ Complex carbohydrates: Some grains i.e., wheat, etc.
- ❖ Meat: mostly red meats
- ❖ **Salt**
- ❖ Caffeine
- ❖ MSG
- ❖ Alcohol
- ❖ Large Meals
- ❖ Sleep: All aspects of sleep have set my episodes into motion
- ❖ Falling asleep, waking from sleep
- ❖ Stress (good)
- ❖ Stress (bad)
- ❖ Dehydration
- ❖ Fasting
- ❖ Sitting too long
- ❖ Changes in the weather
- ❖ Fatigue
- ❖ Heat
- ❖ Cold
- ❖ EMFs
- ❖ Exercise: Episodes may develop soon after or the next day
- ❖ Rest after exercise: May set an episode into motion
- ❖ Medications
- ❖ Saline Drips
- ❖ Glucose Infusion: If an IV is needed, Mannitol can be used.
- ❖ Oral or Intravenous
- ❖ Corticosteroids
- ❖ Muscle Relaxers

- ❖ Beta Blockers
- ❖ Tranquilizers
- ❖ Pain Killers (analgesics)
- ❖ Antihistamines
- ❖ Puffers for Asthma.
- ❖ Antibiotics
- ❖ Eye Drops to Dilate Eyes.
- ❖ Contrast Dye for MRIs.
- ❖ Lidocaine
- ❖ Anesthetics
- ❖ Epinephrine
- ❖ Adrenaline
- ❖ Over-the-counter medications.
- ❖ Cough Syrups
- ❖ Eye Drops
- ❖ NSAIDs

Completing the Trigger Chart:

- ❖ Fill in the date.
- ❖ Begin recording your activities, food, drink and medications in the top section. Start at the time you wake up. Include all food eaten in a meal. Record what you are doing, i.e., sitting, eating, reading, exercising, walking, cooking, shopping, etc.
- ❖ Record how you are feeling, i.e., good, very thirsty, constipated, confusion, sleepy, unsteady, legs are weak, total paralysis, etc.
- ❖ Put a check mark in, (or fill in) the box that best describes your condition, i.e., normal, weak, more weak, partial paralysis, more partial paralysis, or total paralysis.
- ❖ Continue this through your day, it is not necessary to do it at night, but you may want to include paralysis, numbness, etc., if it is happening at night.
- ❖ The bottom of the chart will become a graph and it will aid in seeing the times of symptoms.

In the completed chart below, we can see that two and one half to three hours after eating breakfast and taking septra, an antibiotic and a calcium tablet, the patient begins to experience weakness and then paralysis. It is a good chance that the medication or something eaten at breakfast was the cause.

If this person eats the same thing every day and takes the

calcium every morning, and the only new thing is the septra it would be safe to assume the antibiotic caused the episode.

By four pm the episode has stopped. At five pm muscle weakness begins after an hour of being up and preparing dinner. This may be from exercise intolerance or due to something eaten at lunch.

If someone eats the same lunch everyday but does not always help with dinner, it could be safe to assume the exercise caused the weakness. The same could be true in reverse.

At seven pm, overall weakness takes hold for the remainder of the evening. This may be from the food eaten at dinner or a continuation of the weakness from the earlier activity.

During the night there are three episodes of total paralysis. Since sleep is a trigger, it may be impossible to stop the episodes throughout the night.

Evaluating the Data

When looking at your completed charts, it is best to first check the periods of paralysis. Then check the activity, medications taken, or food eaten two to three hours before that time. Was anything new? Was any activity out of the ordinary?

- ❖ Check period of paralysis or weakness:
  - ➤ Check two to three hours before.
    - ▪ New medication?
- ❖ New food, drink?
  - ➤ New activity?
    - ▪ More than usual?
    - ▪ Longer than usual?
- ❖ If answer is not clear: Continue to chart for a few days. If there seems to be a pattern:
  - ➤ Change only one thing at that time:
    - ▪ Remove sugar or
    - ▪ Cut medication dose or
  - ➤ Stop or reduce the activity

- Less than usual
- Shorter than usual

❖ Check again after a day or two. If the symptoms of paralysis are reduced or better, you may have found the trigger. If not, add the thing you removed or reduced back into the meal, etc. Then repeat and change something else:

❖ Change only one thing at that time:
  ➢ Remove sugar or
  ➢ Cut medication dose or
  ➢ Stop or reduce the activity
    - Less than usual
    - Shorter than usual
❖ Repeat until you find the trigger or triggers.

Some suggestions for how to avoid the triggers once they are found:

  ➢ On feet too long?: Break the activity in several shorter periods on feet.
  ➢ Cannot eat sugar?: Stop and try sweeteners, honey, stevia, etc.
  ➢ Cannot eat certain food?: Find replacement or do without.
  ➢ Cannot take medication?: Cut dosage, stop taking or get a replacement (under supervision of medical professional).
  ➢ Sitting too long?: Get up every hour or less and move around.
  ➢ Sitting too long?: Exercise in chair.
  ➢ Dehydrated?: Drink more water, set timer.
  ➢ Hungry?: Eat several smaller meals.
  ➢ Too hot?: Wear looser, cooler clothes, use neck cooler.
  ➢ Too cold?: Add clothing layers, use a blanket, drink hot drinks.
  ➢ Cannot drink caffeine?: Drink decaffeinated drinks.

As the triggers are discovered and eliminated the attacks of paralysis and other associated symptoms will begin to decline. The quality of life will improve. The information will be recorded and can be shared with the doctors and used as a tool during the diagnosing process.

Trigger Chart

Date	6am	7am	8am	9am	10am	11am	12pm	1pm	2pm	3pm	4pm	5pm	6pm	7pm	8pm	9pm	10pm	11pm	12am	1am	2am	3am	4am	5am
Food, Drink, Meds, Activity																								
Symptoms																								
Conditions																								
Total Paralysis																								
Partial Paralysis																								
Total Weakness																								
Partial Weakness																								
Numbness																								
Normal																								

Blank charts to print can be found on the PPN web site at: www.periodicparalysisnetwork.com

Discovering Your Triggers

Date	6am	7am	8am	9am	10am	11am	12pm	1pm	2pm	3pm	4pm	5pm	6pm	7pm	8pm	9pm	10pm	11pm	12am	1am	2am	3am	4am	5am
Food, Drink, Meds, Activity																								
Symptoms																								
Conditions																								
Total Paralysis																								
Partial Paralysis																								
Total Weakness																								
Partial Weakness																								
Numbness																								
Normal																								

Monitoring the Symptoms

Once many of the triggers have been established and a diagnosis has been obtained (or not), it will be necessary to continue to observe and monitor the symptoms and the triggers. As we have discovered from my experience and that of others with Periodic Paralysis, the triggers may change over time or what may have seemed to be the cause, may not actually be the cause. It is important to keep track continually in order to regulate and control the symptoms.

For instance, at first it may appear that sugar eaten in a cookie is the culprit causing attacks of muscle weakness or paralysis. Later it may be discovered that it was actually the white flour or the chocolate in a cookie that may have caused the episode. Accidentally, it may be figured out that a person might be able to eat small amounts of sugar in a gluten-free cookie. Then after eating the gluten free cookie every day for three days, a paralytic episode occurs. This may be that too much was eaten. So, it may be that small amounts of sugar may be eaten occasionally, just not every day.

It is a fine line that an individual with Periodic Paralysis must walk every day. We must move through life as if we are walking a tightrope. I have heard it said that when we figure out what our triggers are, we must treat them as if they are allergies, something we must avoid. However, it becomes a problem when those things are important elements needed in the body such as salt or sugar.

In discussion with other individuals, we also have discovered that surprising things may actually cause an attack. We may believe we are doing everything correctly and avoiding all triggers and then we suddenly slip into full body paralysis. This happened to me recently. I tripped on my oxygen cord and landed on my knees. I scraped up one of them, but otherwise felt fine. Three hours later I was in full body paralysis.

After discussing this with a friend and wondering what had caused this attack, he reminded me that adrenaline is released when the body is stressed or experiences some trauma. I realized that although I did not notice much when I fell except a small scrape to my knee, my body had recognized it as trauma, released adrenaline and three hours later I was paralyzed and for the following several days.

Now I will remember that if I fall again, no matter how small or uneventful it may seem, I must prepare for the possibility of slipping into paralysis. I will be sure to take some potassium and rest and hope it will either not happen or be as serious as the last time. Better yet, I need to be more careful, now that I know if I fall, I will go into paralysis (or break a bone knowing I have severe osteoporosis).

Monitoring or keeping track of triggers is important because it seems as if they are always changing and maybe they are or maybe it is the amount of something we are using, but also it may be that we have misinterpreted one trigger for another. We must use the charts to keep track of symptoms and possible triggers and put them together in a journal. The information in the charts and journal will be recorded and can be shared with the doctors and used as a tool during the diagnosing process or for treatment options.

Chapter Twenty-Three
Relieving Your Symptoms

"WALKING A TIGHTROPE"
Introduction

As discussed in previous chapters of this book, we know that individuals with Periodic Paralysis, suffer greatly from many symptoms such as partial or total paralysis, heart arrhythmias or muscle weakness brought on by any number of triggers such a sugar, stress or carbohydrates. This chapter contains the most important components for the relief, treatment or management of those symptoms. Due to the fact that I am unable to take any type of medication, this plan is based on and uses mostly natural methods and substances in order to reduce the attacks of paralysis and other symptoms.

Calvin and I created our plan after a great deal of research and much trial and error over a period of several years. Calvin and I have both written this chapter. He writes from the point of view of the discoveries he made trying to save my life. I write from the point of view of what I discovered as my life was saved and my health improved

Avoid All Known Triggers

The most obvious thing that can be done is to avoid the triggers known to cause symptoms. Some are very obvious, and others may take some time to discover. (Sometimes you may never know what sets an attack into motion.) Chapter Seventeen discusses in great detail the most obvious and common triggers and Chapter Twenty-Two discusses how to discover the triggers that set off a paralytic attack or other symptoms. Referring to those chapters will be helpful to know what to avoid. The following are reminders of some of the more common triggers.

Medications/Over-the-Counter Medications

It is best to remember that most medications including over the counter are triggers. If you are taking prescribed medications, it is important to discuss this issue with the doctor. Do not attempt to stop taking prescribed medications without the care of a physician. Many pharmaceuticals may produce very serious complications if stopped all at once. Tapering off slowly is the best method, however, even slowly withdrawing from a medication may cause unexpected symptoms. If a person needs to begin a new medication it is best to begin with one quarter of the amount prescribed until it is known if the body will tolerate it. Sometimes there is a delayed reaction, and it may take a few weeks before symptoms occur.

Stress

Avoiding stress of all types is extremely important. This is difficult because it includes "good" stress. Strong emotions such as excitement, fear, panic and anger should be avoided because they cause the body to produce adrenaline, also known as epinephrine, and release it into the bloodstream. For some individuals with Periodic Paralysis the release of epinephrine triggers paralytic episodes because it lowers the amount of potassium in the blood. Illness or injury in the body also causes stress. Temperature extremes (heat and cold) and fasting or going without eating all put stress on the body and need to be avoided by some individuals. Besides paralysis, adrenaline also produces an increase in the heart rate, blood pressure, blood sugars and irregular heartbeats. [53, 54, 55, 56]

Physical Exercise and Exertion

Exercise is stressful to the body and therefore, epinephrine is released into the bloodstream during exercise or exertion.

Usually, an individual with Periodic Paralysis does not have a paralytic episode during exercise, but upon resting after exercise, paralysis may be triggered. So, exercise or exertion for some individuals should be avoided. [57, 58]

Heat and Cold

Maintaining a balanced temperature in the environment is important for people with Periodic Paralysis. If an individual gets hot or chilled, the body becomes stressed and can trigger a paralytic episode. Being prepared for transition times is the best idea. Some simple ideas for temperature fluctuations may include wearing several layers of clothing or having several layers easily available. Have blankets and throws easily available. Use an electric blanket to heat the bed and turn it off just before slipping in (especially for those who have a problem with EMFs). Or use the clothes dryer to warm nightclothes and slip them on just before crawling into a cold bed or to warm clothes when dressing in the morning. Using a neck cooler when overheated can really help. Keeping one ready in the refrigerator is helpful. Either warming a car or cooling it before entering it can help avoid the drastic changes in temperature during the winter and summer months.

Diet and Nutrition
Make Healthy Lifestyle Changes

Calvin writes: When it comes to good health, what you do not put inside of your body is just as important as what you do put inside of your body. Both Susan and I have had health issues plague us throughout our lives. Some of our health problems are related to our ignorance about what chemical substances do to create illness and disease. Many times, Susan has come close to death ingesting doctor prescribed medications that were supposed to help. They actually caused many of the health crises she experienced. Many of my health problems were linked to poor eating habits and ingestion of chemical substances that affected my health. My health-related issues were more closely aligned to chemical addictions. However, Susan has always been conscientious about what she was eating especially limiting the amount of salt, fat and processed sugar, which can lead to heart disease and diabetes. Who would have ever guessed that the pharmaceutical drugs doctors were prescribing lead to a breakdown of her entire system?

We have learned many lessons from our misfortunes and mistakes. We both now eat in similar ways and have found common ground about how to be as healthy as we can. There is enough information published over the Internet about what not to eat. There are plenty of articles about the serious health effects of consuming processed foods, salt, sugar, caffeine, nicotine, alcohol, street drugs, additives, preservatives, artificial sweeteners, and all other synthetics and unnatural chemicals. If you are consuming any of these substances, it is our advice to stop immediately. It is possible to live life without uppers and downers and everything else designed to alter mood. Most of the illnesses and diseases we hear about today can be prevented and possibly cured just by refraining from ingesting foreign substances. Most cancers are caused by poor lifestyle choices. Most heart disease and diabetes is caused by uninformed and poor judgment. Once you have stopped putting poisons inside your body, how do you know what is safe and healthy to eat?

We have adopted several sayings when it comes to eating.

"Eat to live rather than live to eat."
"Eat 70 percent alkaline and thirty percent acidic."
"Eat from the farm and not the factory."
"If it's delivered through a window then it's not food."
"Go on a diet if you want to gain weight."

"Physical exercise tones muscles, proper nutrition tones cells."

The 70/30 rule is the most important of the group. We have it posted on our refrigerator along with the acid and alkaline ratings of particular foods.

It will take a great deal of self-discipline to make healthier lifestyle choices. People generally do not make personal changes unless they are faced with some painful consequences of doing something unhealthy. If you are having difficulty ridding yourself of poor lifestyle choices, you are like many millions of other people. Many people need some type of outside intervention and support to make major lifestyle changes especially when it comes to stopping the consumption of poisonous substances such as nicotine, alcohol, caffeine, salt, artificial sweeteners, processed sugar and foods, animal fat and pharmaceutical drugs. Drugs obtained illegally are especially difficult to stop consuming due to their addictive nature. It has been my experience that I needed to become extremely ill before relinquishing any of my addictions. It was very difficult and painful, but the alternative was to continue consuming poisons and continue to suffer with unnecessary illness and disease.

The things we consume that cause health problems are called triggers. Discovering our triggers is part of the process of regaining our health. I know that wine and cigarette smoke trigger migraine headaches. I have learned that candy bars, soda pop and junk foods cause elevated blood sugar levels and diabetes. I know that eating fat causes my cholesterol and blood pressure to rise. It also causes my heart to work too hard and labors my breathing. It took me many years to break these habits and adopt healthier eating habits. I wish I had taken all of this more seriously sooner as I could have avoided many life-threatening conditions.

People eat more food than they need because they are starved of the nutrients the body needs to conduct metabolic processes. The more junk food we consume, the hungrier we become simply because junk foods are not real foods. Junk food addicts are hungry all the time. Anything that is processed and packaged at a factory is not real food. Most people know what we do when we get hungry.... we eat. It is a vicious cycle that can only be stopped by a serious change in lifestyle or death.

Over the past few generations, we have forgotten the main purpose of eating. The main purpose of eating is not to feel good but rather to provide our bodies with the nutrients needed to remain healthy and alive. Without the right nutrients, our bodies suffer, and we become dysfunctional. The corporations that process, package, and sell junk foods tell us that their products are filled with nutritious substances or at least deny their products cause any health problems. Government agencies are complicit in their lies due to improper or non-existent oversight. The corporations know it is much less expensive for them to pay lawyers to fight claims that it is to take precautionary measures to ensure food quality and safety. The government turns a blind eye, and the people suffer from serious illness and disease. The junk foodstuff factories present their goods to the public in the same manner the cigarette companies did before people woke up to the fact that consuming tobacco products in any form will cause cancer. The only way to protect yourself and your family is to stop purchasing processed and package junk and instead buy unpackaged and unprocessed real foods.

Another guideline of differentiating between real food and non-food items is "if it's delivered through a window then it's not food." Everything you purchase to eat that gets shoved through a drive-up window has absolutely no nutritional value and will contribute to illness and disease. If we wanted to get serious about health and nutrition in this country the single-most important thing we could do, would be to shut down all fast-food delivery systems. Of course, this will never happen because most people have the right to choose what they consume even if it is something that is causing them harm.

The good news is that most of the negative effects of poor nutrition can be reversed if caught in time. The solution is simple, but the process is extremely difficult and uncomfortable. It takes a lot of time to prepare healthy meals. It takes time to plan and to prepare foods that are healthy. To move from a junk food diet over to eating real food takes a change in lifestyle. The change requires a commitment until new eating habits can be formed and lifestyle choices ingrained in daily routines. Another benefit Susan and I have discovered is a reduction in our food bill as a result of eating natural foods and not eating anything that comes with a label.

Some of our health problems are not curable but we believe they are manageable by the things we consume. Potassium shifting can be partially controlled by the types of things we consume. Highly acidic chemicals and foodstuff can trigger unusual potassium shifting. The relationship between potassium shifting and metabolic acidosis is very real and should be taken very seriously as to avoid life-threatening heart complications. The goal is to consume much more alkaline and much less acid.

Eat a Proper pH Balanced Diet
"Eat to live rather than live to eat"

Susan writes: A few years ago, when I was dying from the effects of metabolic acidosis, and I was unable to take any medication, Calvin began to search for ways to save my life. He had discovered that the pH balance in my body was unbalanced with too much acidity.

He set out to increase the alkaline in my body. He found a website with a chart containing the pH balance of the most common foods. With the chart in hand, he hurried to the store and bought as many of the foods containing alkaline, he could find, mostly vegetables. Then he found our juicer and made a vegetable and fruit drink for me every morning, he prepared fresh vegetables for my lunch and made a fresh salad for my dinner. He cut out almost all foods with acidity. It was difficult for me, so he decided to eat the same diet with me. Soon I was doing better. I grew stronger, the attacks of paralysis decreased in number and severity and by the time six months had passed, we both lost twenty pounds and our cholesterol levels were decreased and sugar levels were down in the normal ranges.

While attending a visit with one of my diagnosing doctors, we told him about the diet and how it had helped me. He said that we were now, "Eating to live and no longer living to eat". He was so right!

What we had discovered was the body has a natural pH balance. It is 70% alkaline and 30% acidic. Any deviation from this may cause an imbalance. Any imbalance in the body causes stress and may trigger symptoms or paralysis. If the body becomes too acidic, metabolic acidosis may occur, creating hyperkalemia. In Chapter Nineteen, in the section Metabolic Acidosis/Lactic Acidosis, the seriousness of becoming acidic is explained.

Too much alkaline in the body can also be a serious problem causing dehydration. With this in mind, each meal eaten should contain 70% alkaline food and 30% acidic food. There are several good websites on the Internet with charts listing foods high in acidity and high in alkaline. These sites also have instructions for how to follow the diet and recipes for preparing healthy dishes. Links to these sites can be found on our website Periodic Paralysis Network. [59]

Unprocessed Foods
"Eat from the farm, not the factory"

The best way to follow a pH balanced diet is to remember to, "Eat from the farm; not from the factory". This is because most junk food and processed foods are packed with substances, which are acidic or naturally more acidic. Meat is also a more acidic food. Another way to remember how to shop in order to keep the body pH balance is to stay out of the center isles in the grocery store. The good and healthy foods are always on the outer lanes of the store.

That being said, it is best to remember the word "balance". It is easy to be afraid to eat too much alkaline and forget to eat the 30% acidity. With that in mind, and remembering an individual's triggers, some food with acidity is permitted. [60]

Organic Foods

We suggest that when purchasing the food for the pH balanced diet it should be organically grown and processed as much as possible. There are several reasons. The most important is to avoid additives, hormones and pesticides, which can possibly be triggers. If not triggers, they may cause illness and indirectly be triggers for paralytic attacks.

Most cows and cattle (and other animals we eat) are given hormones and antibiotics, unless organically raised. The dairy products and meat from these animals will contain a certain amount of them. If antibiotics or hormones are triggers for an individual, he or she may not be aware that those will be found in the milk, cheese or meat they eat. Without realizing it they may be ingesting them, thus creating episodes of paralysis and not knowing why.

Distilled Water

The same thing applies to our drinking water. The hormones, antibiotics and other medications passed from humans and animals into our water supply are remaining even after the water is purified. Individuals with Periodic Paralysis may not realize they are actually ingesting these medications, hormones and antibiotics in drinking water. For this reason, we suggest using a distiller to process drinking water. It is the only way to have pure drinking water, unless the water is from a good well, which has been tested and found free of all contaminants. [61]

Nutrient Extractor

Extracting nutrients from natural food sources is much more affordable and convenient today with the use of a nutrient extractor. Nutri Bullet is the kitchen tool we use to turn raw vegetables, fruits, nuts and seeds into liquid drinks that help optimize metabolism, overall health and pH balance on the alkaline side. [74]

Balance
"Sugar and Spice and Everything Nice"

"Balance" is the most important word in our plan. If just one thing is out of balance, it can mean the difference between life and death in some cases. Besides the 70/30 balances in our diet, the other elements in our body must be in balance also, especially the elements or minerals (sometimes called electrolytes). This is due to the fact that Periodic Paralysis is a mineral metabolic disorder and when the minerals are out of balance, paralysis will occur. Some of these elements are calcium, magnesium, sodium, potassium, chloride, and bicarbonate.

That being said, however, salt (sodium) may be a trigger for paralytic episodes for most individuals. Due to that fact many of us avoid it like the plague. If we do not eat any salt, then our body will get out of balance and episodes of paralysis or other symptoms may develop. So, we must carefully ingest some sodium for that balance.

This also includes natural sugar and some fats and oils. These are also needed in our body, but care must be given to how much we eat of them in our diet and which types. Natural sugars in fruits would be a better choice than white processed table sugar. Olive oil is a better choice than vegetable oil. Monounsaturated fats and polyunsaturated fats are a better choice than saturated fats.

I discovered these things the hard way. After many months of not eating salt, sugar, carbohydrates and fats and oils, and experiencing great improvement with almost no paralytic episodes, I suddenly got very ill and began to have more episodes of severe paralysis. I became extremely weak and overall, quite ill. After researching it, I discovered I was probably suffering from too much alkalinity and an imbalance of electrolytes, and my body needed some sugar and some fats. I decided that I needed to carefully re-introduce these things back into my diet, one at a time to monitor for problems. I began to feel better, the paralytic episodes decreased, and I regained my strength. I am still very careful, but I now enjoy better balanced diet. "Balance" is the key!

Supplements

Calvin writes: Let's face the facts. No matter how many fruits, vegetables, nuts, and grasses we consume, we still will not get all the vitamins and minerals our bodies need to function optimally on a daily basis. This leaves us with the question of whether or not to take supplements? The whole notion of taking dietary supplements runs contrary to everything I have said about eating natural substances originating directly from the farm and avoiding processed foods made in a factory. Dietary supplements are a product of some form of factory processing. But like all other absolutes; there are exceptions to the rules.

Taking dietary supplements might just be the exception to the rule because the potential benefits outweigh the deficits depending on the supplement. Supplements come in all shapes, sizes, forms, and containers each with multitudes of claims. How do we separate out fact from fiction? Research is the only way to identify honest from dishonest claims. Many people take supplements in the form of a pill and other people use liquids and powders.

We have chosen to take our supplements in powder form along with a glass of fresh vegetable and fruit juice made with our juicer. This works for us but might not work for everyone else. It is a personal choice. We read labels and verify claims using the Internet. We avoid preservatives and unnecessary additives. We avoid capsules and hard-shelled pills. We avoid non-organic vitamin and mineral sources. Research helps us make informed and healthy choices. It all takes time and a commitment to living a healthier lifestyle.

We have discovered several trusted Internet based businesses with quality supplements that can be bought in bulk such as potassium bicarbonate, potassium citrate, calcium citrate, and magnesium citrate. Susan is unable to take any antibiotics because it causes muscle paralysis, so she uses herbs to treat bacterial infections and takes probiotics to help avoid infections. We are learning to use natural herbs to help boost our body's natural immune system. The businesses with quality supplements which we trust can be found on our website Periodic Paralysis Network. [59]

Stay Well-Rested

It is extremely important for individuals with Periodic Paralysis to stay well rested. Otherwise, an individual's body becomes stressed and stress equals paralysis. A full night of sleep is essential. Unfortunately, many are affected by paralysis at night because different phases of sleep are a trigger. Falling asleep, during sleep and waking up may trigger a paralytic episode. It is best to do everything possible to make those times, stress free, comfortable and temperature controlled to make it less likely to trigger an episode.

There are many methods that may help in falling asleep, getting better sleep and staying asleep. It is best to experiment to discover what will work.

Stay Well Hydrated

Being chronically ill leaves individuals more susceptible to dehydration, which is when the body loses more liquid than it takes in. Less water and fluids affect the balance of the electrolytes and prevents the organs from working properly. This creates an imbalance, and this creates stress in the body. As we know, stress can trigger paralysis.

The most important way to stay hydrated is to drink plenty of water.

Treating Muscle Paralysis
"Potassium, Glucose or Nothing?"

For most individuals diagnosed with Periodic Paralysis or with symptoms of Periodic Paralysis, they know which type they have. It is either Hypokalemic Periodic Paralysis, which is low potassium levels or Hyperkalemic Periodic Paralysis, which is high potassium levels. They can discover when the level of potassium in their blood is too high or too low by

217

using a cardy meter (discussed later in this chapter). It is best to use the meter to know for sure what the levels are before medicating or taking potassium when symptoms begin.

The individuals with low potassium levels causing their paralysis have different medications prescribed for their respective symptoms and different types of potassium in different forms. Their paralysis is fairly well controlled. The individuals with high potassium levels causing their paralysis also have medications to help alleviate their symptoms. They do not take potassium, because they already have too much, and this would cause serious paralysis and metabolic acidosis. They can take glucose to help control the high amounts of potassium in their blood. Eating carbohydrates or trying to move around can also be helpful.

Individuals with Andersen-Tawil-Syndrome or Andersen-Tawil-Syndrome "like" Periodic Paralysis must be extremely careful when taking potassium. Because, they have periods of high potassium and low potassium, it is essential to use a cardy meter to measure the amount in their blood when they begin to feel symptoms. Doing this, will assure that an individual will use the correct method by either taking potassium or eating some carbohydrates or by doing nothing.

Types of Potassium

When considering which type of potassium to use, it is important to understand the most common types, potassium bicarbonate, potassium citrate and potassium chloride. Potassium bicarbonate is a salty substance with no color or smell, and it neutralizes acidity. Potassium citrate is also a salty substance. It is potassium bicarbonate, which has been combined with citric acid for faster absorption. It reduces acidity. Potassium chloride is also a salty substance created from a combination of potassium and chlorine. It will increase the acidity in the body. [62, 63, 64]

It comes in many forms which include, salts, powders, liquid, and tablets. Some tablets may be released over time, or some are easily dissolved. Liquid forms need to be diluted in water. The soluble tablets ad powder or salt forms need to be dissolved in water. Tablets should be swallowed whole with 8 ounces of water after meals. [65]

How does someone know which type and form is best for him or her? We are not medical doctors, so we avoid offering advice about the type of potassium supplement to use. That needs to be discussed with your trusted medical advisor. However, that being said, the various forms and types are discussed here for a better understanding and decision-making.

After researching and knowing that I have chronic metabolic acidosis, I chose to use potassium bicarbonate because it neutralizes the acidity in my body. I use the salt form because and I can dilute it in water for quick absorption. I take it when my potassium levels are low. I must be careful with the amount I take because I easily swing into high potassium levels.

Although most individuals with Periodic Paralysis will get prescriptions for potassium, some may choose or need to purchase their own potassium supplements. If you purchase your own form, be sure to use natural sources of potassium from a reliable natural organic source. The businesses with quality supplements which we trust for our needs can be found on our website Periodic Paralysis Network. [59]

Use Oxygen During Periods of Paralysis
"The Elephant on the Chest"

Oxygen should also be used for anyone with Periodic Paralysis when in a paralytic episode because very often, an individual develops breathing issues. It can become difficult to breathe and it may feel like an elephant sitting on the chest. Breathing sometimes stops during an episode. Oxygen levels may drop, and the individual may develop hypoxia, or inadequate oxygen levels. This can lead to respiratory arrest and death.

Oxygen should be used for individuals with Andersen-Tawil Syndrome or Andersen-Tawil Syndrome-like symptoms who are in paralytic episodes. An oximeter may not indicate the correct oxygen levels because of chronic or acute dilatation of the heart. This is an enlargement of the heart cavity. Death can occur. [66, 67]

Meditation and Mental Imagery
"I Am at Peace"

Paralytic attacks can be very frightening. They can last anywhere from a few minutes to several hours to days at a time. They can involve part of the body or the entire body. They may be severe or mild. Complications can arise such as breathing problems, heart arrhythmias, muscle cramping or choking. It may be difficult to remain calm during those times.

I know the fear involved and have spent many hours in full body paralysis, which involves not being able to see or speak or move in anyway. I experience choking, heart arrhythmias, chest pain, fluctuating heart rates (slow and fast) fluctuating blood pressure (high and low), difficulty breathing (slow and fast) and stoppage, severe muscle cramping, jerking, and pain, and fluctuating body temperatures with sweating and chills. All during this, I am still able to hear everything going on around me. On many occasions I was sure I was dying.

Over time, I have learned to relax to the best of my ability and just let it happen. I spend my time listening to the television or radio, whichever may be on, or the conversations going on between the people around me. I have also learned to meditate.

When not in paralysis, I have taken time to learn how to meditate and use imagery. I practice this so it will come easy to me during an episode. I close my eyes and relax as I repeat, "I am" while I breathe in and "at peace" while I breathe out. I do this for several minutes.

Then I visualize being in my favorite place in the forest of pine and aspen trees, on a dirt path strolling beside a bubbling creek. I see squirrels and birds and an occasional deer. I see beautiful wildflowers of all colors along the path. The sky is always blue, and the sun is always shining, the temperature is warm and feel a slight breeze on my face. I continue to walk along the path and see new flowers, birds, trees and animals. I may meet someone on the trail. I may find things along the way.

Soon the episode has passed, and I am able to open my eyes and I am able to begin moving once again. This has helped me to get through some very rough times. Anyone can adapt this to their own preferences, such as walking along the beach at the ocean or enjoying a boat ride on a lake.

Conclusion

We believe this chapter to be one of the most important in our book because it contains our techniques based on research and trial and error for maintaining a "balance" in all aspects of life for individuals with Periodic Paralysis. With this method, some control may be regained in life by reducing the number and severity of the paralytic episodes and other symptoms and the debilitating complications experienced. We believe that by following the steps in this plan, which uses natural methods and common-sense ideas, the cruel symptoms of Periodic Paralysis will be relieved for everyone who seriously attempts to stay balanced in order to 'walk the tightrope'.

Chapter Twenty-Four
Monitor Your Vitals

"THE TOOLS FOR THE JOB"
Introduction

Calvin Writes: Diligent monitoring of vitals will help in the management of Periodic Paralysis (PP). Once you understand that potassium induced muscle paralysis is not a neurological disorder (something most medical professionals fail to understand) then you can begin to understand the dynamics of this metabolic disorder. There is only one sure way to know how your body is functioning and that is to use medical devices to measure things such as oxygen level, body temperature, blood pressure, heart and breathing rates, potassium levels, pH levels and blood sugar levels. Without this information it is unsafe to make any interventions. Without this information, we are engaging in a guessing game, which could trigger serious life-threatening conditions. Taking hundreds and thousands of milligrams of potassium to treat hypokalemia to boost potassium levels does absolutely nothing except to overload the kidneys and might possibly cause them to fail. The kidneys work to manage serum potassium levels.

Serum potassium typically consists of only 5 percent of the total amount of potassium inside the body. Approximately 95 percent of the body's potassium resides inside of cells. The mechanism that controls how much potassium gets retained and how much gets released from each cell is part of the cell wall structure. Potassium works in conjunction with the other elements such as magnesium, calcium and sodium. Along with potassium, these are the basic building block of life.

The body works to maintain a pH level of 7.35, which trends towards the alkaline side of the pH scale. The body will strip minerals from muscle and bone in order to maintain an overall pH level of 7.35. If this level fluctuates even a tiny amount, then serious health complications arise, and serious organ failure and death will follow shortly thereafter. It is very complicated and the best we can hope to do is gain an understanding of the internal mechanics of metabolism and how they are affected by biological and environmental events in order to help manage the degree and frequency of potassium induced muscle paralysis.

As I mentioned before, medical devices and tests are necessary to understand the inner workings of the body. After the medical community has given up trying to help you understand what is causing your muscle paralysis (typically after labeling you with conversion disorder, referring you to a psychiatrist and feeding you psychotropic pharmaceutical drugs) you and your caregivers are left alone to figure this thing out on your own. I believe that most people with this condition just give up at this point in time and continue to consume the smorgasbord of medications prescribed by the doctor never questioning the fact that many, if not most, of these pharmaceutical drugs are causing the disease to progress at an ever-increasing rate. The evidence of this is in the increase in the intensity and frequency of paralytic episodes.

Not many people question the opinions of the medial professionals. Their opinions, even when entrenched in fiction and imagination rather than fact-based medical test outcomes, are rarely challenged. The god-like stature they are granted in our culture contributes to unnecessary deaths due to medical malpractice. The proof can be found by looking at the numbers of medical malpractice claims flooding the halls of our courts. I imagine there are millions of more medical malpractice claims that never make it to the office of a lawyer or inside a courtroom. When Susan and I pursued a medical malpractice claim against our local hospital and several medical providers, the lawyer told us that it would cost us tens of thousands of dollars and getting other medical professionals to testify against their tightly knit group of other medical professionals would be next to impossible. It appears there is a code inside the medical community and the first rule is that you do not question the wisdom of another doctor and under no circumstance do you testify in court regarding their medical incompetence.

What we are left with in the end is a choice between self-diagnosis and treatment or to continue along the path of taking antidepressants and other pharmaceutical drugs that damage one organ in order to treat another organ. Which path you choose is a personal choice. We are here to lay out some alternatives to traditional methods and means of regaining some level of personal health and quality of life. There is no known cure for potassium induced muscle paralysis. There are ways to manage the ravishing effects that do not involve pharmaceutical drugs.

When someone is experiencing unusually high blood pressure, having waves of hot flashes, pulse is beating harder than usual or there is some other event going on that is out of the ordinary, it is comforting to have some ways to identify the source of the problem. High blood pressure can mean a number of things and can be caused by a multitude of events or conditions. To know what is causing the rise in blood pressure is the only way to know how to treat the high blood pressure. The same holds true for other events. Chest pain can be caused by many things some of which are as serious as a heart attack and as minor as excess gas in the gut, which was brought about by drinking too many carbonated beverages. In order to identify and manage any health condition, it is important to know the cause of the condition. Outside the range of a life-threatening symptom, there are tests that can be performed at home that help identify the causes of the discomfort or in this case, muscle paralysis.

Learning to trust your own judgment is an important part of managing this disease. Keeping written records helps to ease some of the panic and fear usually associated with the onset of muscle paralysis. Having a caregiver who is capable of conducting the necessary tests and monitoring you while you are in a paralytic episode is critically important. Taking this entire situation very seriously is very important. Getting other people to take your condition seriously is another matter. From the perspective of most onlookers, a person in a state of full body muscle paralysis is faking the condition. This misconception is what misleads most medical professionals into diagnosing the condition as conversion disorder. They misunderstand the secondary importance of conducting medical tests. The primary purposes of conducting medical tests are to identify the cause or causes of a problem and then apply treatment options. The secondary purpose of conducting medical tests is to rule out possible causes. As more tests get conducted and negative results are returned, valuable information is gained. Just because a cause cannot be identified by medical tests does not mean the cause resides inside the imagination. There is so much we have yet to learn about our bodies, metabolic processes and this disease. But, after so many tests are conducted and so many negative results get returned, the natural inclination of medical professionals is to conclude the cause of the mysterious muscle paralysis is psychosomatic or resides in the imagination of the patient. As despairing as this is to most people suffering with unexplained muscle paralysis, this is a starting point for hope and to gain some degree of personal control. The ultimately goal is to improve the quality of daily life. Once the traditional medical options have been exhausted either by doctors misdiagnosing the condition and giving up or insurance companies refusing to pay for any further testing, you are left to fall back on your own resources. But some comfort can be had in the knowledge that there are people who take this disease very seriously and who are willing to share all the information they have about diagnosing the condition and managing the symptoms.

Putting together some at-home medical testing devices will give you some control over the unknown. It will also help any caregiver understand when to reach out for help and when to wait. Calling an ambulance every time someone has a paralytic episode is extremely upsetting for everyone involved especially after many trips have been made to the emergency room (ER) and the outcomes are always the same. The emergency people will eventually begin to ignore any sense of urgency especially when they are not allowed to administer saline IVs and inject massive amounts of potassium. Telling the ER to only monitor your condition without doing any interventions will further cement the idea that you are suffering some form of psychosomatic disorder and another referral to a psychiatrist will follow. Mental Health will be called in to evaluate the situation and a prescription for psychotropic drugs and prolonged therapy will be recommended. It is a vicious cycle, which gets repeated until a patient either moves or passes away from a sudden onset of hearth arrhythmias, or some other complication triggered by abnormal potassium levels. The death certificate will fail to reflect the actual cause of death and the disease will move forward with the next generation in the dark.

Once you and your caregivers stop calling an ambulance with the onset of each paralytic episode, you can begin to take vitals in a calm and methodical manner and record those readings. These numbers will help you see the larger picture about the inner connectivity between things such as blood pressure, temperature, oxygen levels, respiration, pulse, serum potassium levels and urine pH levels. As you adopt a diet high in alkaline and low in acidity and begin to rid yourself of the other drugs and chemical substances such as processed foods, stimulants and depressants, you will begin to make connections between symptoms and some of the things that contribute to the frequency and degree of paralytic episodes.

Several pieces of medical equipment can be very handy for measuring your vitals. These include: a cardy meter, a finger pulse oximeter, blood sugar monitor, stethoscope, wrist blood pressure monitor, a thermometer and a digital pH balance reader. These items are necessary for caregivers to monitor vitals primarily because the person in paralysis is unable to communicate. The vitals serve as the communication tool. Keeping written records is very important especially when making connections between individual events.

For several years, Susan and I recorded her vitals many times throughout the day on charts and graphs that we developed along the way. A graph is an easy way to identify patterns. As an example, Susan took measurements of urine pH throughout the day. Morning readings typically were highly acidic in the six range and evening readings typically tended to be more alkalinic in the seven and eight range. As we gathered these readings over an extended period of time patterns emerged, and abnormal readings became more apparent. If a person has a urine pH reading of 6 every morning for several months and suddenly one morning gets a reading of 4, this will warrant further inquiry as to why the reading altered to such a huge degree. It may be that the person consumed a meal on the previous day that was highly acidic including a lot of meat and very few vegetables. It might also indicate that person was dehydrated. It might also indicate a condition of metabolic acidosis was in progress and might be correlated to an episode of muscle paralysis.

The number of possible connections is too numerous to outline but with the readings listed on a graph it is possible to draw connections and draw possible conclusions about what was causing the spike of acidity or alkalinity. Compared with other vital readings a story begins to unfold about the inner metabolic processes. The same holds true for the measurement and recording of other vitals such as blood pressure, temperature, blood sugar levels, oxygen levels, respiration, heart rate and the input and output of fluids. It is time consuming and tedious work but most people suffering with Periodic Paralysis have no other treatment options. The few over-the-counter prescriptions medical doctors prescribe often cause symptoms to worsen. Some even cause other life-threatening conditions. Susan is unable to take any form of antibiotics or 99% of any other type of medications. We have learned ways to treat conditions such as bladder infections with herbal remedies and work in a preventative mode most of the time.

It will be overwhelming at first looking through the list of medical devices and supplies needed to manage Periodic Paralysis. A well-stocked medical tool kit will cost somewhere between five hundred and one thousand dollars. Some of the equipment is obtainable through a medical provider depending on his or her willingness to write prescriptions. Most insurance companies will argue against the necessity of patients having such equipment and be unwilling to pay for testing equipment and supplies. They will deny many requests and refuse to pay for claims without proper documentation demonstrating specific needs. We had to purchase all these devices with our own funds but have never regretted having them. These devices relieve a lot of uncertainty and help both patient and caregiver cope with very difficult circumstances and help with making informed choices. The more we knew about metabolic processes the better our decisions could be on how to manage and provide treatment options. These devices will help you take better control over your own health.

The Tools and Supplies

Cardy Meter

The cardy meter is not recommended or approved by the manufacturer or Food and Drug Administration to be used as a device to measure serum potassium levels in humans. With that said, there really is not any other piece of medical equipment that can be used at home by non-professionals to measure serum potassium levels. Now, with the disclaimer out of the way, I must include another caution about using the cardy meter at home. The cardy is an extremely sensitive and sophisticated piece of equipment that is much more difficult to use than the other medical devices included in our arsenal of at-home medical devices. I prepared several You Tube videos demonstrating the use of the cardy and how to calibrate the meter for accurate results.

After you order the cardy and it arrives, you should take time to read through the directions thoroughly. You should practice with the cardy dozens and dozens of times before getting comfortable with the results. After several days or weeks of practice it will become easier to take samples and get readings in a relatively short time. It generally takes me two or three minutes to get a reading from start to finish. You should not rely too heavily on individual results when making decisions about whether or not to take potassium supplements. We learned to use readings gathered over a period of time to identify patterns and develop a baseline. Once a baseline is established, abnormal readings or unusual fluctuations in serum potassium levels become easier to identify. The main goal of taking all vitals, in addition to getting individual readings, is to compare all the various readings, which will give you a larger picture of metabolic processes.

In the very beginning after Susan received her cardy, we used saliva to measure potassium. We soon learned that saliva readings fail to accurately reflect potassium levels in the blood stream. Each bodily fluid (saliva, blood, urine) has chemistry all its own and the pH of each fluid can fluctuate greatly from the other fluid samples. When using saliva to get potassium readings, Susan's numbers were in the high range. The samples taken throughout the day fluctuated. There did not seem to be any recognizable pattern. When we began using blood rather than saliva to measure potassium levels, the samples stabilized with smaller fluctuations. Susan's numbers range anywhere from the high 3 range into the low 5 range. We discovered that Susan experienced both hypokalemia and hyperkalemia. She also was having paralytic episodes when her numbers were in the 4 normal ranges. We learned that a person could experience muscle paralysis even when their serum potassium levels registered in the normal ranges. The term used to describe this anomaly is normokalemia. After taking several months of daily readings, we learned that Susan was having muscle paralysis episodes even while her serum potassium levels registered in all three ranges: high, low and normal.

As we discussed previously, determining what constitutes normal, is riddled with errors. For the general population that is generally healthy and free from disease or illness, ranges of normal can be generally established. For someone with a serious illness or disease, especially one that causes the body's metabolism to fluctuate at a high degree, there is no such thing as normal. It is my advice to take the serum potassium reading in the context of other vitals. Using the cardy meter to determine a particular dosage of potassium is unadvisable. Potassium that is ingested will not have any immediate impact on serum potassium levels. Taking potassium supplements will be effective when incorporated into a diet high in alkaline and low in acid-based food substances on a regular daily basis. Potassium bicarbonate has an easier time crossing wall of the intestine and will also help counter the effects of metabolic acidosis.

All instructional videos, charts and graphs can be located on our Periodic Paralysis Network website and also on our Facebook page. You will also find links to our You Tube videos and other resources.

All of the other medical devices we use to take measurements of Susan's vitals are much less complicated to operate. Here is a list of the medical devices we use to measure Susan's vitals:

Digital Oximeter

When Susan was experiencing her very worse symptoms, she was barely able to rise from a sitting position without her oxygen level dropping below 85. Normally, oxygen levels range around the high 90's. Her heart began to race, pulse doubled, and she felt faint. Muscle paralysis soon followed. With the help of some very kind and very aware technicians at Lincare, we were able to obtain a prescription from Susan's medical provider for oxygen therapy. After a few short days of continued oxygen therapy, Susan was able to stand without incident. She continues to monitor her oxygen levels throughout the day because a drop in oxygen typically means Susan will begin to experience muscle paralysis. With the use of oxygen, Susan's heart and lung function stabilized. The oximeter also has a pulse reading, which is critically important in knowing how hard the heart is working. These readings combined with a blood pressure reading helps Susan identify potential problems.

pH Meter

An electronic device that measures the acidity or alkalinity of a liquid is called a pH meter. It has a glass probe, which when placed in the liquids creates an electronic volt, which then registers a number like a thermometer from 1 to 14.

We used this to measure Susan's urine levels throughout the day in order to detect too much acidity, which can lead to metabolic acidosis. We also used it to measure some of the foods, juices or even medications dissolved in water that Susan was ingesting and were surprised to learn of the acidity levels or alkaline levels contained in each.

Blood Sugar/Glucose Meter

It is important to measure blood glucose or sugar levels in the blood. High blood sugar levels can cause a drop in potassium levels causing hypokalemia. Adversely, high potassium levels or hyperkalemia decreases the blood sugar levels. This is another method of knowing if potassium levels are likely high or low based on the sugar levels. This can help with Susan's diet in attempt to avoid the highs and lows.

The blood glucose meter kits also have the stick for pricking the finger, which can be helpful in getting the blood for the cardy meter.

Wrist Blood Pressure Cuff

Blood pressure can go up and down during episodes of paralysis. As we know from previous chapters, blood pressure can increase during hypokalemic episodes and decrease during an episode of hyperkalemia. Blood pressure can increase during a hypokalemic episode and decrease during an episode of hyperkalemia. This can be very dangerous and must be monitored during episodes and can give a clue as to whether we are dealing with high or low potassium for Susan.

The wrist blood pressure cuff displays the blood pressure reading as well as the pulse or heart beats per minute and if arrhythmias are present. This can be helpful to know whether paramedics need to be called.

The wrist cuff is an easier and more convenient tool to use rather than the other type that must be wrapped around the upper arm and a stethoscope is needed to listen for the beats. It is best to not move the person during an episode, so the wrist type works the best.

Digital Thermometer

Using a digital thermometer for measuring Susan's body temperature is the only option during an episode. There is really no other way to measure for a fever. Since illness or infection cause stress to the body, which in turn causes potassium levels to drop, it is important to check for that possibility as a cause. We have discovered that many times Susan is in serious paralysis over an extended period of time because she has a bladder infection or other illnesses.

And so, a digital thermometer, blood sugar meter, wrist blood pressure cuff, and digital pH monitor and cardy meter are all of critical importance when stocking a toolbox with at-home medical devices. Having these devices and keeping written records of readings helped us become organized and focused. One of the most difficult things for any provider to experience is watching someone slip into full body muscle paralysis. These tools will help control some of the panic and chaos that often accompanies an episode of potassium induced muscle paralysis.

These tools and links to companies where they can be purchased are listed at the Periodic Paralysis Network web site.

Chapter Twenty-Five
Finding a Doctor Who Cares

"NOT AN EASY TASK BUT POSSIBLE"
Introduction

So many people with all forms of Periodic Paralysis struggle with finding doctors who can and will help them with both a diagnosis and proper treatment. They go from doctor to doctor and disappointment after disappointment, misdiagnosis after misdiagnosis and mistreatment after mistreatment. This can go on for many years with the misinformation following them from physician to specialist. Often, this will lead to a diagnosis of hypochondria or malingering and a referral to a psychiatrist. Many of the patients become depressed and begin to doubt themselves after being prescribed medications for mental disorders that invariably make the symptoms worse or different, thus creating the need for yet another referral to yet another specialist.

This vicious cycle can continue for years as the symptoms worsen and the patient becomes more disabled and debilitated. Family and friends tire of dealing with the situation and many friends are lost, marriages end in divorce and family members withdraw their support. The patient is left in more pain and despair and the humiliation can be unbearable. Many are never diagnosed and never receive the treatment they need and deserve.

I myself saw over thirty different physicians in six years before I was diagnosed at the age of sixty-two after a lifetime of illness, disability and loss of friends, family and a marriage. For the most part they were rude and did not understand what was happening to me. Most of them were frustrated and believed it to be all in my head.

At one time, I was trying to find a new doctor because my previous doctor suddenly moved out of town. The new doctor I chose told me on my first and only visit, "You are too sick, I will not take you as a new patient". I started crying and cried all the way to the insurance office. I reported him and was told that he did not have the right to do that. They called it "cherry picking", but they did refer me to another doctor. Through some extensive research we discovered that this doctor and 80 other doctors practicing medicine in the local area were the shareholders of the Medicare supplemental insurance company and it appeared they were systematically refusing to treat patients with more serious and chronic illness. Medicare was paying this group of doctors a set amount of money each year, which was easily depleted by more costly procedures. They were engaged in systematic delay and denial of referrals to specialists outside of their group. It appeared to be fraudulent but there was not any oversight being done by state or federal regulatory agencies.

After my diagnosis I have seen eight more doctors, all of whom do not know how to help me, including one who is a specialist in Andersen-Tawil Syndrome. I have been in contact with a physiologist who studies ion channelopathies who would like to help me and my family but is not sure how. I have spoken with one of the neurologists who misdiagnosed me, who has now apologized for missing some important findings in my labs and the opportunity to diagnose me two years earlier.

I also was able to finally locate a few doctors who have been willing to work with me (two more left town after seeing them for a short while) and have read the information I provided for them about Periodic Paralysis and done some research on their own. They do not deal directly with my PP symptoms, however, but with the things they know about, such as, diabetes, oxygen therapy and referrals to specialists as I need them.

After all my experiences with finding doctors who will work with me, I have devised a commonsense plan that can assist anyone to locate a primary care physician (PCP) who will be willing to work with them before they ever step into the physician's office. There will be no more insults from a person who should be showing compassion and no more leaving the office in tears and despair.

This is presented in an outline form so it can be used as a checklist.

Warning!

Avoid at all costs any doctor who seems at all skeptical about Periodic Paralysis. Once you see the "blank look" with glazed eyes, the "shoulder shrug", and the "I don't know about this." comment. Run; do not walk, as fast as possible, from this medical professional. Chances are the comments he puts in your records will follow you for a very long time and may taint other doctors' view of you. Once there is any kind of resistance, it is time to move on.

Finding a Doctor: The Plan

> - Ask your present doctors if he or she is willing to work with you.
> - Ask your present doctors for referrals to other doctors who may know about PP.
> - Call your insurance company.
>   - Tell them your story.
>   - Ask for a case manager to assist you.
> - Call internal medicine doctors' offices; ask if they know about PP.
>   - Neurologists
>   - Endocrinologists
>   - Nephrologist
>   - Ask to speak to the office managers.
>   - Explain your story to them.
>   - ♦ They can speak to the doctor for you.
> - Check on the Internet.

> ➢ Ask on the PP message boards.
> ➢ Check PP websites for lists of PP doctors.
> ➢ Check on clinics in the area.
> ➢ If no insurance check local health department.
> ➢ Think "outside the box".
> ➢ Search the Internet for the university hospitals near you.
>   - Search for doctors who are specialists in channelopathies.
> ➢ Contact the nearest MDA office to get a referral.
>   - BUT: Be very careful
>   - Many MDA clinics and doctors know nothing about PP.
>   - If they do, they do not always know enough to help.

If you do not have a diagnosis but suspect you may have Periodic Paralysis and you already have a doctor, then the most obvious place to begin your search is to ask him or her if they would be willing to work with you. If not, it is time to find a new Primary Care Physician. You have hired your doctor to work with you and if he or she will not, then you have the option to fire them and hire a new one that will.

If you have a good doctor who has decided to move on in his or her career, you may ask your present doctor for the name of a physician who knows about Periodic Paralysis or who would be willing to work with you. If he or she gives you a referral, be sure to have them confer with the new doctor about your disease and provide him with as much information as possible before your first visit. You may also want to provide information of your own ahead of time.

If you are not that lucky, the next thing you can do, if you have insurance, is to call your insurance company and request a "patient advocate" or "case manager". Most insurance companies have employees whose job is to help their clients who have "more than the average" or "out of the ordinary" medical needs.

Once an advocate is assigned to you, you will need to explain your situation and Periodic Paralysis and explain your need to find a doctor who knows about the disease or who will be willing to work with you. It would be wise to seek out neurologists, internal medicine doctors and endocrinologists. You may need to see more than one doctor before you find the "right" one for you.

If your insurance company does not have patient advocates and has a restrictive list of particular doctors and specialists covered in their program, again, you will need to explain your situation and Periodic Paralysis and explain your need to find a doctor who knows about the disease or who will be willing to work with you. They will sometimes do the work for you.

If not, you can search through the lists of neurologists, internal medicine doctors and endocrinologists and call each office and ask for the office manager. You will need to explain your situation and Periodic Paralysis and explain your need to find a doctor who knows about the disease or who will be willing to work with you. In most cases, the office managers will speak to the doctor or doctors about your case and get back with you if the doctor is willing to see you.

If your insurance is not restrictive, you will have to check your local phone book or the Internet for neurologists, internal medicine doctors and endocrinologists in your area and proceed with the phone calling until you find one who will work with you.

Another good option, if your insurance is not restrictive and requires no referrals, is to check out the clinics in your area. The one I attend had 85 doctors and are connected to a local hospital. There should be at least one doctor willing to work with you.

You can proceed as explained previously; call and speak with one of their representatives. Explain your situation. The representative will go through the list of their physicians and chose a few that may work for you. The doctors will be consulted and one or two may agree to see you. It may be wise to spend time with each to decide the "best fit" for you.

Without insurance, seeking out help from your local health department can be productive. Also, your local services for disabled will have some possible options for finding a local doctor. You may be able to secure a social worker. He or she may do the work for or with you.

Thinking "outside of the box" can bring some surprises. I was so frustrated and about to give up on ever finding a local doctor who could diagnose and treat me, when I had a wild idea.

One of our local television stations offers a wonderful service every Tuesday evening during their two-hour news coverage. A local physician, and a guest specialist of her choosing, take calls from viewers and answer medical questions.

I called and asked if she knew about Periodic Paralysis. I was shocked when she told me she had a patient who had it and that the patient saw a local neurologist who treated her. She gave me the name of the neurologist. I made an appointment and after two visits was diagnosed! (I must explain that I had all my medical records in hand with years of medical testing ruling everything else out and a referral from my nurse practitioner.)

The next option I offer must be used with caution. You may search the Internet for specialists. Seeking out these specialists in the field of Periodic Paralysis or Andersen-

Tawil Syndrome, may lead you to some severe disappointment. There are several across the United States and a few around the world. Many do not see patients and are involved in research only.

In our experience, the specialists will only diagnose based on genetics or a very "pure" form of the disease. (This may be based on the fact that most of them are researchers, and their funding is based on working with only those who are genetically diagnosed. This leaves out a high percentage of us.) We have found their view can be extremely narrow and we have been surprised that their knowledge of the disease can be severely lacking in some areas. Their only option for treatment is limited to medications that do not work for many of us. If you have other conditions co-existing with your Periodic Paralysis or do not have a known genetic code, you will be sent packing in tears and humiliation. It may not be worth the time or money you may spend to travel to another state or country.

The Muscular Dystrophy Association (MDA) is an organization that treats patients with muscle diseases, including all forms of Periodic Paralysis. In order to see their doctors, you must already have a diagnosis or be referred for a diagnosis by a doctor. However, in our experiences many of the doctors who have information about Periodic Paralysis at the MDA Clinics, do not know much about it or Andersen-Tawil Syndrome. We have discovered that many offices around the country do not know about Periodic Paralysis. If you call for a referral or information, you will probably be told that they do not know what you are talking about. I have had to call many MDA offices around the country for patients to tell them that they do indeed treat Periodic Paralysis and Andersen-Tawil Syndrome patients. I refer them to the information at their own website.

It has been admitted to me by employees of the MDA that

their doctors do not always know much about Periodic Paralysis and that perhaps I can teach the MDA doctors about Periodic Paralysis and Andersen-Tawil Syndrome. Thus book, in part, was written with that in mind and is hopefully a good tool to do that.

Also, we have been told that although you may already have a diagnosis, you must see their doctors and be re-diagnosed before you will receive any treatment or benefits offered. It is my understanding that if the MDA doctor does not agree with your previous doctors due to their lack of knowledge of the disease or their narrow view based on old facts and research, you may lose your diagnosis. That being said, there are some very good MDA doctors and some of our friends with Periodic Paralysis are having some success with the ones they are seeing. And most of the information on their web site about Periodic Paralysis is helpful.

Some Other Things to Consider When Selecting a Doctor

Calvin Writes: Shopping for a doctor is similar to planning a healthy diet. It takes time to find the person who will best serve your individual needs. When looking for a doctor, you should talk with other people in the community who have had previous experience with that particular doctor. You should also look at things like the office environment. Ask yourself a few questions. When you enter the office for an appointment does it feel safe and clean? Does the office staff treat you with respect and do things seem organized? You should expect the doctor to keep appointments in a timely manner. You should expect the doctor to spend more than 30 minutes with you during each visit and spend some of the time listening to your concerns. Ask yourself if the doctor makes you feel important or does the doctor talk down to you treating you like your opinion doesn't count? Does the doctor talk with you about your diet and insist that you eat nutritious foods and eliminate the bad habits that are making you ill?

Does the doctor suggest treatments for conditions that are not made in a pharmacy? Does the doctor write a prescription before conducting a thorough examination?

You should stay clear of doctors who only know how to write prescriptions and perform surgeries. A doctor can be honest without insulting or blaming you and help you get on the right path towards proper nutrition and health. If the doctor or staff makes you feel uncomfortable while you are there, then turn around and look for another provider. When you get home, get online and write an honest evaluation of your experience where other people can review.

As more people come forward with symptoms, eventually the medical establishment will take this disease seriously and begin to treat people with symptoms with credibility and respect. Getting a prescription or surgery are not always the best options. Force your doctor to give you options that are not written on a prescription pad or open up your body with surgical devices. There are many more things that can be done along the lines of nutrition that can be tried before shoving pills down our throats or looking for a diseased organ to remove with a scalpel. The most important thing you can do is to carry a copy of all your personal medical records. These records contain information about your personal medical history. You should be the one deciding which records a doctor will receive and which records will be avoided due to medical inconsistencies or misrepresentations.

Conclusion

Many of the people with genetic codes, which have been located do have good doctors and receive good treatment and proper medication for their particular forms of Periodic Paralysis. They are very lucky. The medications help them, and they can lead nearly normal lives as well.

We understand, however, it is difficult to find a doctor who will work with those of us who suffer from the effects of Periodic Paralysis, if we have not yet been diagnosed or those of us with variants for which no genetic code has been discovered yet, even if we have been diagnosed clinically (based on symptoms) or for those of us who have other diseases which co-exist with our form of PP. The truth is, very few of us will get any real help from a doctor even if we find one who knows about the disease and is kind, sympathetic and empathetic. This is due to the fact that most of us are unable to tolerate the known medications and the doctors do not know how to help us.

So, although I have a primary care physician and several good specialists, Calvin and I are still left to deal with my episodes of paralysis and my other symptoms with no real help from the medical field. They do not know how to help me, but treat me well and look after the things they can, like my heart problems, power wheelchair, oxygen, diabetes strips, labs, etc. I appreciate and understand their lack of knowledge of such a rare and baffling disease.

They trust us with the plan we have created after much research and trial and error.

Chapter Twenty-Six
Getting a Clinical Diagnosis

"HIT THEM BETWEEN THE EYES WITH THE FACTS!"
Introduction

Calvin Writes: Most of what goes on inside of our bodies we are unable to see. One role of science is to uncover these mysteries and in cooperation with governmental agencies and commercial businesses and organizations apply the discoveries to improving quality of our everyday lives. Scientists have established ways to unravel these mysteries through scientific methods of inquiry. Many important discoveries begin with an idea and end up as established fact after going through the rigors of scientific testing. The tests get repeated over and over until the outcomes are predictable. Only then are we allowed to reap the benefits of remedies and cures in the form of pharmaceutical drugs, surgeries and an expanded awareness about the inner workings of our bodies. It is a remarkable process that has evolved over time and captures our personal and collective imaginations. The process is necessary to sort out differences between facts and opinions about certain medical conditions and treatments.

In the case of Periodic Paralysis, the scientific community is in the beginning stages of inquiry, testing and treatment. There are many unanswered questions about the disease and very few ways to treat or manage symptoms at this time. Most people suffering with the disease are left alone to find ways to manage their condition with very little help from medical professionals, family and friends. To make matters worse for people suffering from this life changing disease, they are often misdiagnosed with other conditions.

When a medical provider is unable to properly diagnosis a medical condition, they typically blame the patient and attribute the symptoms to psychological psychosomatic origins. In other words, because the condition is so difficult to diagnose, people with the disease are often seen as suffering with a mental illness. Many patients are treated with medications, which perpetuate symptoms and an early end to life. It is a real-life tragedy for many people. Fortunately, most people have a certain level of resilience and survive the prescribed treatments and mistreatments but not everyone suffering with Periodic Paralysis will ever know the causes of their muscle paralysis. The medical establishment is in the infantile stages of the identification and treatment of Periodic Paralysis.

Diagnosis Through the Process of Elimination

Getting a diagnosis of Periodic Paralysis requires patience, resources, and access to competent medical providers and services. The correct diagnosis usually occurs through a process of elimination.

Partial or complete muscle paralysis usually causes a person to seek out medical attention. The initial response of a medical provider will be to run a series of tests including taking samples of bodily fluids, complete physical examination, and conducting some specialized tests of the major body organs including the brain, heart and lungs. As more standard tests get performed and negative results returned, a competent medical provider will begin to narrow in on a specific range of diseases such as Periodic Paralysis as the culprit of the disease. However, most medical providers do not have expertise, experience or even desire to identify and diagnose Periodic Paralysis. Most general parishioners will pass the mystery off to specialists.

As the patient visits different specialists and results return negative results, the disease typically gets misdiagnosed. The patient typically does not respond to prescribed treatments and the symptoms continue to worsen. Eventually many patients are seen as suffering from some form of mental illness and prescribed medications that make symptoms worse. It is difficult for most people to recover from this position of misdiagnosis, mistreatment and mistrust.

There are ways to identify and manage Periodic Paralysis symptoms and ways to avoid making things worse than they have become. The first step is to establish the known facts about the causes of the disease and facts about how to manage the symptoms. We need to rely on science to help unravel this puzzle. The tools are available for anyone to use but unfortunately most medical providers do not know how to use their own tools. Getting the facts is the key to understanding and managing this disease.

The Plan
"HIT THEM BETWEEN THE EYES WITH THE FACTS!"

Susan writes: We met with a technician for medical equipment when we were trying to get oxygen because I was having trouble breathing. She told us the best way to get the help we needed, and a diagnosis was to, "Hit them (doctors) between the eyes with the facts". That is just what we did!! Based on that idea I have created the following plan for others to use to gain a diagnosis. I am presenting it in an outline format to make it easy to follow and to use as a checklist. The story of my own diagnosis follows in this chapter.

❖ You must **gather all the facts**:
  ➢ It is important for **everything else to be ruled out**. Your PCP and a neurologist do these, because most of the symptoms resemble neuromuscular disorders. The tests ruling everything else out might include but are not limited to:
    ▪ Lab work of all types,

247

- Blood
- Urine
- MRIs,
  - Brain
  - Spine
- Spinal taps,
- X-rays
- EEGs
- EMGs
- EKGs
- CMAPs
- Muscle biopsy
  (Some of the tests above may show changes that can be markers for PP).

❖ Most doctors diagnosing PP want lab work showing either:

➢ Paralysis during shifting in normal ranges

➢ Paralysis during shifting in low potassium and/or,

➢ Paralysis during shifting high potassium

- This is done by obtaining serum potassium levels
  - May need to be done several times until a baseline is established
  - Then during episodes every 5 to 10 minutes...not just one blood draw...there is no way to see the shifting otherwise.
  - It may be necessary for hospitalization in order to do this while in the paralysis.
  - May need to be done for more than 24 hours until each is documented, during the episodes.
  - If the shifting is in the normal ranges, it may never show up during tests, unless it is done every few

248

minutes.
- ♦ 50% of PP patients may not have potassium shifting out of normal ranges
- ♦ ATS patients may shift all three ways.
- ➤ However, the latest information for diagnosing PP based on potassium levels in blood serum is as follows:
  - ▪ The potassium in the blood does not always shift above or below normal ranges in 50% of patients experiencing muscle weakness or paralysis or it shifts so quickly that it cannot be measured. Doctors need to diagnose a patient with Periodic Paralysis based on the patient's symptoms, specifically, heart symptoms on an EKG and the muscle strength or weakness and history of episodes of paralysis.
- ➤ *** The information above needs to be shared with your doctors. Most do not understand these concepts. ***
- ❖ There needs to be periods of paralysis, either total or partial, which can be documented (or progressive, gradual, fixed muscle weakness, all other things ruled out).
- ➤ Videotaping is the best way to do this.
- ➤ It may be necessary for hospitalization in order for doctors to see an individual while in the paralysis.

Warning!
Under no circumstances should an individual provoke his or her symptoms or an episode of paralysis by omitting medication or ingesting foods or perform activities, which are known

> triggers. **This is a very serious thing to do and can lead to death. Please read Chapter Twenty-Nine for more information on this subject.**

* ❖ ECGs or EKGs consistent with "ion channelopathy", Periodic Paralysis or Andersen Tawil Syndrome. For specifics see Heart Issues in Chapter Nineteen.
  * ➢ Needs to be done while in the paralysis so it may need to be done for more than 24 hours until each is documented, during the episodes.
    * ▪ Holter Heart Monitors are the best method.
* ❖ Oximeter (oxygen) recordings
  * ➢ Indicating, levels dropping during paralysis.
  * ➢ If in an advanced case of PP, it may show hypoventilation.
* ❖ Genetic testing is available
  * ➢ Not necessary, but helpful for treatment and prognosis
  * ➢ See below for Specifics for Genetic Diagnosing of PP
    * ▪ 30% of all people with PP do not have identified mutations.
  * ➢ See below for Specifics for Genetic Diagnosing of ATS
    * ▪ 30% - 40 % of all people with ATS do not have identified mutations.
* ❖ Gather all previous medical records.
  * ➢ Be sure to ask for all doctors' records from each appointment you attend.
  * ➢ Get all lab records, x-rays, hospitalizations, etc.
* ❖ Chart the triggers for the episodes.
  * ➢ See "Triggers" in Chapter Seventeen and "Discovering Your Triggers" in Chapter Twenty-Two"
  * ➢ Documenting an increase of episodes after eating carbohydrates or red meat, after exercising or after taking

certain medications is important for being able to control the episodes and letting the doctor see what the triggers are for a diagnosis.

❖ Documenting a reduction of episodes when using potassium is good. This can indicate the loss of potassium after shifting and may indicate low potassium levels.

❖ Gather a team of doctors. (Knowledgeable about PP or willing to learn)
  ➢ PCP
  ➢ Neurologist
  ➢ Electrocardiologist
  ➢ Nephrologist
  ➢ Endocrinologist
  ➢ Counselor or therapist
  ➢ Others as needed for symptoms
  ➢ MDA doctors if possible

❖ Gather as much medical information as possible from family members who may have symptoms similar to Periodic Paralysis. It has a hereditary component.
  ➢ If one suspects Andersen-Tawil Syndrome, gather as much medical information as possible from family members and note the characteristics/symptoms. Create a family flowchart with this information. Adding pictures can be helpful in demonstrating the characteristics.
    ▪ See example of a family flowchart in the appendix.

Diagnosis For Andersen-Tawil Syndrome

Andersen-Tawil Syndrome can be diagnosed clinically. This information is found in "Andersen-Tawil Syndrome" in Chapter Thirteen.

Genetics and Periodic Paralysis
"A GENETIC CODE IS NOT NECESSARY"

I will not write about the genetics involved in Periodic Paralysis except to say that anyone interested can locate that information using a computer and the Internet. This is because I do not believe it is necessary to be diagnosed with a known mutation other than it might be helpful for treatment issues in some cases. The reason for my conviction is written in Chapter Twenty-Nine in Part Four.

How I Got My Diagnosis
"THE BIRTH OF THE PLAN"

At the age of sixty-two I was newly, clinically diagnosed with Periodic Paralysis (PP) on February 7, 2011. The type I was diagnosed with is Andersen-Tawil Syndrome. As time has passed, I was tested genetically, and it was discovered that I do not have the known mutation for Type 1. So, the type I have is a variant of Andersen-Tawil Syndrome Type 1 or an Andersen-Tawil Syndrome-like Type of Periodic Paralysis.

As discussed in previous chapters, I have had episodes of partial and total paralysis for many years. During the episodes, my potassium shifts are low (hypokalemia), high (hyperkalemia) and normal ranges (normokalemia). Due to several misdiagnoses and a lack of proper diagnosis and treatment for over fifty years, I have become totally and permanently disabled with weak muscles throughout my body including those involved with my vision, digestion, breathing and my heart. I must be on oxygen constantly and cannot exert myself in any way. The electrical workings of my heart are defective. I have had a heart loop monitor inserted in my chest to monitor the tachycardia and arrhythmias, which include long QT interval beats. I now spend my days in a recliner, unable to walk farther than across a room. I must use a motorized wheelchair for anything farther. If I did not have the help of my husband, I would have to live in an assisted living program. I was misdiagnosed for many years.

Through the past years of my physical decline, I have had to give up my career as a special education teacher, my hobbies to include hiking, walking, swimming, exercising, fishing, camping, traveling, shopping, cooking and baking. I had to sell, and move away from, a beautiful home in the mountains of Utah. I can no longer drive. I have lost many friends, because I could not keep up with them or entertain any longer. I have lost contact with family members who did not understand or did not want to watch my decline or who thought I was a hypochondriac. I have lost the connection I once had with my grandchildren because I can no longer keep up with them or continue a meaningful relationship with them. The relationship with my husband has changed from husband and wife to caregiver and patient. Most of the over thirty doctors I have seen in the past six years have treated me poorly and like I was mentally ill.

I have spent the past several years working diligently to get a diagnosis and treatment for the ailment that cruelly stole the quality of my life. The most difficult part of this, for me, is knowing that I may not have become this seriously ill if just one of the over thirty doctors I have seen in the last six years in Oregon and the many years before, would have taken me seriously.

Once I realized what I actually had, the struggle became even more difficult trying to convince my doctors. By this point, everything else had been ruled out, but no one wanted to diagnose me. I heard I was "too old" to have it. I was ignored. I was dismissed and told to go have a "good time" as long as I was in Portland, after driving two hundred fifty miles for the results of a muscle biopsy (The test did show myopathy, change in shape and size of muscle fiber but I was told it was normal). I was given lidocaine after telling my primary care physician (PCP) I could not have it during a mole biopsy...it caused an episode of paralysis, but I was treated as if I were a naughty child behaving badly. I was left alone in the room in paralysis. I was in metabolic acidosis, twice in front of my PCP and sent home rather than to the hospital. My heart was in tachycardia, and I could not breathe. After discovering that I was having long QT interval heartbeats on a Holter Monitor (a marker for ATS), this was dismissed by my PCP, even after being told it meant I could go into cardiac arrest at any given moment. After two months, I had to request a referral to an electrocardiologist. The referral took two more weeks to get from my PCP and the insurance company.

All during this time, I continued to decline as I had more and more severe total paralytic episodes. I had tachycardia and palpitations of my heart and I was having difficulty breathing. Sometimes my breathing would actually stop for a few seconds at a time. It felt like an elephant sitting on my chest. It was very frightening. Soon the difficulty of taking breaths in and out began to happen when I was not in paralysis. I found it more and more difficult to breathe. Every time I stood up, ate a meal or exerted myself in anyway, the breathing got worse, and my heart would speed up until it was beating 130 to 140 beats per minute, even while I was eating.

My husband became so concerned with the lack of caring being displayed by my PCP and our insurance company, that he walked into a medical supply company and told them what was happening and asked if they could help me to get oxygen because I could not breath. After speaking with him for a few minutes, the manager told my husband that she would give all the information he had carried in with him, to one of the technicians and that they would see what they could do for us. She told my husband that they find it is best to get all the information together and then, "Hit them (doctors) between the eyes with the facts".

They came out and hooked me up with a recording oximeter. It was discovered that my oxygen saturation levels were dropping dangerously low during my episodes of paralysis, and it was apparent that they were low every time I exerted myself in any way. The technician took the information to my PCP, and she had no choice but to sign a referral for me to get oxygen. At that point, we began to look for another PCP and decided to change insurance companies to avoid the need for referrals.

A month or two before this point, I was in despair over trying to find a doctor who knew about Periodic Paralysis. Then on the evening news, I saw their weekly feature of offering direct calls to doctors with any medical question. I quickly picked up the phone. After a wait of only a few minutes, I was speaking with one of the physicians. I asked her if she had heard of PP or knew of any doctors who might know about it. As luck would have it, she herself had a patient with it. She gave me the name of the neurologist the patient sees.

I went to my PCP with this information and talked her into giving me yet another referral. The neurologist eventually diagnosed me with "probable" Periodic Paralysis. He wrote a letter telling my PCP that I needed to see an electrocardiologist right away. It was several months before I got the referral. He described my heart condition, by that point as serious with no treatment, but insisted I needed to have a heart monitor implanted. He also set up a renal specialist to help diagnose what he believed was Andersen-Tawil Syndrome based on all the information being presented to him by my PCP, my neurologist and me. I did get the diagnosis while in the hospital for the implant after going into paralysis and being observed by the doctors. They are giving me a saline drip and lidocaine during the procedure, and it apparently caused the paralytic episode. My diagnosis was actually based on an accident.

The following is the letter I wrote to my family about my final diagnosis:

(Letter Begins)

"Hello Family and Friends.... I made it through one of the toughest days of my life... I had a heart loop recorder inserted in chest with only lidocaine to numb it, because I cannot tolerate any meds. I told them the lidocaine would send me into paralysis, so they used a type without epinephrine and felt assured it would not cause paralysis. As luck would have it (and I knew it) 1/2 way through the procedure, I went into paralysis. By that time the device was already implanted. The doctor and rest of the team were watching my heart doing its thing (tachycardia, arrhythmias) saying things like, "Look at the huge T-waves" and reading off numbers that I did not understand and ohing and awing. He proceeded to explain my disease to them. Then when I was able to answer questions, they all began to ask me questions about it...remember.... what I have, Andersen-Tawil Syndrome.... only 100 other people, worldwide, have been diagnosed with.

As they were ready to take me to recovery, I noticed an IV drip in my arm. I got horribly upset and asked what it was. They told me "saline". I swore and told them I was not supposed to have that. They then removed it. What I did not know was that it had been on me the entire procedure. I thought they had just hooked it up and then took it off after I told them that.

I went back to recovery and was doing fairly well, except for slipping in and out of small paralysis episodes.

My heart doctor had put together a "team" for the rest of the procedures they were going to do for a confirmation of how my potassium shifts and how to treat it. The plan was to put me in ICU and have a kidney specialist direct the testing and an intensivist (intensive care specialist) to monitor all signs and symptoms and be there to treat my symptoms which could include my heart stopping.

I called Shari to tell her how well I was doing and tell her the plan to pass on to everyone.

Just as the kidney specialist showed up to tell me the plan and ask me a few questions, I began to have trouble answering his first question. I slipped into the worst episode of paralysis to date. My heart began to beat at a sustained heart rate of 130 to 140 bpm for over the next hour. My blood pressure was at 168/80. I felt like an elephant was on my chest. I could feel and hear my heart racing and the horrible pain from it. I could not have any pain meds or any meds to slow my heart because it would have made it worse. Everyone was in astonishment watching the heart monitor and not knowing what to do. Calvin was so afraid, and I thought I was dying. I could hear everything but was unable to open my eyes or speak. I could not move, just hear everything and feel all the pain and pressure. The doctors kept saying they had never seen anything like it and the nurses kept touching my hands, arms and face, telling me they were sorry they couldn't help me.

(The saline drip and the lidocaine apparently caused this...if you have PP/ATS never let them put a saline or glucose IV in you and avoid lidocaine.)

My heart finally began to slow down over the next hour. I was finally able to open my eyes and could speak a little. Finally, I was doing very well. The doctors decided to proceed as planned and told us the plan to put me in ICU and load me with carbohydrates to start the paralysis again and then test my potassium levels through the paralysis process, etc.

They got me upstairs and had me ready to begin the next phase. Calvin left to go home and get some much-needed rest. The kidney specialist came in at that point and said, "We have decided not to proceed with the testing and are sending you home now." I asked why? His reply floored me..."We don't need to do anymore testing...there is no doubt you have Andersen-Tawil Syndrome (ATS). Everything we have read tells us that you could die if we do the testing we were going to do, if you have ATS. We are going to give you diamox to treat your paralysis symptoms, but because you have ATS it may not work for you... but we want to try". I thanked him and told him I already knew that but was taking the chance for the little hope I had that the meds might help me...otherwise there is not much else I can do for a better quality of life.

I already had the diagnosis of Periodic Paralysis (PP) from my neurologist, but now I had the diagnosis of the type of PP.

He told me how humbled he felt to be diagnosing me. He said he was just an ordinary MD... nephrologist...not like the big and powerful doctors who wrote all the info on PP and ATS back east. But after seeing what happened and going over all the facts and by the process of elimination and studying all the latest research, I had presented to them and the family flowchart I had put together with all the family medical history and all of your input... including Kathryn's toes! He felt he had no other choice. He told me I had done all the work and had done an excellent job of presenting it all to them. Without that, I might never have got the ATS diagnosis also. He had never heard of ATS before, none of them had, but they had been researching and studying it.

Thank you, Family members, for answering the little questionnaires I sent out and all your input and patience with me over the years.

He has dictated a report which each of you will get. **You** *can then give it to your doctors. My children have a 50/50 chance of having it and of passing it on. All of you must get checked. The Long QT interval heartbeat is nothing to ignore.*

Thank you all for your best wishes and kind words and thoughts. "

(Letter Ends)

Chapter Twenty-Seven
Assembling and Directing the Team

"GETTING PROPER TREATMENT"
Introduction

In Chapter Twenty-Five we share our plan for finding a doctor who cares and will be willing to work with an individual who has Periodic Paralysis. In this chapter we will share a plan for receiving the appropriate care and treatment needed and expected from doctors and other medical professionals. Based on our experiences with doctors and other medical professionals, we have created the following plan for others to use to assemble a medical team and to direct the team. I am presenting it in an outline format to make it easy to follow and to use as a checklist.

The following is such an important message that we have chosen to interject it again to begin this chapter concerning working with doctors and seeking appropriate care.

Warning!

Avoid at all costs any doctor who seems at all skeptical about Periodic Paralysis. Once you see the "blank look" with glazed eyes, the "shoulder shrug", and the "I don't know about this." comment. Run; do not walk, as fast as possible, from this medical professional. Chances are the comments he puts in your records will follow you for a very long time and may taint other doctors' view of you. Once there is any kind of resistance, it is time to move on.

The Plan

Once you find a doctor who is willing to work with you:

- ❖ Follow plan in Chapter Twenty-Six for securing a diagnosis, if needed.
- ❖ Make sure he or she has all your medical records.

❖ Provide her with everything you can find written on Periodic Paralysis.
  ➤ Keep up on the latest treatments.
    ▪ Share with doctor.
❖ Follow the plan for "Walking the Tightrope" on this website as it applies to you.
  ➤ Give a copy to your doctor.
❖ Ask for referrals in order to develop a "Team".
  ➤ Neurologist
  ➤ Electrocardiologist
  ➤ Nephrologist
  ➤ Endocrinologist
  ➤ Physical therapist
  ➤ Counselor or therapist
    ▪ Have them write a letter stating you do not have a conversion disorder or are not faking it.
  ➤ Others as needed for symptoms.
    ▪ MDA doctors if possible.
      • Ask for a referral to your nearest MDA office
  ➤ Contact your nearest MDA office to get a referral
    ▪ BUT: Be very careful. (See previous chapter)
❖ Seek out Community Services
  ➤ Transportation
  ➤ Home Health Care

You are the leader of your medical team so it important for you to "hire" only doctors who will work with you and for you as you direct the team in your best interest.

Once you have found a caring doctor who is either knowledgeable about Periodic Paralysis or willing to learn about it and work with you, follow the plan in Chapter Twenty-Six for securing a diagnosis if needed.

If you already have a diagnosis, make sure the doctor has all your medical records. Be sure to sign all release forms for each doctor you have seen, for all labs, tests of any kind, hospital visits, etc. for your new doctor. He or she will need all your records, especially the ones, which include your diagnosis and lab work and testing which proves it. Put all of this information in a file. Add any and all new information as you get it. You may also gather your own records by going to the doctors, hospitals and labs yourself and collect the records for yourself and then pass them on to your doctor. This is the best way to ensure derogatory written records do not get passed from one doctor to another. It is important to take control over the accuracy of the information being shared about you.

Provide your doctor with all the latest information you can find about Periodic Paralysis, especially about the type you have or believe you have. A copy of this book would also be helpful to share with him or her.

It is best to remember that doctors have very few treatment options for serious illness outside of administering pharmaceutical drugs or performing invasive surgeries. For individuals with Periodic Paralysis, this means there is little that they can do for those who cannot take medications or cannot have anesthesia for surgery. So, it will be up to you to explain these things to the physicians and present them with your own plan. Follow the Plan from Chapter Twenty-Three as it applies to your particular symptoms and type of Periodic Paralysis. You will need to experiment until you find what will work for you. Document your triggers, symptoms such as high or low blood pressure and oximeter readings, Cardy Meter readings, episodes of paralysis and how you are following the plan and share your progress with the doctor.

Ask for referrals as needed to specialists. Do not be afraid to ask. The most common ones needed may include a neurologist mostly to rule everything else out, but not needed after that; an electrocardiologist to treat the heart issues, especially the electrical issues which includes the arrhythmias and tachycardia or bradycardia; nephrologist if kidney issues are involved; endocrinologist who treat metabolic disorders of which Periodic Paralysis is; physical therapist who may be able to assess the muscle weakness and can order walkers, canes, wheelchairs, etc., as needed and a counselor or therapist to assist with the depression and anxiety, which may be involved. There may be other specialists necessary depending on the medical issues which develop such as a pulmonologist for breathing problems and the need for oxygen. Do not forget to get the records from each visit and all labs and tests and add these to your file.

You may also need home health care, respite, loaning of medical equipment or assistance with transportation, etc. so you may want to research the community services available for individuals who are disabled or seniors in your area. Have your doctor assist you with this. You may need referrals.

Ask the primary care doctor to write letters, which state that you, in fact, have Periodic Paralysis. Ask the therapist or counselor to write a letter explaining that you do not have a conversion disorder. Use these letters when dealing with the specialists, paramedics if an ambulance must be called and emergency room (ER) staff in emergency situations.

Ask the doctors to assist with getting oxygen and equipment such as a blood sugar meter and strips, which can also be used with the cardy meter or ordering a cane, walker or wheelchair. Request a standing order for testing for metabolic acidosis and other possible complications.

Conclusion

As written in Chapter Twenty-Five, very few of us will get any real help from a doctor even if we find one who knows about the disease and is kind, sympathetic and empathetic. This is due to the fact that most of us are unable to tolerate the known medications and the doctors do not know how to help us.

So, although I have a primary care physician and several

good specialists, Calvin and I are still left to deal with my episodes of paralysis and my other symptoms with no real help from the medical field. They do not know how to help me, but treat me well and look after the things they can, like my heart problems, power wheelchair, oxygen, diabetes strips, labs, etc. I appreciate and understand their lack of knowledge of such a rare and baffling disease.

They trust us with the plan we have created after much research and trial and error.

Chapter Twenty-Eight
Directing the Paramedics

"NO IV OR TOURNIQUET PLEASE"
Introduction

Chapter Twenty-Seven discusses how to assemble a medical team and then how to direct that team in order to get appropriate care for dealing with the issues of Periodic Paralysis. The team may include many specialists. It is important to build a medical file by gathering all medical records and current information about Periodic Paralysis. Always remember that you are the team leader. Receiving and directing one's proper medical treatment does not stop at the doctor's office door. Individuals with Periodic Paralysis find themselves dealing with paramedics many times before and after finally getting a diagnosis. It is essential that you be able to direct the team that will appear at your door ready to hook you up to an IV.

The best way to do that is to prepare ahead of time for medical emergencies.

The Plan

- ❖ Create a file folder:
  - ➢ A card with the names and phone numbers of your doctors
  - ➢ A list of medications I cannot have.
  - ➢ Information copied from the Internet or this book explaining your form of Periodic Paralysis.
  - ➢ Information on how to treat your form whether hypokalemia or hyperkalemia.
  - ➢ Information about long QT interval heartbeat or other arrhythmias.
  - ➢ A letter from your therapist explaining that you do not have a mental illness or conversion disorder.
  - ➢ The documents with your diagnoses if you have one.
  - ➢ A list of my other diagnosed conditions, i.e., diabetes, osteoporosis, restless leg syndrome
  - ➢ A list for your emergency care
- ❖ Call and set up an appointment to meet with your local paramedics.

❖ Go to your nearest ambulance company or fire department to discuss your particular situation.
❖ Provide them with as much information as possible about your type of Periodic Paralysis.
 ➤ Provide them with information from your file folder.
 ➤ If you live alone give them a key to your home or let them know where a key is to get in to help you.
❖ At home put the emergency list on a bulletin board or refrigerator.
❖ Carry copies of all the information with you at all times.
 ➤ In folder.
 ➤ In purse, wallet.
 ➤ In medic alert bracelet.
 ➤ In car glove box.
 ➤ Pin to car visor.
 ➤ In badge holders, attached to chain around neck.
❖ Know when to call an ambulance.

Meeting with your local paramedics is probably the best way to begin preparing for medical emergencies. It may take a few phone calls to discover which are the correct fire department and/or ambulance company for your neighborhood. Set up an appointment or discuss your issues with the chief paramedic or fire chief over the phone.

Provide them with as much information as possible about your type of Periodic Paralysis or the type you believe you have. Provide them with information on how to treat you. Be sure to include a list of the medications you cannot have. Give them copies of all of your important medical information. Make sure to give them copies of the letters written by your doctor or counselor backing up your diagnosis or possible diagnosis and information indicating you do not have a conversion disorder and that you are not a malingerer. If you live alone, be sure to either give them a key to your house or let them know where one will be in an emergency.

Since the paramedics may not have had any training about your condition or new ones may show up or in case they have forgotten, making an emergency list of the things the paramedics need to know as soon as they enter your door is the single most important thing you can do. It needs to be posted on a bulletin board or on the refrigerator in plain view. Although you may have a spouse, friend or family member there with you, you may not be able to speak and those with you may forget to relay important information. Having it written down and posted will be helpful for everyone involved.

As suggested in Chapter Twenty-Seven, you should have a folder with your entire collection of medical information and information about Periodic Paralysis. The emergency list should also be in the file, on the top. The folder should be in an obvious and easily accessible place known to everyone in the family.

Making several copies of this information and carrying a set with you would be a good idea. You may end up in an emergency somewhere out of your home and paramedics may arrive who will know nothing about you. If carrying your entire file with you is not practical, then make sure to at least have your emergency list handy. You can carry your medical information or the emergency list with you in several ways: in a folder, in a purse or wallet, in a medic alert bracelet, in a car glove box, pinned to the car visor or in a badge holder attached to a chain bracelet secured around your neck. You need to be creative but also realistic. Be sure it is in an obvious and easily seen place.

When making the emergency list, remember that you may be alone and may not be able to speak. Think of the things they will need to know. First, they cannot put you on a glucose or sodium IV. If they take a blood sample, they cannot use a tourniquet because it can make the potassium levels appear higher than they are.

A copy of the emergency list I have designed for myself can be found in the Appendix.

(List Begins)

"My name is Susan. I am sixty-three years old, and I have a very rare disease called Periodic Paralysis. The type I have is Andersen-Tawil Syndrome Type 2. Potassium shifts in my body if I am hypokalemic, hyperkalemic or normokalemic. I become totally paralyzed when the potassium shifts from my organs and goes into my muscles. I am unable to move in any way and am not able to speak or open my eyes. I look like I am asleep, BUT I can hear everything going on around me. I can hear everything being said.

I may be able to move my index finger on my right hand. If you ask "yes" or "no" questions, I may be able to answer. Up and down is "yes" and sideways is "no".

My husband, Calvin, knows exactly what to do for me, so listen carefully to what he says and follow his directions. If he is not with me or is unable to speak or help me please follow the outline below:

If I must go to a hospital take me to (name of medical center).

My doctors are: (name/s and contact information of medical providers).

- *Primary Care Doctor*
- *Neurologist*
- *Cardiologist*
- *Renal Specialist*

❖ *Please talk to me and tell me what you are doing to me*

and for me.
- ❖ *Please make sure I am comfortable.*
- ❖ *Please make sure I am reclining but not lying flat.*
- ❖ *Please be sure my oxygen is on and working.*
- ❖ *Please cover me with a light sheet or blanket because I get cold.*
- ❖ *Please make sure my head and neck are supported. My head will fall to the side and can hurt a great deal.*
- ❖ *Please do not try to move me when I am paralyzed. Damage can occur to my muscles and joints.*
- ❖ *Please do not put me on an IV. I cannot have saline or glucose. If one must be used, mannitol may be ok.*
- ❖ *Please do not give me any medications of any kind to include antibiotics.*
- ❖ *Please do not give me any type of anesthesia, to include lidocaine.*
- ❖ *Please do not use a tourniquet if blood is to be taken to check my potassium levels.*
- ❖ *Please do not put any food or liquid in my mouth, I will choke because I cannot swallow.*
- ❖ *Please watch my breathing it may stop or be very shallow.*
- ❖ *Please watch my swallowing. I may choke.*
- ❖ *Please monitor my heart. I have a heart loop monitor in my chest. I have long QT interval heartbeats, arrhythmias, tachycardia; bradycardia and my heart may stop beating. I may go into cardiac arrest.*
- ❖ *Please do not be alarmed if I have myoclonic jerks or fasciculations. It may mean that I am hyperkalemic, and it is not a seizure.*
- ❖ *Please have patience. I will come out of it eventually. It may last 15 minutes to several hours or I may go in and out of it.*
- ❖ *Please be ready with a bedpan or be ready to help me to the bathroom. I will have to urinate urgently after I come out of paralysis but will still be too weak to walk by*

Living with Periodic Paralysis

myself to the bathroom.

Other conditions: List your conditions

> ◆ *I have a Medtronic Reveal XT Heart Loop Monitor implanted in my chest…do not give me an MRI*

My medications:
- *potassium bicarbonate as needed*
- *oxygen therapy 2 liters 24/7*

Personal Contact Information:
- *Susan Quentine Knittle-Hunter*
- *Address*
- *Phone number*
- *Date of birth*
- *Emergency contact"*

(List Ends)

When to Call an Ambulance if You Have Periodic Paralysis

After understanding and studying Periodic Paralysis and Andersen-Tawil Syndrome, we have learned that an ambulance does not need to be called every time I become paralyzed. When I have an episode of paralysis, I will usually be fine in a few hours. Calvin carefully monitors my vital signs and potassium levels and watches for serious problems. However, if I have trouble with my blood pressure, my breathing, and my heart or with choking or swallowing, then an ambulance may be necessary.

When dealing with hyperkalemia (high levels of potassium) the following may be helpful. I have been told, if the level is 6.0 or more than emergency treatment may be necessary.

This can be determined from cardy meter readings and symptoms. These symptoms include a weak heartbeat, problems with breathing, nausea and a loss of consciousness. Hyperventilation may indicate metabolic acidosis has set in. A rapid heartbeat may indicate that the potassium levels are dangerously high.

When dealing with hypokalemia (low levels of potassium) the following may be helpful when trying to make a decision about calling for the paramedics. If the potassium level is below 2.5 as indicated on a cardy meter and there are problems with high blood pressure, chest pain, slurred speech, confusion, breathing, arrhythmias, choking or swallowing emergency care may be necessary.

My Experiences with the Paramedics

On four different occasions I rode in an ambulance to the hospital due to symptoms of Periodic Paralysis, however, at the time I had no idea what was wrong. It was very frightening. Calvin and I assumed the problem was my heart because of the tachycardia and chest pain involved. On one of the occasions, total paralysis was also involved as well as muscle contractions throughout my body that made it look like seizures. During that trip, one of the paramedics gave me some glucose by mouth. He told me I was hypoglycemic. Within a few minutes, my body was jerking, especially my legs and feet. They were beating against the back door of the ambulance. By the time I got to the hospital, I was worse than when the ambulance arrived at my home. I assumed it was due to the glucose.

On the other three trips I did not get the glucose. The ambulance was called due to total paralysis, arrhythmia and tachycardia. On all four occasions, I was hooked up with an IV as I lay in the ambulance in the driveway. We sat there for quite a while before we left for the hospital. It was a long, slow drive to the hospital because we lived in the mountains about ten miles outside of town. I arrived at the hospital in worse condition than when I left my home. It was not until I realized I had Periodic Paralysis and began to study everything I could about the condition that I discovered why this happened.

I should never have been given IVs of glucose or dextrose (sugar and water), or saline or sodium (salt and water). Apparently, the IVs had worsened my condition on each occasion. We now know that glucose and saline given intravenously are triggers for individuals with Periodic Paralysis. If an IV is needed mannitol may be used in diluted strengths. [68]

Besides the important information about IVs, it is also important to understand that improper use of a tourniquet and the clenching of the fist can result in false lab results for potassium levels. If the pressure is too tight and the time too long of the tourniquet it can falsely raise the level of potassium in the serum blood results. [69, 70.]

It is important for anyone with Periodic Paralysis to know the above information and to have it written available in case an ambulance must be called. I keep this information in my folder and on my emergency list along with everything I know is important and that the paramedics must know when coming to my aid in an emergency. I approach it as if I will have no one with me to explain my needs. I keep it near the door and take it with me when I leave home. The information you should have in your folder is discussed earlier in the chapter.

Due to the previous mishaps, I have taken time to call my ambulance company and the fire department and explained my condition to them, so they will understand ahead of time and be ready to assist me appropriately. At first, the person I talked to, began to laugh at me and scoff about my calling with information ahead of time. She said it was not necessary for them to know anything before the ambulance is called. I began to cry in frustration and told her that she could laugh and scoff if she wanted to, but she had better pay attention to what I was saying. I told her I had a very rare disease that only one hundred people worldwide have been diagnosed with, and I had some very serious health issues that required special attention. I told her if I was not treated appropriately, I could die.

She got very quiet and serious and then began to ask me questions. After listening to my answers and the other information I offered, she told me she would have a meeting with the EMTs and paramedics and train them about Periodic Paralysis: Andersen-Tawil Syndrome and my special needs and what to do when they get a call to help me. I told her to instruct them to look at my file and listen to my husband's instructions. He will know my potassium levels (we have a cardy meter) and they had to trust what he says.

I explained that they have to monitor my breathing; make sure I do not choke and monitor my heart due to the tachycardia, and arrhythmias, watching especially for the long QT interval heartbeat. They are not to hook me to an IV and they are not to give me glucose or any medications. They are not to use a tourniquet or have me make a fist if they need to take my blood. They should look through the folder for any other info they may need before reaching the hospital.

Since that conversation, I did have one more trip in an ambulance to the hospital. I was having breathing difficulties. On that occasion I was taken to another town at Calvin's request. He knew I would get better service and care. At that time, we were prepared. My emergency list was posted on a bulletin board just inside our door and my information folder was next to it on the counter. Calvin presented the paramedics with the information as they walked in the door. After taking my vitals and observing my breathing, the decision was made to transport me to the hospital. It was nearly an hour-long drive, but the paramedics knew not to give me an IV and so things went much better than on the previous rides to the hospital.

Calvin and I recently moved to another state and found new doctors. The first thing I did was to call the fire department and was connected with the fire chief. I told him about my medical issues. He took down all my information and then asked where the paramedics could find the information they would need to know when they arrived in an emergency. I told him and he noted that information for future emergencies. I now feel a little more secure, in knowing that I did what I could to try to get appropriate treatment the next time I may need an ambulance.

Chapter Twenty-Nine
Directing the Emergency Room Staff

"AVOIDING THE PITFALLS"
Introduction

Chapter Twenty-Eight outlines how to deal with and direct the paramedics in an emergency situation. It is important to be prepared before an ambulance team appears at the door ready to attach an IV to someone with Periodic Paralysis. In most emergencies the patient will be transported in the ambulance to the hospital and be seen, evaluated and treated in the emergency room and possibly be admitted to the hospital if the situation is serious enough. Just as it is important to be prepared for the paramedics, it is equally important to be prepared for the emergency room and to be able to deal with and direct the staff for the best and safest treatment possible.

Avoiding the Pitfalls of the Emergency Room

It is extremely important for an individual with Periodic Paralysis and their family members and friends to know why and when to call an ambulance, which is outlined in the previous chapter. That is, if the potassium level is low or high as indicated on a cardy meter and there are problems with blood pressure, breathing, heart, choking or swallowing, emergency care may be necessary.

Then, in order to avoid the pitfalls of the emergency room and to be certain to get the best and safest treatment when arriving at the hospital, it is necessary to be prepared in advance. This is much the same way as preparing for the paramedics but more detailed.

After I received my diagnosis and due to several previous mishaps in the emergency room (ER) and the hospital, I took a trip to the hospital with all my records. I had them copy all my information. This is for four reasons. First, to prove my diagnosis; second, to teach the doctors about Periodic Paralysis; third, to educate the doctors so they will know how to treat me the next time I am in a crisis and fourth; to clarify all the lies and misdiagnoses.

While there, I explained that they have to monitor my breathing; make sure I do not choke and monitor my heart due to the tachycardia, and arrhythmias, watching especially for the long QT interval beat. They are not to hook me to an IV and not to give me glucose or any medications. They are not to use a tourniquet or have me make a fist if they need to take my blood. They should look through my file and/or folder for any other information they may need. It is also important for them to know listen to your significant other (if you are lucky enough to have one), who will be your voice, if you cannot speak or explain things to them.

Since that conversation, and now having everything in place for the next emergency, I feel better about the possibility of having to ride in an ambulance and being admitted to the hospital if needed in the future.

The following plan is in an outline form for easier understanding and to use as a checklist.

The Plan

❖ Call hospital administration office.
  ➤ Explain your problem.
❖ Tell them the history of visits and the problems during them.
❖ Tell them about your fears due to the previous visits.
❖ Explain your diagnosis or possible diagnosis.
❖ Explain your plan to bring in all your records for your file.
❖ Ask how you can speak to the supervisor of the ER.

❖ Call the ER supervisor or make an appointment to meet with him/her.
  ➢ Explain your problem.
❖ Tell them the history of visits and the problems during them.
❖ Tell them about your fears due to the previous visits.
❖ Explain your diagnosis or possible diagnosis.
❖ Explain your plan to bring in all your records for your file.
❖ Meet with ER supervisor or representative in person.
❖ Bring your significant other or a friend or family member.
❖ Present your records with detailed information including the name/s and number/s of your medical providers and also information about Periodic Paralysis.
❖ Copied from the Internet.
❖ The types.
❖ Andersen-Tawil Syndrome?
❖ Hypokalemic Periodic Paralysis?
❖ Hyperkalemic Periodic Paralysis? (How to take your labs, how to treat your symptoms, how to diagnose, if not done yet done).
❖ Your diagnosis reports (from doctors) if you have them
  ➢ List of medications you cannot have.
❖ No IV.
❖ No medications that paralyze.
❖ No meds that cause long QT (if it applies).
  ➢ List of medications you take.
  ➢ List of other medical issues.
❖ Possibly diabetes, heart problems, etc.
❖ Records of previous labs and tests which helped with the diagnosis or ruled other things out to include but not limited to:
❖ EKGs.
❖ Holter monitors results.
❖ EMGs.
❖ EEGs.

❖ Muscle biopsy.
❖ Sleep studies.
❖ Pulmonary study.
❖ Physical therapy.
❖ Letter from therapist clearing you of mental issues.
   ➢ Good to be seeing a therapist to help deal with failing health and to provide moral support.
❖ Possibly a standing prescription from your doctor:
   ➢ If muscle weakness or paralysis
     ▪ Blood serum labs for potassium
❖ Have hospital records copied by the records department or ER personnel.
❖ Explain anything else you believe is important.
❖ Share a copy of this book.
❖ Always carry a well-labeled plastic folder with copies of the above information in case you find yourself out of your local area in an emergency.

Direct the Team

You, your spouse or relatives must direct your care in order for you to be safe. If you find yourself in the ER for an extended period of time or admitted to the hospital, be sure to continue to "teach" new staff at shift changes of all the above information. Remember that it is most likely that none of the doctors and nurses and support staff have any knowledge or understanding of Periodic Paralysis. Have them read through your file or check your information posted in the system. Share a copy of this book with them. Continue to refuse the IVs and medication, which they insist on giving, if you know it is something that you must not have. In exchange for an IV drink plenty of water. Do not allow the ER staff to insert a catheter just for their convenience. They oftentimes do this just so they do not have to help patients to the restroom facilities. You could save yourself a serious infection or damage caused by the insertion of a catheter. Although in pain, refuse the medications, unless you know they will not affect you. Refuse to take tests, which may include dyes or contrasts if they cause you to go into paralysis or which may create arrhythmias or long QT interval heartbeats. Find out what procedures or treatments are being advised and discuss what may be involved that could be of harm to you. Is the test or procedure worth the risk to you? You have the right to refuse any tests or treatments or procedures. Discuss options. Do not be afraid to question anything and everything.

Part Four:
Emotional, Psychological and Social Expectations

Chapter Thirty
Seeking a Genetic Diagnosis

"KNOWING THE GENETIC CODE IS NICE BUT NOT NECESSARY"
Introduction

Part One of this book contains my medical history related to Periodic Paralysis. Part Two discusses all aspects of Periodic Paralysis from what it is to what it is not. Part Three covers the management of the symptoms using natural methods. Part Four deals with the emotional, psychological and social aspects of Periodic Paralysis.

In my opinion, based on information gleaned from many sources; from speaking with many individuals with Periodic Paralysis and by using my knowledge and skills obtained as I earned my degree in psychology, I believe the process of seeking out and obtaining a diagnosis for Periodic Paralysis is so stressful emotionally, psychologically, socially, physically and financially for an individual suffering from this rare, horrendous and misunderstood metabolic disorder, it can actually lead to death by mistake or by mistake after attempting to provoke or create the symptoms for testing or by a lack of proper treatment or by suicide. I have therefore decided to begin this section of the book with this serious subject.

I believe that a genetic diagnosis is a nice thing to have but not something that is necessary to be diagnosed and appropriately treated because only about half of all individuals with Periodic Paralysis actually have a known genetic mutation. An individual with Periodic Paralysis can be diagnosed clinically when all other possibilities for a diagnosis have been eliminated and when his or her symptoms are documented, just like any other disorder or medical condition. At that point, treatment should begin, or a lack of treatment, depending upon the type of Periodic Paralysis. There should be nothing more or nothing less involved. However, that is not the case for those of us with Periodic Paralysis as has been experienced and written about in the first three sections of this book.

The first part of this chapter is about the issues of seeking out a genetic diagnosis. The second part is the actual story of a young man who died accidentally very recently in an attempt to get a clinical diagnosis after sending his blood for genetic testing and getting frustrated with the long wait.

Struggling For a Diagnosis

Most individuals spend twenty to thirty years searching to give a name to the condition that stole the quality of life from them. By the time an individual discovers Periodic Paralysis they are extremely ill and have been treated cruelly by many doctors and have been wrongly diagnosed with mental issues and are depressed. They have probably lost a promising career, have a failing marriage or are divorced, have lost family members and friends and are near bankrupt. They lack self-esteem and are emotionally, and psychologically drained. Many are alone and desperate for answers.

They will find the listservs and discussion boards where they will attempt to find answers and support from others like themselves. They will learn quickly that a diagnosis is essential in order to be accepted into the loving and supportive arms of some of the groups... not just a clinical diagnosis based on their symptoms, but a genetic diagnosis based on a genetic mutation in the DNA, which will have letters and numbers.

Without the genetic code they discover that although they have the same symptoms as the others, they do not belong. So, someone who is already desperate and as far down as anyone can go emotionally, psychologically, socially, financially, and physically will then be ostracized again and be left to fend for themselves. This is based on my own story and the story of others who come to our website where they do find help and support regardless of a diagnosis.

I lived through this experience. After being clinically diagnosed and as I waited for over a year for my DNA results, after sending my blood out of the country, I wrote the following essay. While I believe a genetic diagnosis would be nice, I know that nearly half of all the individuals who suffer daily from this cruel metabolic disorder do not have a known mutation, which has been discovered yet and I believe it is important that everyone sending their blood for research and a diagnosis needs to know that.

Everyone who finds the Periodic Paralysis boards and websites (except ours) on the Internet is encouraged to send a sample of their blood to be studied in research genetic testing. They go through quite a bit of trouble to find someone to draw the blood and must pay for it out of their own pocket because insurance will seldom pay for it. Then they have specific packaging and mailing requirements to follow. Although they say it is free for the study once the blood gets there, it cost me nearly two hundred dollars to just get it there. (Most of us do not have that kind of money so many cannot do it.) After waiting for over a year, one day half of the individuals or less will they get their "rejection" letter.

They become depressed and assume that they do not have Periodic Paralysis and feel shame for even believing they may have it. However, the letter simply says that they did not find any of the "known" mutations in their DNA. (Remember only about fifty percent of them will have a known mutation because the remainder of them have not yet been discovered) But, their family members, friends and their doctors become skeptical, as do the people on the support boards. They find themselves at "square one" and become even more ill over the stress and are ready to give up.

Some of these desperate individuals may end up dead from not being able to get proper treatment and others from committing suicide for not being believed and falling into despair.

"THE RED BADGE OF COURAGE"

Day after day people with Periodic Paralysis contact me on the Periodic Paralysis Network. Most every story is the same. Each one has periods of paralysis due to potassium shifting. They are very ill with varying degrees of gradual, permanent muscle weakness and problems breathing. They have had the symptoms as long as they can remember but they are unable to get a clinical diagnosis due to the attitudes and lack of proper education of their doctors. These people are unable to get the medical help they need and are seeking support and information. Most have broken spirits and have lost everything including careers, family and friends.

There is another group who contacts me. These people also have periods of paralysis due to potassium shifting. They are very ill with varying degrees of permanent muscle weakness and problems breathing. They have had the symptoms as long as they can remember but they have a clinical diagnosis. This means they are diagnosed based on their symptoms; however, they have not been diagnosed genetically. The genetic mutation, the basis for their symptoms, has not been found yet.

These people are either unable to join some of the Periodic Paralysis boards, listservs or social groups on the Internet, or if they are allowed to join, they are treated rudely or ignored. This is done by the other members and by the doctors who "lurk" on these boards.

It seems that if one does not have an identified genetic

mutation, he or she does not "really" have Periodic Paralysis. His or her periodic paralysis episodes and potassium shifting, and other symptoms and suffering are somehow not as equal as those who have a genetic marker.

Men and women without genetic markers are just as ill, if not more ill because they have gone untreated for many years and need treatment just as much as those that do have markers. Most of them are in dire need of support and help. That is why they join these boards.

What is happening to them is unconscionable. I know because I was one of them. On several occasions I desperately needed help. I asked specifically if one of the doctors could please answer my "life and death" questions about when to call 911 based on potassium levels and symptoms. I never heard back from any doctor and only a few members in my own situation responded. On other occasions members actually challenged me on issues or questions I asked. I sunk into deep despair after months of this, especially when I noticed that when the possibility of a doctor appearing on a TV show was discussed, a doctor was responding within a few minutes of the post, wanting information about it. Apparently, being on TV was more important than helping sick people.

It was clear that the people who were ill and needed help were not getting it nor were they going to on those boards. It was also clear that a divisive distinction was set up between the "haves" and the "have-nots". This is part of the reason we created the Period Paralysis Network.

One morning after hearing about a conversation on a Periodic Paralysis board, about the genetic markers, I became fed up. Apparently, a woman was unable to get a genetic diagnosis based on the fact that a doctor would not do it because he would be "stepping on the toes" of another genetic researcher and the basis of the decision was research money. Without the diagnosis, the woman was unable to get the medications and treatment she and other family members needed.

I wrote this following note to my friend who was still a member and being abused daily. Her genetic mutation has not been found yet although her blood had been sent to the genetic specialist four years before. She has yet to receive any notification from them.

> *"I want this madness to stop...so I am just going to make a small comment or two.... To all the doctors involved and the others with PP who wear their mutation numbers as a "badge of honor": bottom line...Who gives a flying f--k? We are all sick with varying degrees of periodic paralysis, some of us are dying...get over it doctors and forget the genetic mutation...*
>
> *TREAT US...we need help... Not all disorders or diseases need a genetic test before they are treated. Others wear their "badge of honor" while the rest of us must wear a scarlet letter...either, "H" for hypochondriac, "F" for faker, "M" for malingerer or "C" for conversion disorder. We also have another badge posted on our back that must say "KICK ME", especially when I am down. But what most of us has to wear is a RED BADGE OF COURAGE to face the message boards, doctors and our families everyday... Please stop this madness....*
> *You may quote me on this...*
>
> *Susan Q. Knittle-Hunter"*

Aleksandr's Struggle

An example of what can happen when an individual is seeking desperately to get answers and a diagnosis in order to erase the doctors' claims of mental illness; is trying to save his job, attempting to get proof for his family and hopefully a diagnosis for appropriate treatment and is then encouraged to send his blood to another country and then must wait for too many months or years is as follows.

Aleksandr Batutenko (Sasha) was a young man who suffered greatly with the effects of Periodic Paralysis. He lived in the Ukraine. He had a wife Nadezhda, and two children. The following was written by Aleksandr's wife, Nadezhda using some of Aleksandr's own words pulled from his journal. It has been translated.

> *"This article is dedicated to the memory of Aleksandr Batutenko, a person who was not afraid to tell others about his rare disease.*
>
> *The rarer the disease of the patient is, especially of the ones who live in this country (Ukraine), the less possibility there is that it will be diagnosed correctly, despite the fact that some of such diseases not only worsen the quality of life but also lead to death. They can be hereditary. Just imagine the situation: the doctors one by one consider the disease to be a mental disorder, although the patient is totally of sound mind. Unfortunately, in most cases such patients become unsociable and avoid speaking about their disease even with those closest to them.*
>
> *This article is dedicated to the memory of a person who was not afraid to search for people with the same problem and to raise questions about his ailment in the general public. It did not save him, though. Aleksandr Batutenko has died in the beginning of December. He has left two children. His brother and sister also have children. And all of them might have the same horrid fate if at long last Ukrainian neurologists do not learn about the disease.*

We had known each other since we were 14 years old, – says his wife Nadezhda Kalinichenko. – I came to Lebediw from the Russian Federation together with my parents; spoke a lot with a subtenant who lived in his flat. Sasha was a musician; he was always entertaining his friends. That is how we had met. He played almost all instruments: the accordion, the piano, the violin, and the pipe. The rock group "Edelfeis" created by him and his friends was famous both within the region and beyond it. Later its participants grew up and their field of interests changed. Sasha worked as a carpenter. He did any carpenter work assigned to him. Sometimes he worked as a tree feller, although this job is connected with big physical loads, sang in the church choir. We got married in 2004. We were regular visitors of Nikolaevskii Church. Later on when Pokrovskii Church was restored, we started to go there. Before I married Sasha I knew that he was seriously ill and nobody knew what he suffered from.

Once every nine months he had a paralytic stroke. For three to four days he could not move but could speak and was mentally completely alert. He could breathe although sometimes he experienced difficulties with breathing as well. He had had such strokes since he was 13 years old; all in all he had more than 30 of them throughout his life. He was hospitalized for a few times during such strokes and examined but usual examinations did not help discover the reason for the strokes. Except from the stroke times everything was normal. That is why later he refused to be hospitalized. From one side, doctors did not know how to cure him, from the other it was easier to look after him at home. Doctors considered his disease as a mental one but we were sure that it was not correct. The strokes were very stable till 28 years. We knew what was going to happen almost hour-by-hour.

I think I started to get ill in the early childhood, long before the first paroxysm which happened when I was 13, - wrote Aleksandr in Internet searching for people with the same symptoms.

Once I noticed pain in the calves when I was learning to ride a bike. I was only 4 at that time. All of a sudden, I felt pain. The pain was in the muscles, which are used for biking. It kept increasing and, in an hour, or two the muscles were awfully seized with pain even when I was just trying to make a movement. It was unbearably painful to move even fingers. Due to incompetence and maybe unawareness my parents did not pay attention to what has happened and started to "treat" me with a blue lamp, an instrument that was an essential constituent of a medicine box in any family at that time. I was "warmed" like that for a day or two till the pain stopped itself...

After that time, I was afraid to bike for long and to confess to my parents that my hands and legs hurt me. Sometimes spines, cervical muscles, collar zone muscles, and clavicle muscles hurt too. But I did not feel the paresthesias or as they are also known "the feeling of pins and needles" in arms and legs unless I had a paroxysm.

In the summer in our country house after waking up I found out that I could not move any limbs and lift my head, although I felt them. It was a very terrifying feeling. As if muscle tonus has disappeared. My muscles did not obey me but at the same time I could feel everything: cold, pain, warmth, touches. Being terrified I called for help. I did it without any problems: the voice did not change. My parents were very upset about the incident and thought I was afraid of something. They kept telling this suggestion to all the doctors who had examined me. As a result, I have been suffering according to official diagnosis from psychiatric disorder instead of neurological disturbance. The doctors think I have hysteria, obsessive-compulsive personality disorder and none of them wants to change the diagnosis. Neurologist and psychiatrist asserted that the problem should disappear as I grew up. But it did not happen. The strokes were happening sometimes more often, sometimes rarer.

From 2005 till 2012 a psychiatrist officially saw me. But I stopped seeing him because I did not receive any qualified help or examination. True, he suggested making additional examination to confirm the diagnosis "schizophrenia", but I refused.

During complicated paralysis strokes my brother saved my life twice. He noticed at the 11th hour that my head was buried in the pillow, and I could not lift it independently to breathe freely. Sometimes my stomach stopped working and on the third day of paralysis I began vomiting. My lungs stopped working; I was suffocating because of slime that had accumulated in them. My family was helping me to cough up, pressing the chest with hands.

It is complicated to describe this state. The worst is the third day when the body is totally exhausted and dehydrated. Bedsores are burning so much that I cannot lie calmly even for a minute. The ones who are taking care of me cannot stand it for long because I keep asking to turn me over every minute. When the stroke is going away it, usually after three days, almost within an hour the ability to strain muscles of legs and arms returns at the same time and I can walk although with great difficulties. The whole body hurts so much as if it has been beaten and broken apart. But all of that appears not important because I am able to move again!

Each time Sasha was learning everything from the very beginning, - tells Natasha. – To walk, to move, to do some work. At the same time during the strokes, he did not lose sensitivity. He felt warmth, cold, touches and pain... We had children. Sasha loved them very much.

We did not stop trying to find out what his disease was. Finally in 2006 we knew the biggest part of his diagnosis. A famous neuropathologist from Sumy, Leonid Rostislavovich Betterlikh, examined him and managed to make the correct diagnosis. It turned out that Sasha had Hypokalemic Periodic Paralysis (paroxysmal myoplegia) or unifamilial paralysis. It is inheritable.

When I came back from the hospital I immediately started to ask in detail about my relatives, – wrote Aleksandr. – And for the first time in my life I knew that my mum had an aunt, born in 1933, who led an unsociable way of life. She did not let anyone near her and did not want to speak to anyone and she had "some problems with legs". She met with us unhappily but agreed to listen to us. As soon as she heard that I have had strokes from 13 years, – she us told about her problem.

She was also ill from 13 years old. Once she woke up in the morning and could not get up from the bed. She could not move anything at all. Their cow had just dropped a calf at that time and she wanted to see it very much. But she spent a month and a half in the bed trying to overcome gradually leaving weakness of her muscles. After the stroke she felt totally broken. The strokes kept

295

repeating usually in cold weather. Sometimes she could not even put on clothes or comb her hair. She was asking her family members to help her, but they thought that she was a little bit off her center.

When she was young, the disease caused her especially hard states. The weakness took usually around a month or even longer. She studied in the Western Ukraine. The doctors there made diagnosis "chorea". Later on the strokes continued when she started to work. She came back to our city in 1982 and local doctors arrived at a new diagnosis of "rheumatoid state". The paralysis strokes kept happening in Lebediw as well where she worked as a stock manager. She traveled with tourist vouchers to Odessa. There she started to feel somehow better. She was regaining strength. Now she has great troubles while walking. She suffers from heart problems (doctors call it "pre-heart failure"), gout in the legs and backbone.

Maybe the state of Aleksandr would get better with time too. But at that time each stroke could lead to death and was making life complicated:

The strokes prevented me from my favorite occupation. Because of the disease I am not able to drive, as I cannot be fully sure that there won't be any attacks while I am driving. I have only one day-off in a week and I have to spend it sitting, or sometimes even lying in the bed waiting muscle tonus to resolve.

It was hard to explain my state at work that is why the management made the conditions so that I would quit the job myself...

This is the reason why I was extremely motivated to find out how to prevent the strokes and ideally to cure them completely. The difficulty is in the following: Hypokalemic Periodic Paralysis (paroxysmal myoplegia) can be of three types. It depends on the quantity of potassium in the blood.

It was necessary to make analysis of blood exactly at the time of a stroke, - tells Nadezhda. But the treatment depended on these results. In normal state the results were absolutely normal. To prescribe medicine-containing potassium, if a person has it, can be a problem because too much can kill him. But Leonid Rostislawowich prescribed him one drug, which could be used in all forms of myoplegia. It helped him a lot. The next four years there were no paralysis strokes although sometimes he still felt bad.

All this time Sasha was trying to find people who had the same health problem. In order to make the disease known not only for single doctors but also for all neuropathologists it was necessary to prove that such cases are not unique in Ukraine. This would allow organizing seminars on official level, open specialized clinics. Both we with Sasha and his brother and sister have children, who might have the same problem in prepubescent years. It was important to find a way to make DNA test to identify the mutated gene and to determine if our children have it too. And if they had it to start their treatment to prevent the dangerous strokes.

In Ukraine, a country where only few people know about the disease, such tests are not made. But we managed to contact International Association of Periodic Paralysis and to register there. The registration in this association and the official diagnosis "myoplegia" made by a neuropathologist are necessary conditions for the DNA-test in Germany. German professor Frank Lemann-Horn does it free of charge. True, it takes a year...

The German doctor makes the analysis free of charge as a charity, – explained Aleksandr on the online forum. – It is worthless to expect or to demand that it would be done faster. The analysis is quite complicated. Till now the doctor has singled out 50 genetic mutations, which lead to periodic paralysis. It is known for sure that if your variant of mutations has been singled out before then you can expect your results within a year. But if you have a rare mutation, which has not been discovered yet, you might wait even longer. But it does not mean that the examination won't be carried out and you will be forgotten. The doctor himself is interested to find new unknown mutations. There was a case when the result took 9 years! But according to statistics 60-65% of Europeans receive their results within a year, some of them within three months...it is also worth mentioning that the mechanism of sending the serum from the territory of Russian Federation to Germany is not tuned. It is connected with the official prohibition to send out biological samples and blood components outside the country. The only way to send your DNA is to receive the permission from the Ministry of Health, and then to deliver it by the international courier. Serum as you may know cannot be sent in such a way, as it has to be delivered within 24 hours. DNA is more stable. That is why before sending it has to be singled out from the blood (from lymphocytes of peripheral blood). That is what I have done. Although Ukraine does not prohibit sending outside the country biomaterials and blood components, courier FedEx does not guarantee delivery within 24 hours. It took them 3 days to deliver my DNA to Ulm. After the sample arrives, secretary of doctor Lemann-Horn sends confirmation via e-mail.

We have sent the DNA around half a year ago, – tells Nadezhda. – We received confirmation of the delivery

298

and are still waiting for the result. Sasha felt that it should be done more quickly. During the last year we have met another famous neuropathologist in Sumy and although he has a private clinic, he got interested in Sasha's disease and examined him for free. We have agreed with him to do the necessary tests during the stroke. Sasha provoked it artificially, by not taking the medicine when the first sign of the stroke appeared. The stroke started on the first of December. It happened unusually, fast. Sasha was fully paralyzed within an hour. We took him to Sumy in the morning and did the necessary analysis. It had to be ready on Monday, on the 3rd of December. But when we came back home, his lungs started to stop working and he could not breathe independently. We took him to the hospital where he received oxygen. They tried to give him the usual medicine but the stomach was not working and everything was going back. And on Sunday he was gone...

But all the groups in social networks, which he has created, are active. They contain all the information about this disease, its symptoms, and procedures necessary for sending the DNA for testing and so on. He managed to find a few people who suffer from the same disease in Ukraine and in Russia. We hope that in the near future doctors will appear who will get interested in this disease, will visit the seminar of the American Association of people who suffer from Periodical Paralysis and will be their representative in Ukraine. It would allow not only to spread the information about Periodic Paralysis (paroxysmal myoplegia) among patients and doctors, its symptoms and treatment, but also to raise awareness about the disease on the official level.

And probably then people who are ashamed of their

"psychical" disease would receive correct diagnosis and treatment. All the more so as this disease disables people.

Aleksandr has created the group in Face book called "Hypokalemic Periodic Paralysis Net", in Vkontakte "Пароксизмальная Миоплегия или Periodic paralysis". The pages of these groups contain all the information collected about this disease."

Thank you Nadezhda for sharing with us.

Unfortunately, Aleksandr's struggle was much the same struggle those of us with Periodic Paralysis face, no matter where in this world we live, from the United States to the Netherlands, to Denmark, to Wales, to Australia and to the Ukraine.

Let us hope that we can all learn from his life and death. Especially, let us hope and believe that the medical professionals around the world will read about his struggles in life to be taken seriously, diagnosed in a timely manner and treated appropriately and vow that no one else will have to struggle as he did.

In his death may the doctors recognize the symptoms of Periodic Paralysis, diagnose it clinically in a timely manner and treat those of us with Periodic Paralysis appropriately both in body and mind. And let us also hope that his death may call attention to more research into treatment by doctors and a possible cure for Periodic Paralysis.

The Periodic Paralysis Network will be connecting with Aleksandr's Face Book group in order to share our information with the people of the Ukraine. Let us hope that we can all learn from his life and death. Especially, let us hope and believe that the medical professionals around the world will read about his struggles in life to be taken seriously, diagnosed in a timely manner and treated appropriately and vow that no one else will have to struggle as he. Let us hope that we can all learn from his life and death. Especially let us hope and believe that the medical professionals around the world will read about his struggles in life to be taken seriously, diagnosed in a timely manner and treated appropriately and vow that no one else will have to struggle as he did. Let us hope that we can all learn from his life and death, Especially, let us hope and believe that the medical professionals around the world read about his struggles in life to be taken seriously, diagnosed in a timely manner and treated appropriately and vow that no one else will have to struggle as he did.

The Truth for My Family Soon

I do not believe we need a genetic diagnosis to be recognized as having any of the forms of Periodic Paralysis, because we can and should be diagnosed clinically based on symptoms in a timely manner for proper treatment and management. However, knowing the genetic code is something we may still pursue due to the possibility of learning more about treatment and the possibility of a cure some day in the future.

That being said, I have just been accepted into a clinical genetic study at one of the leading colleges of medicine in the United States, through their human genetics program. It is specifically for people who have been clinically diagnosed with Andersen-Tawil Syndrome and later the genetic testing came back as negative for ATS. It is a study for my entire family. It is their plan to draw some of my blood to do full exome sequencing (clinical testing) and to rule out the known genes for Periodic Paralysis first. I understand there are 7 of them. I have had only the main three ruled out, in my prior research study, but there are apparently more rare genes, which have been discovered in the last year or two, they want to rule out before enrolling more of my family members. So, if nothing is found in my testing of the known genes, a few other family members will be added to the study. They will provide either blood or saliva for comparison looking for new mutations.

We may or may not have some answers soon about the genetic mutation affecting my family. However, I am not worried or concerned about the outcome for myself. I know I have Periodic Paralysis. My doctors know I have Periodic Paralysis. I have a clinical diagnosis. I am managing the symptoms. However, the one thing that I would like to see as an outcome would be to have a genetic code found for my family members who are working with doctors who will not give them a clinical diagnosis.

If anyone is interested in having full, clinical, exome sequencing genetic testing completed for themselves or family members, the testing can be ordered by your doctor and though expensive, many insurance companies will pay for it, especially if it is recommended for those of us without any treatment options.

Chapter Thirty-One
Emergency Room

"BE AFRAID, BE VERY AFRAID"
Introduction

This part of the book involves the emotional, psychological and social aspects of living with Periodic Paralysis. Due to the many feelings, I experience when I hear the words "emergency room", including but not limited to fear, pain, embarrassment, shame, disbelief, frustration, humiliation, anger and learned helplessness, I believe that this chapter about the emergency room very much belongs here. When an individual is in extreme distress physically and in need of emergency care, he or she should be able to receive quality medical care and be treated with respect. In the case of others and myself, who have various forms of Periodic Paralysis, that has not been the case.

On four different occasions in the emergency room and a few subsequent hospital stays, I have been mistreated, misdiagnosed, yelled at, laughed at, scoffed at, lied about, lied to, ignored, mis-understood, made to stay in pain from an IV, developed an infection from an IV, put on a catheter without needing it, called names, put through testing or procedures that caused arrhythmias including long QT interval heart beats, had information withheld, had information dismissed, important data was overlooked or ignored. Twice Calvin had to physically remove me before they killed me. After telling them not to do it, they gave me medications in an IV. The doctors and nurses did all this. The support staff, however, always treated me well.

My Experience With the ER

The following is difficult for me to write. Going through my medical records is stressful due to all the negative things written about me, the misdiagnoses, the unkindness I endured, the opportunities missed by the doctors to treat me appropriately, the horrible reactions to the medication I suffered and the fear I have been left with when I think about returning to the emergency room (ER). I have contemplated how I was going to write this and after much thought, I have decided to tell the experiences in as much detail as I can, so the reader can understand my frustration and fear. By sharing my experiences in this manner, I hope to help others avoid what happened to Calvin and me in the ER and hospital. After writing my experiences, I will outline a plan to help others avoid the pitfalls of the emergency room.

I found myself in the emergency room (ER) of my nearest hospital on four different occasions due to symptoms related to Periodic Paralysis. Three of those times I was taken by ambulance and the last time my husband drove me. Three times I was admitted for further observation. Each time I was released, I had no diagnosis or a misdiagnosis. Each time I was given medications that made me worse. Each time I was mistreated. My hospital records are filled with lies and misleading statements, misinformation and misdiagnosed conditions such as "pseudo" seizures. These have followed me since my first visit to the ER and continued to interfere with getting a diagnosis and proper treatment. It has been a life-threatening and continuing nightmare that could have been avoided if someone in the ER or the hospital had taken me, my husband and my symptoms seriously in the very beginning. Had this disease been caught earlier, I would not be as ill as I now am. I must presently be on oxygen 24 hours a day and my heart is seriously damaged.

My first ambulance ride and hospital stay were on September 30, 2008, as the result of heart palpitations (felt like it was beating out of my chest), tachycardia, arrhythmias and chest pain, early one morning. I was sitting at the computer when it began. I took a nitroglycerin tablet, but it didn't help so I took another one. The pain continued so I got up to walk to the bedroom to tell my husband. I could not walk and fell to the floor. I could not move. Calvin heard and then came to help. He called 911. They arrived in what felt like a very long time. We lived ten miles outside of town in the mountains. The EMTs placed me on a stretcher and wheeled me to the ambulance. They hooked me up to an IV and after checking all my vitals, asked me to sign a paper. I found I was unable to hold the pencil. After what seemed like another long period of time, we began the drive to the hospital.

Once at the hospital, I was doing a little better. I was hooked up to all the necessary machines and equipment and all types of tests were performed. After several hours, the doctor walked in and was about to send me on my way, when suddenly my heart went into tachycardia. He changed his mind and had me admitted. During my stay I was continually on an IV which hurt horribly, but they would not fix it (a few weeks later I got phlebitis in my arm due to the IV and twice ended up in the ER to get an antibiotic for it.), and given several medications including Tylenol, ativan, zophran, morphine and ambien. I had severe problems with being able to walk and was having tremors. After they gave me the morphine in my IV, I had an immediate reaction of sudden chest pain and palpitations and passed out. After one night and two days they discharged me, with an unknown diagnosis, but the suspicion that I had chest pains due to my acid reflux although the lab work indicated I had some type of event with my heart. I was given reglan, upon my discharge, a medication for the reflux. Once home I was doing better, but when I took the medication after dinner, I went into tardive dyskinesia, it lasted all evening and through the entire night.

What I know now, from the hospital records obtained recently, is that the labs indicated a possible heart attack or ischemia. Cardiac enzymes were elevated, and testing ruled out pulmonary embolism. The doctor had me admitted to rule out an ischemic cardiac event. Ischemia is an absolute or relative shortage of the blood supply to an organ. It was not ruled out, but the cardiac event was obviously due to my Periodic Paralysis that we did not know I had at the time.

Had we known, I should not have been on an IV due to it causing paralysis to people with Periodic Paralysis. I should not have been given the other medications due to the side effects of them and the long QT interval problem. At the time we did not know what was wrong, but the effects at the hospital should have given them clues about what was going on. They were ignored or misinterpreted.

Unfortunately, the hospital recommended a coronary angiogram to be done after I left the hospital but neither my PCP nor cardiologist ever let me know about it. They both left town within a few months after that and it never happened. That could have been a turning point for me, and I could have received some help, however, I didn't know about it and the new doctors did not follow-up.

In July of 2009, my life changed forever. At that point I had just found a new doctor because my previous doctor had left town for a better position in another state. The first doctor I went to told me I was too sick and that he would not be my physician. I left out office crying my eyes out and went straight to the insurance company. They gave me the name of the doctor who was accepting new patients. I was able to get an appointment with him for the next morning. At first, he seemed like a caring doctor but was upset with the number of medications I was taking, as was I. I was on fifteen medications at the time. I was having ataxia, tremors, tachycardia, and palpitations and having trouble speaking. I told him I was very concerned over all the symptoms and asked if he would help me. He asked me to stop taking a few medications, which I did, and that I was to return to him in the future.

However, on July 27, 2009, I had what appeared to be a seizure of some type. It was about the fourth time in the past 10 weeks, but by far, the very worst. I was unable to speak, walk or move in any way; I was totally paralyzed. I also had tremors and jerking in my muscles. These contractions throughout my body made it look like seizures. However, I was never unconscious. I knew everything that was happening. As before, I was wheeled to the ambulance and hooked up to an IV. My vitals were checked and one of the paramedics gave me some glucose by mouth. He told me I was hypoglycemic. I was lucky I did not choke on the honey-like substance. My heart rate was over 160 and I was given ativan. We finally left the driveway and headed to the hospital. Within a few minutes, my body was jerking worse, especially my legs and feet. They were beating against the back door of the ambulance.

By the time I got to the hospital, I was worse than when the ambulance arrived at my home. I assumed it was due to the glucose. I do not remember arriving at the hospital or what followed until I woke up while Calvin was arguing with the doctors. They told my husband I was having seizures, but that they did not take care of seizures at the hospital and in the ER. They made my husband take me home with twelve tablets of ativan. Records show I did appear "ataxic" and "spastic" during some of my motor exams and the one of the doctors gave his reassurance that, "Sometimes it takes years to make diagnoses, especially when they are difficult and the symptoms presented are so varied, such as in this case".

For the next two days, I remained in this state. I was in and out of consciousness. I was getting worse and unable to function. Calvin, being concerned, called my new doctor and asked if there was any way I could be admitted to the hospital because he could not feed me or take care of me. After a few phone calls and my counselor/therapist getting involved, an ambulance arrived and took me back to the hospital. I do not remember much about that trip. I was admitted. The doctor was very angry and treated me horribly and wrote blatant lies in the records. I could relate all the lies and distortions but have decided not to do so. Since that time, we know that all the medications I was on and the ones the new doctor gave me and the ones from the hospital including the IVs, caused most of the symptoms. These symptoms combined with episodes of paralysis caused symptoms that they just did not understand. But being told to my face that he was referring me to a psychiatrist and that I was "making it all up" was horrifying and frightening when I was so ill.

I was sent home after a day. I spent the next several weeks in bed unable to do anything for myself. During that time, I found another doctor who put me on new medications without trying to discover what was wrong. The medications made me worse. Calvin asked his sister who was living in another state to please come and help with my care. I spent months recuperating and actually never have fully recovered.

At this point we realized we had to find another doctor. I could not find another M.D. and had to settle for another nurse practitioner. She was very helpful and was glad to take me as a patient. By now, we begin to realize that the medications were creating terrible symptoms for me. I got off them as quickly as I could. We realized that almost all the symptoms of ataxia, tremors and problems with my speech had been related to medications. I stopped taking every medication I was on. Most of the ataxia, and tremors, etc. stopped. Then, I began to have episodes of total paralysis. During them, I was unable to talk, open my eyes or move. I sometimes had chest pain, tachycardia and palpitations with them. They were frightening and we believed them to be related to my heart.

Emergency Room

On the evening of February 19, 2010, I went into a serious episode. I was having trouble breathing during it for the first time. When I could speak, I asked Calvin to call an ambulance. They arrived as before and put me on an IV. At the hospital, I was hooked up to the machines and the testing began anew. It was noted that I spoke in a "slow and low voice with flat affect" (my mouth was paralyzed), and that I had "weakness in my lower extremities". My oxygen was at 96% saturation and my heart rate was 116 with a blood pressure of 147/58. They did admit me for observation.

Once admitted, I lay in the bed going in and out of paralysis, each one lasting between about thirty minutes to an hour. I know because all I could do was lay there and look at the clock when I was able to open my eyes as each episode eased up. During that time, the nurse looked in occasionally and told me that the doctor would be there soon. It was at least 3 hours from the first time she told me, that a doctor finally came to examine me. He wrote, "initially, she is conversant but then she goes into an episode of being unresponsive and some mild shaking. It looks in my experience to be a 'pseudo' seizure." He told me that and told me he was going to treat me with ativan. Calvin told him not to do it. After he left, it was administered in my IV. Within a few minutes, I was very nauseous. The nurse brought me something for the nausea. I then threw up and the next thing I remember was waking up about 10 hours later in the morning.

I had no idea where I was. I thought they had moved me to another room. I tried to send my husband an email. When he got it he knew something was seriously wrong. I could not write or spell. He came and took me home before they could give me any more medication. He was afraid they would kill me if that were to happen again. The hospital records say that I, "responded well to the medication", that I was being discharged in "stable and significantly better medical condition after taking the ativan" which, "completely relieved my symptomology suggestive that his diagnosis of 'psuedo' seizures was correct".

This was an absolute lie. The medication knocked me out and when I regained consciousness, I could not talk or walk or do much of anything for myself. I was in and out of the paralysis again. I was able to send an email with a few words and a phone call to me from Calvin confirmed his worst fears. I was slurring my words and not making any sense to him. He came right away. He had to dress me and lift me into a wheelchair. He took me out of the hospital with no discharge plan. The record states that both my husband and I were "agreeable to the discharge plan". This "plan" lasted thirty minutes. This is ridiculous because there was no discharge plan.

That was the last time we dared to call an ambulance or go to the hospital no matter how sick I got for two years. There were several times when I should have been there, but we were very afraid of what they would do and how they would treat us. Two times we know now, after obtaining copies of the labs, I was in metabolic acidosis and really needed to be seen in the ER. I nearly died both times.

I did end up in the ER one last time in April of 2012. I was having serious problems with my blood pressure, arrhythmias, breathing and continually slipping into paralysis without any warning. At that time, Calvin called an ambulance. We were prepared with my emergency list and my medical records and Calvin had them transport me to the hospital that was about an hour away, rather than the one ten minutes away after our past experiences.

The paramedics did not use an IV. They just monitored me on the trip. However, the ER and hospital stay had some problems despite being prepared. Once at the hospital and in the ER, the doctor wanted to put me on an IV. I was able to tell them "No" and promised to drink lots of water if they brought it. I was put on a catheter, though I did not need it. It began to leak so I lay in wet sheets for many hours before another doctor insisted it be taken out due to my problems with recurring bladder infections.

It was decided that I should be admitted for observation when they discovered some problems with my labs and my other issues did not seem to go away. As the doctors and nurses came and went, shift after shift, I had to explain why I could not have an IV or take their medications. During the first night, I began to have a severe episode with my blood pressure going up, chest pain, heart arrhythmias, choking, and in and out of paralysis. The staff ran in and wanted to give me a pain pill. I told them "No." The head nurse came in and yelled at me. He said, "You are the first person to ever refuse a pain medication. What do you want us to do?" I told him through clenched teeth and paralyzed lips, "I am here to be observed so observe me and write down what you see for the doctor." He left the room in a huff.

The next day I was told I needed to have a stress test on my heart. I fought and fought with them, and finally gave in but I told them what to expect. They scoffed at me but were shocked when I went into paralysis and stopped breathing during it. They were afraid to give me the medication to bring me out of it. They knew at that point they had made a mistake and did not want to make it worse. The test indicated, and the doctor told me, that I would probably "drop dead" from an arrhythmia. Then he proceeded to tell me that I needed to have another test using dyes to look for a pulmonary embolism. I told him that the dye would cause me to have an arrhythmia and therefore it could kill me.

Calvin and I decided at that point, that I just needed to go home before they killed me. I would just have to take my chances with an embolism. To this day, I have not had any problems that would lead us to believe I have an embolism. I doubt that in the future I will go to another hospital. It is too frightening.

Calvin and I have moved to another state since my last experience in a hospital. In this new place I have prepared ahead, just in case I need to go in an emergency situation. I have spoken with the fire chief, and I have sent my records to the local hospital. I can only hope that things will be different here in an emergency, but I really doubt it and fear for the day I may end up in another ambulance and emergency room.

No one should be so afraid to go to the hospital. No one should be afraid of doctors. No one should have to take their chances of staying home and hoping they will not die because they fear what the doctors will do to them. No one should fear going to the hospital because they will be given medications they should not have. No one should fear going to the hospital because they will be told they are mentally ill. No one should fear going to the hospital because they will be scoffed at. No one should fear going to the hospital because the doctors will not believe him or her. No one should be afraid to go to the hospital for fear the doctors will lie about him or her.

I know of many others who have Periodic Paralysis and are diagnosed and others who are not diagnosed, who have had similar experiences to mine. This is happening all over the world. They, like me, live in fear of ending up in the ER. This is just not acceptable. ER doctors need to be able to recognize and know how to treat Periodic Paralysis correctly. It is my hope that this book will finally shed some light on this rare syndrome for the doctors of the world.

Chapter Thirty-Two
Doctors

"THE LOOK AND THE SHRUG"
Introduction

It is very sad that the chapter about Periodic Paralysis and doctors and other medical professionals in this book must be placed in this section in a negative way. I have been horribly mistreated and abused in ways that affected me physically, emotionally, psychologically and socially by the very people in our society who are supposed to be healers and supposed to care for us. When I think about the Hippocratic Oath a doctor must take as he begins to practice medicine, I find it difficult to believe that the majority of the doctors I have dealt with over most of my life actually took the oath and understand what it means. I know that they take an oath promising to have 'warmth, sympathy and understanding' for those they care for and that they also promise to do 'no harm' to their patients. Many have failed miserably in dealing with others and me with Periodic Paralysis. My account of how I was treated by the doctors over the past eight years needs to be told.

Thank You

However, I would like to begin this chapter by thanking the three fantastic doctors who were instrumental in diagnosing my Periodic Paralysis and Andersen-Tawil Syndrome Type 2: Dr M. my neurologist, Dr. P. my electrocardiologist and Dr. S. my nephrologist specialist. They are three professional, intelligent doctors, with integrity, who care about their patients and who went the extra mile to study everything they could about Periodic Paralysis: Andersen-Tawil Syndrome (ATS) in order to correctly diagnose me. I will forever be grateful to them for helping me. The story of how I found them and how they diagnosed me follows.

About four years ago I began to have periods of total paralysis. That followed many years of partial paralysis that had been misdiagnosed as Multiple Sclerosis. The episodes got worse and began to happen more often. One morning, while working wither my computer, I typed in the words "periods of paralysis". Suddenly on the screen appeared the words, "Do You Have Periodic Paralysis (PP)?" As I began to read, I started crying realizing I had found the answer I had been looking for over the years. I found there were communication boards where people with this disease discussed it with each other. I joined the boards and read everything I could about PP.

One day, I discussed my symptoms with someone on one of the boards and she told me to check Andersen-Tawil Syndrome (ATS). It is one of the rarest forms of periodic paralysis and she thought my symptoms fit ATS the best. I was shocked when I saw the symptoms and characteristics of the syndrome. I realized that the other members of my family, who had similar problems, and I must have Andersen Tawil-Syndrome.

I copied as much information as I could about Periodic Paralysis and Andersen-Tawil Syndrome and gave it to my nurse practitioner (I did not have a medical doctor at the time as I could not find one who would take me.) It was obvious that as much as she wanted to help me, she was very skeptical about this diagnosis. I recognized the "blank look" with glazed eyes, the "shoulder shrug" and the "I don't know about this." comment. I had seen it many times before by doctors.

She had been very helpful previously, during the year that I had been with her. She did refer me to several doctors and to the state's only health and research university hospital. However, all tests and exams had led to no diagnosis. I had now hit a brick wall.

One evening I was in despair over my failure to find a doctor who knew about Periodic Paralysis. Then on the evening news, I saw the weekly feature of offering direct calls to doctors with any medical question. I quickly picked up the phone. After a wait of only a few minutes, I was speaking with one of the physicians. I asked her if she had heard of PP or knew of any doctors who might know about it. As luck would have it, she herself had a patient with it. She gave me the name of the neurologist the patient sees.

I went to my PCP with this information and talked her into giving me yet another referral. Dr. M., the neurologist eventually diagnosed me with "probable" Periodic Paralysis by the second visit after ruling everything else out. He wrote a letter telling my PCP that I needed to see an electrocardiologist right away. It was several months before I got the referral, but I finally got an appointment. Once again, a reluctant medical provider who was afraid to make referrals due to the hostile response of the insurance company stalled the referral process.

I did not know which cardiologist to see, so left that up to my PCP. I got very lucky. By the time I saw Dr. P., I was armed with as much information as possible about Andersen-Tawil Syndrome. I knew he was the doctor who would understand what my rare long QT interval heartbeat, combined with my probable Periodic Paralysis diagnosis meant. I may have Andersen-Tawil Syndrome. I presented him with all of the information I had. He was very excited about the possibility of diagnosing me and wanted to learn everything he could about it in order to help me.

He described my heart condition, by that point, as serious with no treatment, but insisted I needed to have a heart monitor implanted. He also set up a renal specialist to help diagnose, what he believed by that point to be, Andersen-Tawil Syndrome, based on all the information being presented to him by me, my PCP and the neurologist and his own research on the Internet. This information about PP and ATS was passed on to the kidney specialist.

I did get the diagnosis of Periodic Paralysis: Andersen-Tawil Syndrome while in the hospital for the implant after going into paralysis and being observed by the doctors. Dr S. told me how humbled he felt to be diagnosing me. He said he was just an ordinary MD (nephrologist), not like the big and powerful doctors who wrote all the information on PP and ATS back East. But after seeing what happened and going over all the facts and by the process of elimination and studying all the latest research, I had presented to them and the family flowchart I had put together with all the family medical history, he felt he had no other choice. He told me I had done all the work and had done an excellent job of presenting it all to them. Without that, I might never have got the ATS diagnosis also. He had never heard of ATS before, none of them had, but they had been researching and studying it.

I was lucky to find doctors who went the extra measures to help me as they did. They are actually unusual. They were willing to accept the information I presented to them. They were willing to study it and research it. They remained open minded and willing to learn. Their egos did not get in the way of helping their patient. They are to be commended. They are to be admired and other doctors seeing patients with PP or possible PP should be willing to follow in their footsteps.

My History and Experiences with Doctors.
An Unfortunate but Typical Account for Many People
with Periodic Paralysis.

This Needs to Stop!

During the six years between our move from the mountains in another state and my diagnosis, I had seen 34 medical professionals. The following are the statistics regarding the care I received. Seven left me; they moved away or quit practicing. One refused to see me after the first visit. He said I was "too sick". Thirteen doctors insulted me and treated me poorly, misdiagnosed me and mistreated me or otherwise disregarded me as hysterical, conversion disorder or faking it, said I had pseudo-seizures, was "too old" to diagnose and difficult to deal with, shrugged their shoulders and gave me blank stares and sent me on my way with medications that made me sicker, gave me new symptoms and/or almost killed me. I fired four of them. (These doctors do not include the ones I saw during four emergency room visits with symptoms and misdiagnosis and mistreatment and three hospitalizations with symptoms and misdiagnosis and mistreatment.)

The remainder of the doctors did try to help me in the medical areas for which I saw them. I had to see a podiatrist, an endocrinologist, a gynecologist, a surgeon, two urologists, a physical therapist, a neurosurgeon, an EMG specialist, a pulmonologist, three cardiologists, a rheumatologist, a dermatologist, and a counselor. Some were to rule out other conditions and some treated my many other medical issues. I saw a counselor to help me deal with my failing health and I needed physical therapy to help me with my balance and weak muscles. Some doctors monitored my normal yearly tests, like pap smears. One took care of my foot problems that included, a neuroma, an extra bone in my foot and a stress fracture. Another was treating the severe osteoporosis in my spine and hips. A surgeon discovered my hiatal hernia and treated my acid reflux. Two urologists tested for interstitial cystitis and treated it. A sleep study and breathing tests were done.

Most of those medical professionals did a fine job of taking care of the other issues I had to deal with.

However, the most difficult part of this, for me, is knowing that I may not have become as seriously ill as I am, if the doctors I saw for my Period Paralysis issues in the prior six years and the many years before, would have taken me seriously. Many I saw, pretended to be reading my records and then gave us the blank stare with glazed over eyes as they shrugged their shoulders. They would tell us what it was not, but they could not tell us what it was. Then we were dismissed and told we did not need to return.

The List Outlining the Doctors and My Experiences with Them Over the Past 6 Years.

My Doctors: March 2005 to February 2011

*=Left the area.
#=I fired them.
+=Helped me.
%=Treated me with neglect or rudely.

❖ *T L: Nurse Practitioner…quit after a few months.

❖ % Dr. C…Neurologist…one visit…said nothing wrong

❖ #R M: Nurse Practitioner said I had MS. He dared me to go to a major medical center 250 miles away. He was angry I was looking for a "Zebra". Very angry every time I got symptoms from the meds; he gave me. He would throw his pencil and spoke rudely to me.

❖ +Dr. C…Podiatrist found extra bone in foot and took care of my broken foot.

❖ "%Dr. D…Rheumatologist diagnosed fibromyalgia. Put me on mirapex. He yelled at he, pulled leg really hard and insisted "nothing else was wrong."

❖ *+Dr. S…Neurologist did not think anything wrong but suggested I be seen at a major medical center. R M did not tell me. I found it in the records years later.

❖ *+Dr S…Cardiologist ran tests. He told me I had a small heart and other heart problems. He left shortly after that.

❖ +L N…Cardiologist Assistant took over. She suggested I get a heart ablation.

❖ +Dr. Y…Dermatologist diagnosed Rosacea.

❖ +Dr C…Gynecologist found Osteoporosis.

❖ *+Dr H…Endocrinologist put me on an experimental medication I had to inject in my thigh daily called forteo. Ran a series of tests all test normal. He moved away.

❖ +Dr. L…Surgeon diagnosed hiatal hernia and acid reflux.

❖ +R…Physical therapist.

❖ *+Dr. D M…She really tried to help me. Sent me for more testing at the major medical center 250 miles away. Put me on many medications. She left before I got the results of MRI. So, I did not get the results for another year.

❖ +R W…Counselor to help me with my health decline and to deal with my mother's impending death. Wrote me a letter for the doctors saying, "no conversion disorder".

❖ +Dr. R W…Neurologist major medical center 250 miles away. Said I did not have MS. She ordered an MRI. Got back with me 1 year later about MRI results, small vessel ischemia of the brain.

❖ +Dr. G…Urologist diagnosed interstitial cystitis

❖ + Dr. M…Urologist did several tests including kidney x-ray. I went into paralysis. He wanted to do a procedure-using anesthesia, so we had to decline.

❖ *%Dr. H…MD refused to take me as a patient…said I was "too sick"

❖ #%Dr. S…MD… Had huge seizure-like episode. Treated me horribly. Lied about me in hospital record. Accused me of being suicidal due to assistive directive, being a drug addict, faking. He took my medications away and gave me other more serious medications that caused seizures. I fired him.

❖ #%Dr. T…MD…did not care or try to find out what was wrong. Gave me anti-psychotic meds to help me sleep. I got sicker and weaker and had more seizure- like episodes. I fired her.

❖ %Dr. S…Neurologist was tainted by Dr T. He said I did not have MS and was not having seizures. He provided no help or ideas, but he referred me to a neurosurgeon due to a problem in my neck.

❖ +Dr. A…Neurosurgeon so concerned said I needed to be seen at the major medical center 250 miles away. He could not operate on neck. It would paralyze me. Said to not see any more neurologists in the southern region of the state.

❖ #%L PJ…Nurse Practitioner Seemed to care in beginning. Realized all meds were causing symptoms of ataxia, tremors, tardive dyskinesia, and seizure-like activity, etc. Tried to help, then began to stall, not help, would not follow through, etc. Referrals were hard to get and there were problems with office help. She did not recognize nor act upon important lab information. She walked out when I was in paralysis and I needed her. She did not take us seriously. She almost killed me by not recognizing serious symptoms of my heart and breathing.

❖ %Dr. G...EMG accused me of faking, although discrepancies showed up on testing.

❖ *+Dr. E...A young neurologist at the major medical center 250 miles away, did testing and said, "I do not know what it is maybe we can name it after you". He left before he could give me results of all testing.

❖ %Dr. C...Neurologist at major medical center 250 miles away. Did testing and said, "I do not know what it is maybe we can name it after you." He did muscle biopsy. He did not notice me in paralysis.

❖ %Dr. L... Neurologist at major medical center 250 miles away, did not give me the results of the testing done. After driving 250 miles he told me the biopsy was normal and that I had no neuromuscular diseases or mitochondrial diseases although changes in shape and size of muscle fibers did show on the biopsy. When I questioned it he said we should go have fun while we were in Portland. I told him, "If I could have fun I would not be sitting in his office" and reminded him of the periods of paralysis. He sent us on our way with nothing further to say. Later found out he is in charge of Periodic Paralysis for MDA and that there were other results and a diagnosis for Periodic Paralysis, but he did not tell me.

❖ %Dr. M...Cardiologist and none of my records were there. LPJ had not sent them. He said nothing wrong but did order 24-hour urine catch. It came back normal. He never asked to see my records.

❖ #%Dr. A...A neurologist for MDA. Got a referral after talking to others on message boards that said MDA doctors are able to diagnose and treat PP. Started by telling me I was too old to be asking if I had PP and told me he would not diagnose unless potassium levels were below 3.5 during an episode. When I had test done it was ½ hour too late and showed a problem with creatinine levels, potassium was 3.8; he did not bother to call for 8 days, though he knew the results within 2 hours. Someone in his office called and said results were "unremarkable". We had tried to explain that potassium did not have to shift below normal to prove PP. His info was old. After being treated so poorly, I decided not to return to him. He had too much ego to listen to the most current info on diagnosing PP. He did not care enough to get back with me although the lab was very concerned about creatine levels. He did not care to see all the records I brought to the appointment.

❖ +Dr. R S...Internist I called when on television news. Asked if she knew any doctors who knew about Periodic Paralysis. She told me about Dr. M.

❖ +Dr. M...Neurologist. He took me seriously, believed me and ran a few last tests then gave diagnosis of "Probable Periodic Paralysis". He said I needed to see
❖ an electrocardiologist due to long QT on the Holter Monitor.

❖ +Dr. P...Electro cardiologist. He believed it to be Periodic Paralysis, possibly Andersen-Tawil Syndrome, due to the long QT interval heartbeat, and other symptoms. He said I need a heart loop monitor implanted. He called in a team (Renal Specialist and

Intensivist) to help diagnose me in the hospital while there for heart procedure. (As of 05/19/11...told me he can do no more for me. Does not need to see me again. He will refer me to any ATS Clinic in the country.)

❖ +Dr. S...Renal Specialist...diagnosed "Periodic Paralysis with Long QT. Probably a type of Andersen-Tawil Syndrome". (No other type of Periodic Paralysis has long QT except Andersen-Tawil Syndrome.) This was after seeing me in an episode for over 40 minutes with tachycardia sustained above 140 and with long QT arrhythmias and with my past history, all else ruled out and a family history of all the above and my own characteristics and that of my family.

❖ *+Dr. T...PCP Left the area after a short time.

❖ *+Dr. W...PCP Left the area after a short time. Ordered my wheelchair.

❖ %Dr. R...Neurologist ATS Specialist at a major medical center in another state. He told Calvin and me several things and then wrote opposite things in the report to the referring doctor. Believed PP to be a neuromuscular disease. Because I had other coexisting conditions, he was unsure that I had ATS.

❖ +Dr. O...PCP was a wonderful internist in a great clinic.

❖ %Dr. B...Endocrinologist could not get me out of his office fast enough. Did not want to help me with lactic acidosis

Conclusion

No one who is so ill should have to see thirty-four doctors within six years and be treated so poorly when they are already afraid about what is happening to them and seeking help, a diagnosis and proper treatment. During those six years, I received cruel and unusual treatment. I was mistreated, misdiagnosed, yelled at, laughed at, scoffed at, lied about, lied to, ignored, mis-understood, had information withheld, had information dismissed, important data was overlooked, had things thrown around the room at in front of me out of anger, had my leg pulled at with great force almost pulling me off of a chair, refused to treat me because I was "too ill", accused me of being suicidal because I had an assistive directive, called a "drug addict" and a "faker", ignored while in paralysis, called "too old" and dumped by a doctor because I had Periodic Paralysis and he did not want to deal with me and dismissed by a doctor before he even examined me because I had Periodic Paralysis.

These experiences, during and after the visits to the many doctors and medical professionals were unbelievable and overwhelming and left me with feelings of fear, pain, sorrow, embarrassment, shame, disbelief, frustration, humiliation, anger, despair, self-doubt and learned helplessness. The stress and anxiety were overpowering at times and increased my symptoms. It was a vicious cycle.

One of my favorite doctors, who had to move on in her career after only a short time of treating me, suggested I see a therapist and I am deeply grateful for that suggestion. She believed in a holistic approach, that is treating all aspects of a person. She recognized that I was stressed over my declining health, the uncertainty and the experiences with my past doctors and the specialists I was seeing. I am forever thankful to her for sending me to a wonderful therapist.

My counselor, a licensed social worker, helped me through the past four years of hell. She believed me, believed in me, had faith in me and supported me through each doctor and their mistreatment and saw the consequences of their mistakes. She helped me by writing a letter for me to carry and share with each doctor and the ER explaining that I did not have a conversion disorder and that I was telling the truth about my symptoms. She helped to rebuild my self-confidence and faith in myself. She suggested that I write a book to teach others, especially the doctors, about Periodic Paralysis. This book is the result of her suggestion.

It is my hope that many of the doctors I have dealt with will recognize themselves here and possibly take some time to reflect on their behavior and make attempts to change how they deal with severely ill patients and patients for whom a diagnosis is not always clear. Perhaps they and other doctors will read this book, study all the aspects of Periodic Paralysis and be able to recognize, diagnose and treat it in a timely manner.

Chapter Thirty-Three

Caregivers

I am sixty-two years old and on February 2, 2011, I was diagnosed with Periodic Paralysis. I have had episodes of partial and total paralysis for many years. During the episodes, my potassium shifts are low (hypokalemia), high (hyperkalemia) and within the normal ranges (normokalemia). Due to several misdiagnoses and a lack of proper diagnosis and treatment for over 50 years, I have become totally and permanently disabled with weak muscles throughout my body including those involved with my vision, digestion, breathing and my heart. I must be on oxygen constantly and cannot exert myself in any way. The electrical workings of my heart are defective. I have had a heart loop monitor inserted in my chest to monitor the tachycardia and arrhythmias that includes long QT interval beats. I now spend my days in a recliner, unable to walk farther than across a room. I must use a motorized wheelchair for anything farther. If I did not have the help of my husband, Calvin, of thirty years, I would have to live in an assisted living program. He has become my caregiver.

Through the past years of my physical decline, I have had to give up my career as a special education teacher, my hobbies to include hiking, walking, swimming, exercising, fishing, camping, traveling, shopping, cooking and baking. We had to sell, and move away from, a beautiful home my husband and I built in the mountains of Utah. I had to move far away from my family in order to live in a better climate. I can no longer drive our car. I have lost many friends, because I could not keep up with them or entertain any longer. My husband has lost all of this also.

Calvin is disabled too, but not as severe as me. He does all the shopping, cooking, cleaning, yard work, paying the bills, maintains the house and car and the laundry. He also drives me to doctor appointments, and monitors my vitals to include my potassium levels, blood sugar levels, pH levels, oxygen levels, heart rate, blood pressure and body temperature. He does this to know when to give me potassium if my levels are too low or when try something else if my potassium levels are too high. He does his best to keep me warm and comfortable.

When I go into paralysis, he watches me very closely. I become totally paralyzed. I am unable to move in any way, I cannot speak, nor can I open my eyes. He monitors my vitals during an episode, potassium levels, blood sugar levels, pH levels, oxygen levels, heart rate, blood pressure and body temperature. And, he has to make sure that I am not choking, that my breathing is not too shallow or too fast or that it does not stop. And he has to monitor my heart because I may go into cardiac arrest, and he must be ready to do CPR while he calls 911. He has to make sure not to move me because damage can be done to my joints when I am in paralysis. But he has to make sure my neck and head are not kinked and in pain and carefully adjusts me as necessary. If my potassium levels get too high, he may need to call for an ambulance because that means I have gone into metabolic acidosis, a serious and potentially fatal condition.

As he does all of that he talks to me. He tells me the result of each test. He knows I can hear him and so he reassures me. These episodes may last from fifteen minutes to three or four hours. He is with me and monitors me through the entire episode. As the paralysis subsides, I am very weak and have difficulty speaking. I will usually have to suddenly urinate due to what is called the potassium "dumping". I need to get to the bathroom quickly. He will have to help me to my walker and push me to the bathroom and keep me from falling. Then, depending on the time of day, he will help me prepare for bed.

Calvin has researched every aspect of Periodic Paralysis and continues to do so every day. He has argued with doctors. He has fought with insurance companies. He has driven me 100s of miles to see specialist as I had episodes in the car all along the way. He fought to get oxygen for me, which saved my life. He researched insurance companies until he found one that does not require referrals. He explains everything he can about my disease to those who need to know. He handles all the billing issues. He is with me at every doctor appointment, asking questions and providing them the most recent information about PP and my vitals. He created charts to record every bit of information. He developed a diet for me and helps me to stick with it. He has helped me develop the Periodic Paralysis Network.

Calvin is my hero. I do not know how he does this day after day, week after week and month after month; soon to be year after year. He is an amazing man, and I am thankful to have him in my life. When I tell him how sad I am that things are as they are and apologize to him, he tells me not to apologize. He says, "You would do the same for me ". He is very humble about what he does.

I see it wearing on him at times and wish I could do something for him. I know it must be difficult watching me going through the episodes of paralysis. I know it must be difficult for him to see me so ill. I know it must be difficult for him to see me going downhill physically. I know it must be difficult facing the fact that I am probably dying right in front of his eyes. I know it must be difficult to know that the doctors feel they have done all they can do for me. I know it is difficult for him to fight to keep me alive.

I wish he could take a break from all he must do for me, but he never asks for one. I had hoped we could get respite care from the MDA, but that plan fell through, in an unfortunate set of circumstances. We have no close family. The nearest relative is two hundred fifty miles away. We have no close friends. We have too much income to qualify for respite services through the county or state. The home healthcare nursing services, through my insurance, does not offer respite care.

I realize most people with Periodic Paralysis will not end up as seriously ill and permanently disabled as me. They are lucky. However, I know of several people who live alone and deal with symptoms much like my own. They have no caregiver. It is frightening for them, and safety is an issue. I am not sure how they are able to deal with the issues we face. They need someone to help them. They need caregivers. I hope they will be able to get the help they need through their insurance or their local community. No one should have to go through this alone.

Calvin's Point of View

As difficult as it may seem the most important thing to remember is not to give up trying to locate needed help. When making inquiries over the telephone there might be ten disappointments and one success. The one success makes it worth the effort. Using a home computer connected to the Internet will greatly assist any search efforts. There are numerous federal, state, and local governmental organizations and agencies with the primary purpose of providing services to persons in need. Persistence will produce results in most cases. There are a number of private organizations that offer services to persons in need. In one of our Internet searches, we located a local provider of assistive technologies that was privately owned and operated. They relied on donations and allowed people with low incomes to borrow their equipment. The equipment was returned after the need had passed.

Many people will need to ask friends and relatives to help them in times of need. It is one of the most difficult things

Caregivers

Susan and I have had to do asking for help. We discovered early on that help or support from family was not available and we did not have many close friends. We have depended heavily on assistance from the government. Most people are glad to help if it does not cost them too much in terms of time or money.

There were several occasions when I felt the need to ask for help. It was a very difficult situation for me but even more difficult for Susan. I had to place Susan's needs above my own pride. I was not comfortable asking anyone for help, but I knew that Susan would experience unnecessary suffering if I could not move beyond my stubbornness. The two most memorable times that I reached out and asked for help were turning points for Susan. The one situation was calling Susan's counselor and the other situation involved me driving to the local oxygen supply company and having a very serious discussion with the manager. Both of these women listened to my plea for help and they both provided the help Susan needed to survive. They know who they are, and they will always have my heart-felt gratitude.

Some people might feel a need to join a support group. Some groups meet in person and other groups meet using Internet technology. It is a personal choice the level of involvement someone desires. Susan is a very social person, and I am a very private person. We both have our own comfort zones and respect and understand the other one's needs.

One of the very first people Susan came in contact with through our Periodic Paralysis Network and Facebook web sites is a woman named Kendra. As we learned more about her personal situation living with Periodic Paralysis, we became very amazed how this woman was coping practically alone with daily life filled with episodes of paralysis. We asked Kendra if we could publish a guide she prepared for caregivers. The following is that guide. Thank you, Kendra, for being there for us and being so brave. Kendra is one of the most thorough researchers we have ever encountered and has turned out to be one of Susan's good friends.

"If you find me in Paralysis: A Guide for Caregivers"
by Kendra

On March 18, 2011 (my birthday), I dictated the following guide to empower my caregivers. After 10 years of being frequently paralyzed, March 19 was first day that two caregivers realized I was paralyzed not just asleep. Since then, 3 of my caregivers have found me paralyzed at least 2-3 times each. So, between March 19 and April 20 (when stopped counting) about 7-9 times they found me paralyzed--of course I've been in paralysis many more times than that. We have been using this guide with success.

I've updated the info a few times as I learn more about interacting in that state. I created a copy of the list in Word software so can print certain word in boldface. (Fyi, lost all the bold when copied to this interface.) I printed out a copy of the list and taped it to my bedroom door, encouraging everyone to review it before entering. Hope this will give others a starting point.
~~~
As soon as anyone comes into house, I hear the kitchen door and immediately wake up.

If you enter my room and I do not immediately visibly wake and talk to you, you will know that I am NOT sleeping, I AM PARALYZED.

If you find me in paralysis:

1. Please do NOT call 911. The paralysis will eventually pass, although at times it may take over 4 hours.

2. When paralyzed, my senses and perception are extremely sensitive. Please offer quiet, gentle, patient energy. Please breathe, slow down, lower your voice, wait.
If at any specific time you do not feel able to be calm or do not have time to do the checklist with me, please do NOT come into my room.

3. Check green oxygen tube for water condensed in tubing. Disconnect green oxygen tube from clear nasal canella and dry the green tube. (Ask me or Shawn how.) If there is water in green tube near the connection to clear canella and you do NOT know how to dry it, just turn off the oxygen so that the water does not get forced into my nose.

4. If I am able to talk, please note that I often can only say one-syllable words and only pronounce certain easy sounds, basically only "mmm" (the primordial mmm of our first word, "mama").
* If I cannot talk or make any sound, use the list below to do a visual check of common things that you can help with.
If I am able to talk or make sound, ASK (it's like playing the game "20 questions" :-).
Ask one question at a time. Ask simple questions. Try this pattern if we have clarified it in preparation:

If I can only make mmm sound, give me options for response, ask "yes?"--if I make mmm sound, that means affirm. If no sound from me, that means not yes. Ask "no?"--same ...

5. "Are you thirsty?"
For water, use straw on stool next to bed.

Be sure that my head is turned at least partway to side in case I cannot swallow, so that water does not choke me. Note that I can only take one mouthful at a time for one swallow, and it takes a while for me to swallow.
Offer a second sip of water. Water usually helps me breathe and talk easier, and can often restore my voluntary breathing

6. "Is there pain I can help you with?" See checklist below.
* Are cats lying on my body? If so, move Chandra to foot of bed under covers and move Tor to my left into the cat nest on top of covers.
* Look at the position of my head on pillow: If head is pressing into pillow on side of face, very likely severe pain behind ear where oxygen tube presses and pain on right side of face. If you can, create a small hollow depression in pillow under ear to relieve pressure on face-ear.
If you can (if my paralysis is "floppy" not rigid), slowly, gently move my head, turn just 1 inch toward center. If I make sudden sound, stop and check with me that moving my head is good to do.
* Check position of two small arm-pillows. Position pillow's edge under palm to support wrist and forearm so that fingers "waterfall" over edge of pillow and there is nothing touching my fingertips.

7. "Are you cold?"
* Is my headband completely covering my forehead, especially right temple? If not, reposition to cover and partway cover eyes. (When right temple gets slight cold draft, it can trigger migraine.)
* Are my hands covered? If not, are they cold? If so, cover with small, red top quilt.
With truly boundless gratitude, ~Kendra~"

The Weight of Responsibility
by Calvin Hunter

Being responsible to care for another adult is like accepting the responsibility to care for a vulnerable child. The degree of responsibility depends on how incapable the other person is of performing daily routine tasks. Nothing short of parenting could prepare a person for this role. Susan always played the caregiver role in our relationship especially when it involved her children. She juggled the responsibilities of work and home in a seamless fashion. I do not believe most men understand what it means to be a caregiver until a caregiver role is forced upon them. It really is not in our DNA. We perform other complimentary roles.

Prior to Susan becoming unable to take care of her personal needs, I was always busy working outside the house or involved in some project. Shortly after Susan and I met, we purchased a piece of property in the nearby mountains and proceeded to build a cabin that took up most of our time over the next 20 years. I was good at doing things like that but lacked the skills or even desire to play a caregiver role.

It was not until Susan became incapable of caring for herself that I began to fully understand and appreciate how difficult and stressful it can be to focus 100% of one's attention on another person. It was the most difficult thing I had ever done in my life. I managed to survive the crash course thrown upon me and after several years in the role of caregiver it has become routine. Things might have been better if I had some outside help. Susan's doctors had misdiagnosed her condition for many years and were pumping her full of pharmaceutical drugs. Some of those drugs were addictive and complicated her condition. In addition to taking on the caregiver role, I began to research possible causes of her symptoms. When Susan felt well enough to use her personal computer with the assistance of the Internet, together, we unraveled the mysteries surrounding her life-threatening condition.

Making the decision to stop following her doctor's advice was a tremendous responsibility. The weight of having Susan's life in my hands was crushing at times. My sister Julie came to visit in the beginning and gave us some help for several weeks. Once I realized Susan's condition was not something that was going away in the near future, I began to develop the mental armor needed to survive the personal devastation we both experienced.

There were a couple of professional people involved in Susan's life who gave us the support we needed to get through the darkness. Susan's counselor was like an oasis in the desert and the phlebotomist we met along the way saw that we needed help and gave us that help without reserve. I know she was getting grief by her bosses for being so accommodating.

I have grown into the role, or the role has grown into me. Despite how this entire situation has wreaked havoc on my nervous system, playing this role has forced me to another level of adulthood and responsibility. Life suddenly has a side of seriousness that I was not aware existed before Susan became ill. Susan and I together learned how to manage the situation by eating properly, exercising as much as our medical conditions would allow and to avoid things that trigger episodes and cause us stress. I know what makes me happiest in life and know how important it is to have Susan here to share my life with.

I choose never to allow myself to feel self-pity and stayed away from asking questions like "why us?" I refuse to give up hope and will never succumb to the feelings of helplessness and hopelessness that oftentimes accompany chronic illness. I have gotten stubborn throughout this process and have gained a greater appreciation for our innate ability to understand the context of the individual events that make up the fabric and story of our lives. No matter how dire external events may appear to me, I refuse to give up hope, refuse to feel self-pity and refuse to stop looking for answers.

I believe in Susan's and my abilities to understand this disease and how to manage the symptoms. Together we are living in each and every moment. It has been a challenge for me but a greater challenge for Susan. Even though I have medical conditions of my own, I always remember that Susan's medical conditions are worse than mine. Together we remind each other about the other people we know with this disease who have no caregivers and live alone. The terror they must feel every time an episode of muscle paralysis falls upon them must be enormous. We did not choose this disease but how we meet the challenge is a choice. This is the life Susan and I have together, and we try to make the most out of every day and challenge. I would not trade my life for any other.

First Written Entries

Calvin writes: These are some of the first of many words I would write about my wife Susan and her struggles with Periodic Paralysis. My educational and work backgrounds in the fields of Mental Health, Special Education and Computer Science have given me the knowledge and skills needed to discover what was causing Susan to be so chronically ill. The creative side of my personality afforded me the ability to envision a disease process that was created by a train wreck of inherited and environmental circumstances. Over the past thirty years Susan was left at the mercy of medical professionals many of which diagnosed Susan with phantom conditions and wrote prescriptions that acted in combination as poisons to her system.

Throughout the entire process, I have been shocked by the high levels of incompetence demonstrated by many of Susan's medical practitioners, astounded by the insensitivity of medical insurance companies, and thoroughly disgusted by the lack of oversight of pharmaceutical labs by the Food and Drug Administration (FDA). I have lost all respect for organizations such as the Muscular Dystrophy Association (MDA) and all the medical facilities we have encountered.

Through all this living hell, we have met a handful of dedicated individuals who cared about what they were doing and cared about the people they were treating. Meeting these people during our darkest hours left us with a glimmer of hope that things would improve if we continued to search for answers to our questions about Susan's declining health. Sometimes just a little bit of hope was enough to get us to the next breakthrough which led to an increased ability to manage Susan's condition and improve the quality of her daily life. Only after all hope is lost will we stop looking for answers to difficult questions. I cannot envision that day ever arriving.

Susan and I have often joked about how she feels like a lab rat due to all the testing and probing she has encountered. We have lost count of the number of saliva, urine, and serum samples she has given over the past years. We have acquired many medical devices to collect samples and take measurements. We have kept a written daily record of samplings. Along the way, we have made many discoveries. Sometimes these discoveries came in a flash of insight and other times we had to work for the tiniest bit of new information. Throughout the process I have made many self-discoveries. My diet has changed radically. The stress of all of this was unbearable at times and my life was crushed many times as I watched Susan spiral into a paralytic episode without knowing at the time what was happening to her. She appeared to be in a coma at times.

It was during one of these paralytic episodes that we made one of the most important discoveries. We discovered that Susan was fully conscious and aware of her surroundings while appearing to be totally unconscious. Of course, her doctors at that time ignored this finding and continued along the lines of misdiagnosing her condition as psychological in origin rather than due to a chemical and electrical causes. The discovery that she was aware during the paralytic episodes marked the beginning of the journey of discovery, understanding, and now management of her disease.

Many nights I spent researching new findings and had moments of ecstatic discovery. Each door that opened led us to another door that was closed. We searched together until we found the key that opened the next door. We searched until we found competent medical professionals who took us, and their positions as healers, seriously. And now we want to share what we have learned.

I am by no means a medical professional and have not conducted traditional empirical research. I would hope that somewhere on the planet deep within the walls of some chemistry lab there is a young doctoral student who is looking for a worthy subject for a dissertation. This is new age medicine and holds the keys to modern medical diagnosis and treatment of a wide range of ailments plaguing humankind including Periodic Paralysis. I suspect there are millions of people who suffer from the effects of chemical, electrical and metabolic imbalances mainly brought about by poor nutrition, improper medical diagnoses, and improper treatment of medical conditions with pharmaceutical drugs.

There are many opinions about how to treat Periodic Paralysis; including hyperkalemia "elevated" and hypokalemia "reduced". Periodic Paralysis can be discussed on a variety of levels. Chemists talk in terms of chemical and electrical interactions and imbalances. Health care professionals talk about Periodic Paralysis in terms of affected organs and muscle groups. Dieticians discuss it in terms of calories and carbohydrates. Each specialty has a particular viewpoint, and each specialty has valid points to add to the conversation. Most are just not aware of the seriousness of potassium shifting and metabolic acidosis. Mental health professionals have views that are helpful if framed in the appropriate context, which is addressing depression as a secondary effect of Periodic Paralysis and not in the context of depression being the cause of Periodic Paralysis.

Things get very confusing for people with Periodic Paralysis when the disease is improperly diagnosed as somatic in origins rather than being correctly identified in medical physiological terms. Nothing can replace the value of having "positive thoughts". But having "positive thoughts" does absolutely nothing to help manage chemical imbalances in your body. Use your mental energies to improve your diet and improve your overall health and management of this disease. Chemical imbalances are responsible for many of the symptoms and making adjustments to chemical and electrical balances in your body will do more than anything else to help you manage your disease and improve the quality of daily life.

My understanding of Periodic Paralysis comes from being the caregiver for a person with Periodic Paralysis. My wife, Susan, has Periodic Paralysis. Her symptoms have been there for several decades and have caused many secondary conditions that were misdiagnosed by medical professionals. She has been improperly diagnosed with multiple sclerosis, neuropathy, conversion disorder, diabetes, and quite possibly fibromyalgia. However, fibromyalgia is one of the few conditions that are probably very real because of the restless leg manifestations and the effectiveness of mirapex medication, which supplements dopamine levels in her body. Keep in mind though that involuntary jerking motions can occur as a result of high acidity.

Throughout this process as caregiver, I have spent countless hours researching the causes of her condition. There are not many medical professionals who understand this disease and will probably do more harm than good in prescribing treatments with pharmaceutical drugs. I have found most of these drugs to aggravate Periodic Paralysis symptoms to the point of causing irregular heart waves and metabolic acidosis. Both of these conditions can be life threatening. Prescribing something as simple as oxygen never crosses their minds because they do not understand the disease and the disease process and secondary organ effects. Telling someone to exhale as much carbon dioxide from his or her lungs as possible in a rapid manner while in a state of hyper acidosis seems too simplistic. But in reality, this is the body's way of compensating for highly acidic blood levels.

The comprehension of this disease seems to be outside even the imagination of most medical professionals. They just do not have the skill set or willingness to learn, to be relied upon to diagnose and treat the disease process. At this point in time, we are on our own as caregivers and patients until the science can catch up with reality.

I have learned that I am on my own. I have learned to trust my own judgment but only when my judgments are supported by medical evidence. Throughout the process, I have learned how to use many medical devices including an oximeter, pH meter, cardy potassium meter, digital blood pressure cup, thermometer, blood sugar meter and many other medical devices. The learning curve has been sharp and steep at times. Sometimes I felt like I only had minutes to make decisions about another person who was in life threatening distress. The stress was unbearable at times.

By nature, I am a proactive person. I have learned to not indulge myself in self-pity or self-doubt. I constantly remind myself that this disease my wife suffers from is not about me. She is the one in distress and in need of comfort and treatment. Self-pity is very destructive. I have also learned to stay hopeful because the alternative is despair and inaction. As a caregiver I have learned to remain hopeful even when events appear to be otherwise. The person with the disease needs the care and encouragement to fight on.

Awareness about the disease will help everyone keep the perspective that this disease can be managed even without the help of medical professionals who do not understand mainly because they refuse to listen. As caregiver you will need to be strong and not personalize what is said. And most recently I have learned that I need to allow Susan to experience and express all the emotions she feels no matter how uncomfortable they make me feel. Feelings of hopelessness and despair often accompany the progression of the disease and especially when you both do not fully understand what is causing the condition.

Periodic Paralysis is the new kid on the block with regard to the identification of new-age disease and modern medicine. The dynamics of ion channels and potassium shifting are difficult to understand even by so-called experts. When we talk in terms of ion channel mutations, chemists hold the keys to understand the disease. Hyperkalemic and Hypokalemic Periodic Paralysis are identified alongside these ion channel mutations.

When we shift the conversation to a more practical level of understanding, things get a more manageable. If we talk about Periodic Paralysis in terms of the effects of potassium shifting, alkalosis, acidosis, oxygen deprivation, and paralytic episodes, then things come down to an earthly conversation. I strongly believe in science and also believe that science holds the keys to treatment and possible cure. My goal here is to share some of the information Susan and I have gathered with people in similar circumstances. We have found many other people in similar circumstances left alone by the medical community to perish. There is no known cure but there is hope for a quality life with proper management of symptoms. The end goal is to improve the quality of daily life and also to help caregivers to have some control over events that are life-threatening and nerve wracking. We have found success along the way mixed with a healthy amount of caution.

There are very few people on this planet who understand the fluid dynamics of Periodic Paralysis and even fewer people who can explain Periodic Paralysis in common terms. There are few prescriptions that will not cause paralytic episodes. Almost anything synthetic can cause severe episodes. The person in the Paralytic Episode appears to be unconscious but when questioned after the paralytic episode has passed, they will report being fully conscious and aware at the same time they are paralyzed.

The acid alkaline shifting and imbalance in the body has a great deal of impact on paralytic episodes. The higher the acidity levels the more likely hyperkalemia will occur. The higher the alkaline levels the more likely the hypokalemia will occur. Oftentimes-high alkalinity levels do not get measured in terms of proportionality but rather in terms of an overwhelming amount of acidity. If the pH balance shifts towards an acidity level, then the major health problems such as tachycardia occur. Once the balances are restored then the symptoms to secondary systems leave. This is what makes it so difficult to identify. Shifting occurs and then subsides. If multiple measurements are not taken before, during, and after an episode then no changes in pH or potassium will be noted. If these conditions go untreated then the condition becomes life threatening with the very worse outcome being cardiac arrest and death. The cause of death will go undetected, and it will be recorded in general terms rather than specific causes. Periodic Paralysis is a silent killer.

Finding a medical doctor who understands Periodic Paralysis well enough to diagnose and treat the disease is next to impossible. Typically, people get a diagnosis of Periodic Paralysis because health care professionals just do not know what else it could be. The people who persist in their quest for understanding have better chances of success than those who give up due to the enormity of the task. Susan has undergone thirty plus years of misdiagnoses ranging from multiple scleroses to fibromyalgia. She has suffered crippling osteoporosis due to the effects of the disease and having been given medications that practically took her life.

Traditional medical doctors have 2 tools to treat illness and disease. They are given a scalpel and a prescription pad when they graduate and most of them refuse to consider any alternatives outside of what pharmaceuticals companies disclose. In their defense, the doctors just do not have the time to explore unusual or atypical illnesses and diseases. It is sad but true. Once you accept the fact that your insurance company and your doctor have serious limitations and do not have the time to care about individual patients, and then you can begin to take charge of your own medical care. If you seriously believe you have the disease called Periodic Paralysis, then some of what your read here might be of help in your management of symptoms.

Almost every medication being prescribed by your medical doctor will interfere with your metabolism. For people with Periodic Paralysis this can be devastating. Many classes of drugs cause alkaline to be turned into acid or seriously affect the level of alkaline-acid balance (pH) in your body. You need to believe that artificial substances in your body negatively impact the metabolism of the cells. The only way to prevent this from happening is to stop putting blind trust in the medical community and stop putting poisons inside of your body. Whether we believe it or not, we are in charge of our medical care and life.

Periodic Paralysis is the master of disguise. It mimics neurological, neuromuscular, psychiatric, mitochondrial, cardiological, and autoimmune diseases. Symptoms appear and then disappear. This is what makes it so difficult to identify, diagnose and treat. Many specialists use stringent testing mechanisms that fail to capture the cause of the symptoms. Taking one measure of potassium levels during a paralytic episode is basically useless. Using a patient's age to determine if Periodic Paralysis is possible is misleading. Periodic Paralysis can occur at any time during a person's life. There are only a few hundred documented cases worldwide. How could anyone draw any definitive conclusions about the etiology?

I personally believe Periodic Paralysis is much more widespread than most people are led to believe. Just look at the high number of people who die from sudden heart failure with no real explanation. More than fifty percent of the US population is classified as obese. Diabetes runs rampant as our children are being fed a diet of garbage not fit to be consumed rodents. We are on the edge of a major collapse of our health care system due to the non-food stuff we are putting inside our bodies. When new doctors enter the field of medicine, they are given a scalpel and prescription pad and taught to ignore the real practice of healing and medicine. There are still some aspects of this disease that we do not understand. Maybe you will be the one to connect more dots that will eventually lead to better diagnosing tools and more comprehensive treatments. Susan and I have discovered through trial-and-error valuable pieces of information and understanding with hopes it will help other people cope with this disease. Periodic Paralysis is a very real despite the rebuke of medical professionals.

Chapter Thirty-Four
Friends

"WHAT FRIENDS?"
Introduction

Most people with Periodic Paralysis will not become as disabled as I am and will probably be able to socialize within his or her specific limitations. But, for those of us with more debilitating forms of Periodic Paralysis, having a social life is almost non-existent. Many will lose friends because they will not be able to keep up with the energy it takes to entertain and keep friends. There will be a few who are much like me. Their friends will desert them, and they may spend much of their time alone.

What Friends?

Although I was born with Periodic Paralysis and am now totally disabled, throughout most of my life I have always been a very social being. My formative years were spent in a family with three brothers and too many cousins to count, numerous aunts and uncles and family friends. I had friends who lived in my neighborhood, and I had friends at school. I belonged to a girl scout troop and went to camp every summer. I also belonged to the YWCA and spent time in day camp every summer. I had friends at church and spent much time in church activities. As a teenager, I belonged to a "group" of kids, and we spent a lot of time meeting new kids in other "groups". I spent much of my time socializing with peers and talking on the phone.

As an adult, I spent much of my time with family and my in-laws. I always knew my neighbors. I was active at church. I had jobs over the years and many co-workers became my friends. I always knew the parents of my children's friends. I had a group of friends that I socialized with, some were friends I had as children. When I attended college, I had friends and belonged to study groups.

When we built our home and moved to the mountains, we had a small community of neighbors, about six families, with whom we socialized constantly. We gathered often preparing meals over a campfire, having wonderful conversation and lots of laughs. If we were not entertaining friends and neighbors our mountain home was loaded with family on holidays and weekends.

Early on, I would notice being very tired and weak after our big weekends or holidays. Even a simple dinner with friends would exhaust me. I assumed I just did too much. At the same time, I was getting weaker physically and developing more and more symptoms. The doctors were giving me more medications. I had to stop working. I was deemed disabled.

We began to entertain less and less. We began to go visiting less and less. I talked on the phone less and less. I seldom left the cabin. I had less and less energy. Soon we were not socializing at all except for family gatherings, at which Calvin and the kids were doing most of the preparations. Calvin was usually left to clean up the mess.

I found I had only a certain amount of energy in me to expend each day. I had just enough to do the things I had to do, a little cooking and cleaning and maybe a shower. If I had to shop or do laundry, I was wiped out for a few days afterward. I had not enough energy to do what I needed or wanted to do in a day. This left nothing left in me for socializing, including with family. Talking on the phone even became a chore.

We had to move away from our mountain home with three stories because I could not walk up the stairs any longer. It was a huge house and too much work for me. It broke our hearts, but we left our family behind and moved to a small town in Oregon for a better climate. We had hoped our kids would follow us, but they never did.

We bought some acreage with a small house that needed to be remodeled. Calvin did a nice job, but we were on top of a mountain with no place to go for short walks or exercise. We were very isolated with no close neighbors. One of our closest neighbors made attempts to be social. I had no energy and became even sicker, so we just never did more than visit a few times. Another couple was introduced to us through a relative. We had dinner once and then I was too sick to ever have them over to reciprocate. We met one more couple through a business deal and got together a few times, but then my physical condition prohibited visits.

After my major episode of paralysis in July 2009, we decided to move to town to be closer to the hospital. At that time, we believed I was nearing the end of my life and so decided to move into a senior mobile home park. It was on level ground for easier access, and I used my motorized wheelchair to get around. We found a wonderful home right on the Rogue River and the river flowing by brought me some peace of mind. However, we did not socialize or go to any of the activities due to my health. We knew very few people there and made no real friends.

I was not able to do much more than walk through our house. I spent most of my time in a recliner attached to an oxygen machine in order to breathe. Due to the exercise intolerance the electrical workings of my heart have suffered damage. I am unable to do anything that may cause a rise in adrenalin or epinephrine. Talking on the phone takes every ounce of my energy, so my conversations are short and usually limited to family members. I can no longer cook or clean or entertain. Our friends and acquaintances have stopped trying to make plans with us for understandable reasons. The only person I saw other than Calvin for more than a year was my therapist. She came to our home once a week to help me deal with my failing health and isolation. She has become like a friend and has been wonderful to me.

We have since moved to a small house on two acres of rain forest property in Washington State. We know we do not need to be close to a hospital any longer, so we have returned to a rural lifestyle. We have been here for five months and have made no new friends and have not met our neighbors. Although we have met some wonderful people while we were buying our home and finding new doctors and the other things we have had to do to get settled, I do not have the energy to invite people to our home for any kind of socialization nor do I have the energy to go to activities in the community. The only people I see besides Calvin, unless I go to a doctor appointment or a seldom trip to run errands with Calvin, is the man who delivers my oxygen. We are making the best of the situation and enjoying the peace, quiet and solitude.

And so, as a casualty of Period Paralysis, I have only a few real friends and keep in contact with an occasional phone call. However, I spend most of my time sitting in my chair with my lap top computer. I am able to communicate with the outside world this way without draining my energy. I have nearly 200 "friends" on Facebook. Over forty of them are family members with whom I keep up on the latest gossip and activities and several of them are life-long friends, even a few from elementary school. Some of my "friends" have PP and are in varying degrees of disability. We support each other. Others play games with me. Many of them are genealogy cousins, for whom, I do genealogy research and share information. I spend much of my time writing this book and developing the Periodic Paralysis Network; offering help and support to others like me. I keep on top of politics, have debates with others, share jokes with cousins, and use Skype to talk with my children and grandchildren.

Friends

Next to my husband, my laptop is my best "friend". It affords an entire world of friends for me in what otherwise would be a very lonely life. My advice to others like me is to, if at all possible, they should get a lap top computer or open the one they have and begin to make friends. Join the boards for people with Periodic Paralysis. They will find many people like themselves. They will become friends. They will truly understand you, offer support to you and exchange ideas and information with you. In this world of technology, we are truly no longer alone.

Chapter Thirty-Five
Family

"IT'S JUST THAT SIMPLE"
Introduction

Although families tend to be spread out across the world in modern times, technology can keep families together. Families can still share values, traditions and beliefs. They can share activities and experiences. They can come together in times of joy and sadness. Belonging to a family can provide its members with emotional, psychological and physical support. Each member can help and support one another positively with love, trust, forgiveness, cooperation, respect and honest communication even if there are personal differences. A family can solve problems together and work together. In a family there can be flexibility and cohesion. As a member of a family, an individual should be able to expect from the other members nurturing in times of need, support to deal with stress and a feeling of well-being. Love should be unconditional and support non-judgmental. In a family when one member is ill other family members rally around providing love and care and physical, emotional, and psychological support as may be needed.

That being said, just as it is very sad that Periodic Paralysis and 'doctors' in this book must be placed in this section in a negative way, so is it even sadder that Periodic Paralysis and 'family' should also need to be placed in this section in an unfavorable way. The experiences with my family or lack of experiences, have affected me to my deepest soul physically, emotionally, psychologically and socially by the very people in my life who are supposed to be there for me. These are the very people to whom I have always been there for, when they needed me. And they are the same people that I love very much and am trying to help by writing this book.

Family History and Diagnosis

As previously discussed, on February 7, 2011, I had a heart loop monitor placed in my chest. This was done to keep track of my tachycardia and arrhythmias, including my long QT interval heartbeat with the intention of possibly getting an implanted defibrillator in the future, and to assist in confirming a diagnosis of Periodic Paralysis (PP): Andersen-Tawil Syndrome (ATS). After the procedure, I was going to be sent to the intensive care unit and provocational tests were also going to be performed on me. The tests I was facing were not going to be easy because I would end up paralyzed temporarily and they could possibly elicit deadly heartbeats. I was not able to use any medications, due to the possibility of paralysis or the long QT heartbeat it can cause. I was administered only lidocaine topically and so was very much awake during the procedure. While I was lying on the operating table and Dr. P was inserting the monitor under the skin covering my rib cage, he said to me, "I am so impressed with how brave you are to be doing this." I started to cry and responded by saying to him, "I am doing this for my family." "I have to get the diagnosis for them."

I was willing to go through surgery with no painkillers or anesthesia and the other tests, no matter the risks, because I love my family, every one of them. So many of them have similar symptoms and need a diagnosis to receive the proper medications and treatment. I knew that once I had my diagnosis, the others could get theirs. I had to do it. I kept thinking of them as I became paralyzed on the operating table (from the lidocaine) and later in recovery after I was mistakenly given a saline IV drip. This sent me into the worse episode I had in my life. During the paralysis, my heart rate was over 140 bpm for an hour and then lowered a little for another hour. I feared I was dying, but if it meant a diagnosis was finally possible, I would do it again if necessary. I want all of them to be able to get treatment for their disease before they get as disabled and ill as I am. I did get my diagnosis that day at the age of sixty-two.

As we know, a family is any group of persons closely related by blood, such as parents, children, brothers, sisters, uncles, aunts, and cousins, nieces, nephews, grandparents and grandchildren. A family is a group of persons sharing a common ancestry. A family is two or more people who share goals and values, with long-term commitments to one another. A family is all those claiming descent from a common ancestor, tribe or clan. A family is a lineage that can share a hereditary disease. My family is one of those. We share the hereditary channelopathy disease called Periodic Paralysis: the type is unknown at this time, but the symptoms are like Andersen-Tawil Syndrome. The family I am writing about is the descendants of Lahlee Duggins, my mother. She no doubt had PP, though she never knew it before she passed away a few years ago. She had been misdiagnosed with many things, however, with my diagnosis, it is clear what she suffered from all her life.

It probably came through her father, Louis Duggins, because my mother's sister, and four half-sisters share some of the traits and symptoms as does their children, grandchildren and great-grandchildren. I can trace this disease through six generations. Louis Duggins and his four brothers all died of heart problems, some of them young and sudden indicating the possibility of the long QT interval heart arrhythmia. One was forty-one, he died during a paralysis attack when his heart suddenly stopped, and another was fifty-one. Their only sister suffered most of her life with similar symptoms to my mother and me. My mother and her full sister had episodes of total paralysis and my mother was totally disabled from weak muscles before she died. I have two brothers who are as disabled as me and have episodes of paralysis but with no diagnosis, but we know now that they have ATS as well. Two of my children have symptoms as well as three of my grandchildren. One of my brother's daughters has symptoms as does her children. The children and grandchildren, of one my brothers, have symptoms and characteristics. It is obvious that some who do not believe they have it are carriers because their family members have some of the characteristics.

Family has always been important to me. I am the family historian and have been working on our genealogy for the past forty years. I have three brothers; I was the only girl. My father had twelve siblings and my mother had six siblings. As a child, my aunts, uncles and cousins on my father's side were an integral part of my everyday life. Every holiday and vacation were spent with our extended family. Weekends always included at least one uncle or cousin. Some of my father's younger brothers lived with us after they left home, before they settled down with their own families. We had so much fun at each and every family gathering. We had at least three family picnics a year. We barbecued our hot dogs and hamburgers, ate great food, ate snow cones, laughed, teased each other, played games, sang to the music of our uncles' guitars, went for walks, watched the trains go by, ran up the hill to see when the next one was coming and listened to the adults tell stories of their childhood. On the outside we were a happy and loving family.

However, many of us had health problems. On my father's side there were back problems and diabetes affecting some of the uncles. At least four of them were in constant back pain, including my father. My mother was sick much of the time with many issues, but always put on a happy face. Though a few family members referred to her as being "hypochondriac". As she got older, more and more health issues appeared. We did not live near her family but did have gatherings with her family once or twice a year. Her mother had a stroke at age fifty. Most health issues were not discussed or known on that side because they were Christian Science followers, and no doctors were ever seen.

As children, my brothers and I suffered from growing pains, leg problems, every childhood disease, tonsillitis, one brother had dyslexia and was behavior disordered, one brother had a speech impediment and problems with organization and one brother was the class clown and graduated at age sixteen. I wet the bed until I was twelve, was overweight, had a foot that turned in, could not keep up with other kids on the monkey bars or any sports, could climb up a tree but could not get down, cried all the time, was very uncoordinated, began passing out at the age of eleven and as a teenager began to have pain in my back and joints. My family looked on all of this as normal. We each had problems and our parents all had problems. It was just our life.

As we grew up and left home and began our own families, we began to spread out across the country and were not close like we had been growing up. Priorities changed and many of us lost touch. Our parents' health declined through the years, especially my mother. My health was always an issue and so were two of my brothers during those years. One of my brothers did not seem to have any health issues, though his wife did. As we began to have children, many of them were born with health issues or developed them. As we got older and sicker, we began to communicate more than in previous years. Soon we discovered that many of our symptoms were similar. Two of my brothers and my mother and me, were deemed disabled by the age of fifty-one after years of medical decline. Sadly, many of our children began showing these same symptoms and one of my daughters was deemed totally disabled at the age of thirty-three.

It was clear that this illness was something hereditary. I had to find out what it was. It was now affecting a fourth generation. I was misdiagnosed over and over, but I continued to research our symptoms. It took many years, but I finally came to the realization that we had a disease called Periodic Paralysis. The type we have is a very rare form for which our family DNA is now being studied.

Once I finally discovered the name of the disease that was disabling my family members and me, I set out to get diagnosed. As part of my plan to do this, I created a family flowchart listing all family members and their symptoms over six generations.

I was able to gather the needed information by contacting family members by email and the phone with a survey asking several questions and made a video available for them to see me during paralytic episodes. The following is the note and the questions I sent:

"Hello family members,

Please bear with me. This email may be a little strange and is not meant to scare you. However, the doctors are very close to a final diagnosis for me, which appears to be hereditary. I need to know if other family members have these issues for the medical records. I need to ask a few rather odd questions. I hope you will help me with this. If I get this diagnosis, you will need to know about it. It is a very, very, rare and serious disease and will need to be treated if anyone in your family has it. Even if they have some of the symptoms, they may not have it get serious, but they will need to be evaluated to make sure, due to the heart issues. And, hopefully, to avoid going what I went through if they can get proper treatment.

Do you have a problem with low or high potassium?

Do you have scoliosis?

Do you have webbed or barely webbed 2nd-3rd toes? (Some of us have it; in fact, Shari's son was born with them fully webbed.)

Do you have curved toes?

Do you have a pinkie finger that curves toward the ring finger?

Do you have unusually short fingers?

Do you have a small mouth with crowded teeth?

Do you have small lower jaw?

Do you have teeth missing (born without them or never came in after the baby teeth fell out? (i.e., I never had wisdom teeth and after my eye teeth fell out there were not permanent ones to replace them...so I am missing 6 teeth)

Do you have heart palpitations, fast heartbeat or any kind of heart problem?

Do you have "clubbed" thumbs?

Do you have problems doing things with their hands and arms above their heads?

Do you have periodic muscle weakness or paralysis? (May be just a feeling of a limb going to sleep, especially after sitting for a while.) (May wake up at night with hands numb or trouble walking upon getting up in the morning.)

Do you have periodic extreme, muscle weakness after eating large meals with a large amount of carbohydrates, or sugar, stress, heat or cold, taking medications, exercise or exertion (can be delayed to the next day)?

Do you have problems walking upstairs or uphill?

Do you have weakness, dizziness etc. after fasting?

Do you have episodes of passing out?

Do you have problems with side effects or opposite effects of prescription medications or over-the-counter medications?

Do you have problems with anesthesia or lidocaine?

These things may be very subtle...not real obvious...

I know this all sounds a little crazy, but it is very important to our family and me. If I get this diagnosis, you will need to know about it. It is a very, very, very, rare and serious disease and will need to be treated.

I hope none of these things are a problem for you. That would be great news.

If you want, you may call to talk about this.
Love you, Mom, Grandma, Susie, Aunt Susie"

Many of my family members responded. The answers amazed me and confirmed for me that we did indeed have a larger problem in my family than I had even realized. Much of my extended family also had similar problems. The following is some information sent to me from my mother's

Family

first cousin Linda, about her father, my great uncle whom I never met:

"Dear Susie,

My dad, your great uncle, was 6', slender, and had long legs. He had low set ears and he had many problems with his teeth. He had a strong jaw, which comes from his mother's German heritage. He was sick a lot as a child. His childhood diseases we have no information about because usually his German grandmother used home remedies. I know that he missed so much school he was held back 2 years in a row. He had the worst childhood disease when he was 7. I do remember my grandmother saying he often had a fever and leg pain. Finally, Grandma Mary ignored her mother and took him to the doctor. After this last bad episode, he seemed to improve.

When he was 18 he joined the Army. During basic training his gas mask malfunctioned. After this event he became tired more frequently. He was a driven man always busy and had a hard time sitting still. He worked all day maintaining schools, he would sit down for a few minutes to read the paper when he got home, soon you would find Dad outside weeding the garden, chopping wood, or doing a project. We thought he just was so driven he had a hard time relaxing.

When I was a baby, my dad was between 28 and 30, and he became tired frequently. He had chest pains and episodes of getting out of breath. Dad went to the VA hospital I believe in Portland. He was gone for a while, I know he stayed with family during some of his tests, and I believe he may have been hospitalized. This was sometime between 7/1954 and 12/1957. The doctors at that time did not discover any physical problems but as you know medical science was not as advanced. In fact, the VA was suggesting his problems were in his imagination and wanted to send him to the mental health unit. Dad was not going for that, and I don't believe he set foot in a VA hospital again. Dad continued to have episodes of tiredness, chest pain, and breathlessness. Because he was so active, and his regular physician never indicated there was a problem, his death at 41 years old was a shock. I do remember that he would get very pale in color more often during that last year.

The night before he died, he was laughing and joking with family before we put my great aunt on the bus at 9 PM to return to California. We were home in bed by 10 PM and set to go huckleberry picking the next day. At 4 AM the next morning he began gasping for breath and never woke up. I heard mom asking him what was wrong with panic in her voice. I got up she told me to call for help and I did. She went to get a cold washcloth to revive him. We walked back in the room, and he stopped breathing. We did CPR on him until help arrived, but his heart never started beating again.

When the doctor did the autopsy, he found scar tissue in the chambers of his heart. The scar tissue had been there for years. He determined it was probably a childhood disease that had caused it. He guessed that he had scarlet fever or rheumatic fever, which caused the scar tissue to form. The scar tissue caused his heart to work twice as hard as a normal heart, which resulted in it wearing out twice as fast.

Today that kind of damage is detectible. If he had known he probably would have been stressed and worried about what would happen to Mom and me. The doctor who performed the autopsy believed knowing would not have prolonged his life in fact the added mental stress may

Family

have shortened his time. He died on August 31, 1967, in Castle Rock, WA in the house he, my Grandma Mary, and Uncle Clarence built. It is also the home where my parents got married.

If I can help you in any way let me know. I send my love and good thoughts to you.

Love Linda"

"Dear Susie

I watched two of the videos on You Tube. The second video was a front view of you. At first it looks like you're sleeping and then you gasp as if you are trying to catch your breath. Then your episodes escalated, and at that moment I was transported back to a similar episode. It happened when I was between 7 and 9 years old. My dad would have been between 35-37 years old. I was sick one morning and went into my parents' room to wake one of them up to help me. When I tried to wake my dad, he did not respond. Then he did the same thing with the same facial grimacing and symptoms that followed in your video. Mom and I both tried to wake him. He was often hard to wake up in the morning and complained of feeling groggy.

After seeing this video, it was exactly like the episodes that happened to him. He did wake up and so we just thought he was deep in sleep and over tired. We never gave much thought to them because it just appeared he was one of those people who had more trouble waking up than others.

The fact that you are willing to do this work to educate others is very brave and important beyond what we can measure. You are touching people in a very personal way. Seeing an episode and trying to describe it afterwards to a healthcare provider, as you know, is very difficult. Any family member who has seen these will probably recognize it.

Even if they are unable to face the problem now, this video will be in their mind and may be part of the milestones leading them out of ignorance. Do not be discouraged. I am grateful you are doing this work and have taken on being a pioneer. If Dad were here, he would be cheering you on.

Love Linda"

I wrote the following as part of the chart for my doctors the doctors who are treating and diagnosing my family members.

"This flowchart lists only the symptoms and characteristics of Andersen-Tawil Syndrome for each family member who has or had them. Unfortunately, many other diseases and conditions co-exist or co-existed with the listed symptoms and characteristics for many of these family members. They need to be sorted out and recognized for a correct diagnosis, so the family members who have Periodic Paralysis can get the proper diagnosis. This is imperative so each family member with Periodic Paralysis can receive the proper medications, treatments and assistance from the proper organizations and so they can take part in the studies for Periodic Paralysis.

Some of the other diseases have masked the Periodic Paralysis and have been the cause of misdiagnoses such as fibromyalgia and multiple sclerosis. Odd effects of certain medications have also caused symptoms resembling other conditions such as ataxia and seizure-like episodes. These misdiagnoses have led some family members to be in their 50's and 60's now (and some already passed away) still attempting to find out what has disabled them by gradual muscle weakness, partial and total paralysis and heart problems since their childhood or teen years.

Some of the co-existing diseases include degenerative disk disease; osteoporosis, especially of the spine; arthritis, especially of the spine; peripheral poly neuropathy; type 2 diabetes; restless leg syndrome; asthma; strokes; depression; allergies; migraines; learning disabilities; and cyclic vomiting syndrome.

This family has been plagued with serious health problems and disabling conditions through 3 generations and is now beginning to manifest itself in a 4th generation. Please help this family by considering the strong possibility of Periodic Paralysis.

It has recently been discovered that another branch of this family also has these conditions and characteristics. Due to a time restraint, this family was not added to this report. If needed, this information can be added at a later time."

The flowchart and this letter were instrumental in my final diagnosis, and I hope it will help the others in my family in need of a diagnosis.

My Family Dynamics and a Lack of Understanding

Unfortunately, there are members of my family, who do not understand or who think some of us who are ill are hypochondriacs or malingerers. There are also some members who do not believe they have it, but clearly, they are symptomatic. There are others who do not believe in a hereditary disease in our family, but they are carriers because their children and grandchildren are symptomatic and have some of the characteristics. There are others who stay away because they do not want to watch my decline and that of other family members. There are those who believe we need only to have "good thoughts" and we will get well. Others believe prayer is the answer. Others believe it is best to keep my grandchildren away for fear that the children will see us and be afraid that they will end up like us, by the power of suggestion. I was even given a book by a family member explaining that all my illness was due to choices I had made in a prior lifetime and that I chose and welcomed it on a subconscious level.

This is so disheartening to those of us who are sick and disabled. We are suffering and watching our children suffering with fear for our grandchildren now. We are not liars. We did not choose this. We did not ask for it. Prayer will not cure it. Good thoughts will not make it go away.

Keeping my grandchildren away will not keep it from happening to them if they were born with it. The power of suggestion will not disable them. I am sick and continue to decline and may die soon. Do not stay away too much longer. Please do not keep my grandchildren away; they will miss knowing me due to a baseless fear. They need to know me and understand the disease, because they may have it. Some of you have all the symptoms, please get help now so you do not get as sick as me. Some of you do not understand heredity; it is scientifically based and proven. This disease, Periodic Paralysis: the type as yet unknown is an inherited disease. One has it only if it was passed on to them through one or both of their parents.

To my family:

"I have had episodes of partial and total paralysis for many years. During the episodes, my potassium shifts are low (hypokalemia), high (hyperkalemia) and within the normal ranges (normokalemia). Due to several misdiagnoses and a lack of proper diagnosis and

treatment for over fifty years, I have become totally and permanently disabled with weak muscles throughout my body including those involved with my vision, digestion, breathing and my heart. I must be on oxygen constantly and cannot exert myself in any way. The electrical workings of my heart are defective. I have had a heart loop monitor inserted in my chest to monitor the tachycardia and arrhythmias, which includes long QT interval heartbeats. I now spend my days in a recliner, unable to walk farther than across a room. I must use a motorized wheelchair for anything farther. If I did not have the help of Calvin, I would have to live in an assisted living program.

Through the past years of my physical decline, I have had to give up my career as a special education teacher, my hobbies to include hiking, walking, swimming, exercising, fishing, camping, traveling, shopping, cooking and baking. I had to sell, and move away from, a beautiful home my husband and I built in the mountains of Utah. I had to move far away from my family in order to live in a better climate. I can no longer drive our car. I have lost many friends, because I could not keep up with them or entertain any longer.

However, the hardest losses to deal with are those of my family. I have lost contact with or have a strained relationship with family members who did not understand or did not want to watch my decline or who thought I was a hypochondriac. And, I have lost the connection I once had with my grandchildren because I can no longer keep up with them or continue a meaningful relationship with them or they are being kept away.

Please understand what it is like when I am paralyzed:

"Usually, I wake up in the morning and I am paralyzed. I find I cannot move. I cannot open my eyes. My mouth is open. I cannot breathe through my nose. I have urges to swallow but cannot so there is a choking sound in my throat every few minutes. Sometimes my heart will race or beat irregularly. My breathing stops at times. I do not have any or much feeling in my body. My mouth is very dry. I cannot speak.

As I begin to come out of it, my mouth will start to get saliva, my eyes will open but I can only see what is in front of me, since I cannot move my head. Sometimes my eyes will jerk around when I first open them, usually jerking up. My body will sometimes jerk a little. Sometimes there is a big breath my body will take

Sometimes, I will go back into it. My eyes close, I feel very hot, and all the symptoms return. Sometimes there will be a few jerks as I go back into it.

During all of this I am awake and am aware of everything going on around me. Sometimes I begin to cry, due to the frustration, and fear. I can feel the tears running down my cheeks.

If I have these at times other than upon waking, the symptoms are the same. I get a strange sensation of heat body wide, usually beginning in my back. My eyes will close and then my body goes limp. I may have a few jerks as I am going limp. My mouth will open, and I am in it... unable to move, speak or open my eyes.

Sometimes, I do not go too deep. It is all the same, but I am able to open my eyes and can speak a little with a tight tongue and tight lips. My mouth is still open, however. I cannot move my body.

Once one of these begins, it may last up to 45 minutes to several hours, or can be as short as about 15 minutes, if it is a second or third one in a row.

It takes about 15 to 30 minutes or longer to come out of it all the way. I am always left with lingering weakness for many hours that can linger into days. Speaking is difficult. Walking is difficult. My arms and hands come back sooner than my legs. I begin to get feeling back in my body. I can move my lips. I begin to breathe thru my nose again. It is difficult to speak or move but it gradually comes back. Speech is very difficult; my lips do not want to move. My tongue is difficult to move. I will suddenly have an urgency to urinate. If, at this point, I get help to the bathroom, I am like a rag doll, especially my legs. My arms flail, like a child just learning to stand and walk, balancing herself.

For many hours, I remain too weak to do much of anything but sit up in bed or sit in a recliner. I must use my walker or a wheelchair.

I have a long QT interval heartbeat that can happen while I am in this state. If it does happen, I can go into cardiac arrest and die."

Why would I make it up, pretend, or lie about it? Why would I choose this or make it happen? All the prayers in the world will not make it stop. "Good thoughts" will not keep it from happening. Why would I have given up so much?

Please try to understand the truth of this horrible and debilitating disease. I did not choose it. It is real. You may have it. You may be a carrier. Your children may have it. The sooner you get it diagnosed, the better chance you have of not becoming disabled. I love you and got the diagnosis to help you, your children and grandchildren."

Conclusion

I would like to now address others who have Periodic Paralysis. I am in contact with many people whose family is much like mine. Periodic Paralysis is a cruel disease. It is one that is difficult to diagnose, though it does not need to be. Doctors, for the most part, who do not understand it, look at patients with it as hypochondriacs, malingerers or faking it. If the doctors treat us that way, is it any wonder our families may feel the same?

Some family members stay away or are very limited in their interaction with you, because they cannot face watching your decline. They may feel helpless. Some just do not know what to do or say. Some do not care or are in denial.

Others may not understand, for whatever reason. They may not have read about it. They may misunderstand. They may be stubborn about issues such as hereditary. They may not want to know. They may not care.

Many family members are living in fear that it may begin to manifest in themselves or their children. Others actually have the symptoms but are afraid to face them. They will have to sooner or later. I will be there for them or my website with all the information they may need.

I thought perhaps when I finally got my diagnosis that I had become vindicated and validated to my family. I thought they would believe me and thank me. Except for a few members who already believed me and supported me, I was wrong. The silence remains disheartening and deafening.

The way I handle it is to provide as much information as I can to them. I have the papers with my diagnosis and am happy to share them with those that are trying to get diagnosed. I have developed a web site for them and others to refer to as they have questions. I try to maintain communication with them, however strained it may be. I am here for them and let them know. Beyond that, I can do no more.

The loss of our families seems to be another cruel reality of Periodic Paralysis, and as one of my brothers says, "It's just that simple!!"

Chapter Thirty-Six
Conclusion

"THE NUTS AND BOLTS"
Writing This Book

It is Feb 28, 2013, and I cannot believe that I just completed writing 35 chapters about "living with Periodic Paralysis". It has taken 2 ½ years for me to write. I frankly did not believe I would live long enough to see this day. I truly thought Calvin would have to finish writing it from my outline and notes and his own experiences and memory. I am grateful that Calvin saved my life through his research and sheer determination. If not for him, I would not be here today celebrating such an achievement and a dream come true.

This book actually began after I realized I had Periodic Paralysis and before I received my clinical diagnosis. We created our Periodic Paralysis Network website. I began to write essays and articles to share the information I was learning with others. I was unable to get my questions answered and unable to find the type of help I needed from the organizations and boards in existence, so we created our own. It became clear as more and more people with different forms of Periodic Paralysis joined our group, seeking information and support, that a book needed to be written. Those essays and articles became the basics of and outline for this book. As I stated in my Preface, this book was "invented" or written out of necessity or an urgent need. The fact is when I began writing there were no other up-to-date books written about Periodic Paralysis (PP) and information on the web was scattered and sketchy at best or too difficult to understand for the average person. There was then and is now an urgent need to educate those with the different forms of Periodic Paralysis and their family members on all aspects of the disease including how to manage and alleviate their symptoms. There was and is also an urgent need to educate the medical professionals dealing with those individuals, and their families, to learn to recognize, diagnose and properly treat their patients in a timely manner.

Some of what I wrote was formulated and created in my mind during the periods of time I was partially or totally paralyzed. After regaining muscle strength, I would type my recollections and ideas. I recalled a lifetime of illness and gradual disability, loss of a teaching career, mistreatment by medical professionals, disregard by family members, and a loss of friendships. During the writing of this book, I researched, read and studied everything I could find about every aspect of the different forms of Periodic Paralysis. Due to Calvin's research and his ability to save my life, together, we created the plan for naturally managing and treating many of the symptoms of Periodic Paralysis. This included reducing the number and severity of the paralytic episodes. It also included a pH balance diet, discovering triggers, finding amenable doctors. The periods of paralysis were also times I could recall the psychological, emotional and social aspects of the cruel disease. I believe these to be very important issues of which no one has written, and they needed to be included in this book.

Chapter One through Chapter Eleven became my own experiences, written in narrative and essay format. Section Two became the actual writing about all the aspects of Periodic Paralysis and much research went into what I wrote and all of it is well referenced. Section Three became our overall plan for managing and treating the symptoms, using our own ideas based on our own experiences, experimentation, research and with referencing back up the facts and our ideas. Section Four again based on my own experiences and written in narrative and essay format became the psychological, emotional and social aspects.

As I wrote this book, much of what was written was very difficult to re-live. Some of it was very sad and I cried as I wrote. Some things were funny and made me laugh as I wrote. Some things were embarrassing to admit as I wrote. Other things I revealed made me angry as I wrote. I wanted to yell and scream at times as I wrote. I realized my limits as I wrote. I realized my strengths as I wrote. I discovered people who cared about me as I wrote. I realized who did not care about me as I wrote. I wanted to 'set the record straight' as I wrote. I wanted to 'get things off my chest' as I wrote. I wanted to 'reveal the truth" as I wrote. I wanted to share my experiences as I wrote. I wanted to teach as I wrote. I wanted to change things as I wrote. I wanted to help others as I wrote. I wanted to share with others how I had been violated by medical professionals as I wrote. I wanted to punish people as I wrote. I wanted to thank people as I wrote. I wanted to plead for help as I wrote. I understood the inevitable as I wrote, I hoped I would live long enough to complete the book. Now that I have completed it, I feel satisfied, relieved and proud.

All that is written is as factual as possible. I make no apologies for my honest evaluation and interpretation of what I have experienced. I make no apologies for telling the truth. I have not given the names of any of the doctors or medical professionals or medical institutions in order to protect the guilty and the innocent. I have not hidden the reality of this cruel disease nor 'sugar-coated' it in any way. Many may recognize themselves in this book. It is my hope that positive changes may come from this recognition.

Copyright and Free Use

When I was nearly finished with the writing, Calvin began to edit beginning with Chapter One. Things were fine as he read the chapters through Chapter Eleven. As he began to read Chapter Twelve, he began to get a little worried due to the references I had used. Everything I researched, I found on the Internet, and I cited the URLs for each site. As he was searching for the information about copywriting and looking for the information to make sure it was correct and legal, he found many of the websites were no longer available and many of the others had copyright restrictions.

As I researched and wrote, I was particularly careful not to use information from other Periodic Paralysis organizations. I went the extra mile to find the information and the facts I needed from other sources. I was extremely careful to not use anyone else's words. I went to great lengths to write the information in a format that most people without a medical background could understand. I knew I had not plagiarized anyone. Never-the-less we did not want a lawsuit once our book was published, so we began to research the laws about copyrighting and re-researched the sources.

We discovered some very important things. Ideas may not be copyrighted, nor can facts be copyrighted. Most of what I researched and found and wrote about were the facts about Periodic Paralysis and they were found in the public domain, so there is no problem with copyright laws in that respect. Sequences of words and images, however, may be copyrighted and therefore require permission to be used when writing. My writing does not have a problem with this issue, since I had not used any of the words I found as they were originally written. We also discovered song titles cannot be copyrighted but words to songs may be copyrighted. Knowing this made me have to change a few things I had written. Lastly, if any material, which is copyrighted, is used and referenced for educational purposes, it is considered "fair use" under the copyright law and therefore not subject to a lawsuit.

We realized for a non-fiction book to be deemed credible, reference materials and sources of information for the facts should be cited or referenced in the writing, even if the exact words were not used. Before editing, we had over two hundred and fifty references in the "Works Cited". This became rather cluttered for smooth reading, so we reduced the number. Since all materials used during the research should be listed in a bibliography, much of what was originally referenced, is now listed in the Bibliography. We used Wikipedia quite often as our major source, although many people feel it may not be a credible resource tool. We found that Wikipedia is an excellent reference tool because Wikipedia contains so many references to the source materials used for definition purposes. Wikipedia offers a broad conceptual array of information that fully encompasses other more traditional sources of definitions and information. We found the information contained there accurate and very current. Wikipedia utilizes the best of open-source principles and poses a direct threat to more traditional proprietary approaches to dispersing information for public consumption.

Writing a credible non-fiction book requires knowledge, research and study of the topics discussed. Living with Periodic Paralysis for my entire life and more than two- and one-half years of research, reading, studying, referencing, experimenting, personal experience and hours and hours of typing, retyping, and editing went into the production of this book. We have met all the requirements to write a non-fiction book, which has credibility.

Disclaimers

Due to the fact this book is about a medical condition and medical issues, we must include a disclaimer. This reduces the ability of, or protects us from, being sued for any of the content.

The ideas in this book are based on the authors' personal experience with Periodic Paralysis, and as such are intended to provide only educational information on the covered subject to the reader. This book should not be used as a medical manual, nor should this book be used as a diagnostic tool for Periodic Paralysis. The reader should consult a trusted and qualified health care provider with expertise in Periodic Paralysis.

What's Next?

And now the question is, "What is next?". It is my dream to incorporate the Periodic Paralysis Network into a Non-profit Organization Status. We will become:

The Periodic Paralysis Network, Incorporated

Our Mission Statement (Goal) will be:

The Periodic Paralysis Network, Incorporated exists to assist individuals with Periodic Paralysis by providing a hands-on approach to understanding the disease, getting a proper diagnosis, managing the symptoms, and assisting their caregivers and family members.

In order to do this, we will need to raise money for the following objectives:

❖ Expenses incurred to publish the book: *living with Periodic Paralysis.*
❖ Expenses incurred to maintain the Periodic Paralysis Network website.
  ➢ Providing continual education to individuals with Periodic Paralysis to better understand the disease, to get a proper diagnosis, to manage the symptoms, and to assist caregivers and family members through:
  ➢ The Periodic Paralysis Network, Inc. Website
  ➢ The Periodic Paralysis Network, Inc. Discussion Boards
  ➢ The Periodic Paralysis Network, Inc. web cam educational sessions
  ➢ The Periodic Paralysis Network, Inc. web cam

     support group sessions
- ➢ The Periodic Paralysis Network, Inc. video conferencing
- ➢ The Periodic Paralysis Network, Inc. video classes
- ➢ The Periodic Paralysis Network, Inc. demonstration videos
- ➢ The Periodic Paralysis Network, Inc. videos

❖ Purchasing devices and medical equipment for individuals who cannot afford them in order to better manage Periodic Paralysis symptoms. These include:
- ➢ Cardy Meters and Supplies
- ➢ Oximeters
- ➢ Blood Pressure Meters
- ➢ Blood Sugar Meters
- ➢ pH Meters
- ➢ Thermometers
- ➢ Stethoscopes

❖ Providing financial assistance to individuals needing to travel to specialists of Periodic Paralysis for diagnosis and treatment.

❖ Providing education about Periodic Paralysis to medical schools, paramedics, emergency rooms, hospitals, primary care physicians, neurologists, etc. for better recognition, faster diagnosis and proper treatment.

❖ Researching for better methods to diagnose Periodic Paralysis.

❖ Researching for new treatments and possible cures for Periodic Paralysis.

A percentage of the sale from each book will go to The Periodic Paralysis Network, Incorporated in order to accomplish the above goal and objectives.

I hope I will live long enough to be instrumental in the incorporation of The Periodic Paralysis Network. I also hope I will live long enough to see the goals and objectives become reality. If not, I hope Calvin and my family members will continue this work for those who may need it now and for future generations.

In Conclusion

After sharing my life and experiences, all the aspects of the condition which I know and have learned from research, studying and living with it; our plan to manage and treat the symptoms in natural and common-sense ways based on our own experimentation and the psychological, emotional and social aspects all of which I have experienced; I hope each of you will have a better understanding of Periodic Paralysis. If you have a form of Periodic Paralysis, I hope you can improve the quality of your life by adopting our ideas and know that you are not alone. If you are a doctor or health-care provider, I hope you will be able to recognize, diagnose and treat individuals with Periodic Paralysis correctly, in a timely manner and with the respect they deserve. If you are a social worker or therapist, I hope you will be able to offer the support needed to your patient who has this condition with your newly gained information. If you are a family member, I hope you will now understand the disease and now believe your family members who have this cruel condition and will offer the support and love to them that they desperately need from you. If you are a family member who actually has some of these symptoms but continues to ignore it, please know that the sooner you begin to treat the symptoms, the better you may become and you may possibly avoid becoming more disabled and debilitated. If you are a caregiver, I hope the knowledge gained will be able to assist you in aiding your client or loved one and ease your mind. If you are a friend or relative of an individual with Periodic Paralysis, I hope you will know and understand that your friend or family member still loves you and cares about you and would love to visit and spend more time with you and give you the attention that you deserve, but they physically cannot, and it breaks their heart. If you are a family member or a friend on our discussion board or anyone else who has this condition but cannot get diagnosed, I hope this book will be instrumental in getting that diagnosis. To all the above and to anyone else who reads this book, for whatever reason, please remember that you only fail when you stop trying.

Thank you.

The Afterword

I love John Denver songs and for most of the important things that happen in my life I can relate them to a John Denver song. This also applies to the Periodic Paralysis I must live with each and every day. In the title words of a song sung by John Denver, "Some Days are Diamond, Some Days are Stone."

Yesterday was a "Stone Day" for me. Very few days are "Diamond Days" anymore, but not every day is a "Stone Day" either. They are more like "Precious Stone Days". "Precious Stone Days" are days I am glad to be alive. On those days I cannot do much physically, but I am productive, and I feel pretty good, and I can communicate well, and Calvin is close by. I enjoy those days.

A "Diamond Day" is a day I get to travel somewhere with Calvin. We see new things or things we have seen before, but it is still enjoyable to be with him and enjoying the outdoors. We are usually out in the country or the forest or somewhere out in nature. It can be next to a small creek or an ocean. There can be trees or rolling ranch and farmland.

We are usually recalling the feelings of the days we used to live in the mountains. We are making plans and coming up with ideas for the future. We are attempting to make our dreams come true as we always have for the thirty-two years, we have been together.

On "Stone Days", I realize my limitations. I know how sick I am. I know I am not getting better. I know I am getting worse. I know that most of those dreams and plans and ideas will not come true. They are not going to happen. "Stone Days" are days of reality.

They are days; I am too sick and weak to get out of the recliner or bed. They are days I cannot eat much. They are days I am not productive. They are days when my mouth cannot move well making it difficult to talk. They are days when I feel sadness and regret. They are days when I care little about what is going on around me or in the world. They are days I have to let go. I am no longer in control of anything in my life. I cannot make a choices or decisions.

Thank the gods I have Calvin in my life to take care of me and the things that need to be done on those days.

Today was a "Precious Stone Day". I was able to write this and share it with you. I hope that after reading this book you will begin to have more "Precious Stone Days and even some "Diamond Days".

I wish each and every one who reads this book good health. May your "Stone Days" be few and may your "Diamond Days" and "Precious Stone Days" be plentiful...

Susan Q. Knittle-Hunter
2013

About the Authors

Susan Quentine Knittle-Hunter is a woman who has Periodic Paralysis. She spent many of her 65 years in search of a name for what has gradually weakened her body and caused her to be deemed disabled at the early age of 50. During those years, she raised a family of four children. She attended the University of Utah and graduated with a B.S. in Special Education and a B.S. in Psychology. She has taught children of all ages and disabling conditions in Utah and Wyoming. She has been a consultant on the state level for the States of Utah and Wyoming working with disabled children and adults and their families. Susan has designed several community adult living programs. She has written an instructional manual, *Creating Program Plans for MR/DD Adults*, and has presented workshops using the manual. She was a program coordinator for an adult habilitation program in Wyoming. She authored a book entitled *Cerebral Gigantism, Soto's Syndrome: Sandy's Story "I Wanna Go Home"*, about her daughter's life and death and struggles with Soto's Syndrome. When Susan became disabled herself, she had to give up her career devoted to improving the lives of challenged children and adults.

Calvin Hunter is Susan's husband and caregiver. He has B.S. Degrees in Behavioral Science, Psychology and master's degrees in special education and Information Technology. He has been a consultant and social worker for developmentally disabled adults. He was a resource teacher and taught middle school age learning and behaviorally challenged students. He assisted Susan in designing several community adult living programs and managed the programs. He has written a book about his and Susan's experiences building their home in the mountains called, *Blue Sky Mountain*. Calvin developed his own on-line publishing company and assisted Susan in completing her first book and publishing it for her, as well as his own book. He is now retired and helps Susan daily. He has co-authored, edited and published this book.

Calvin and Susan met 32 years ago in Salt Lake City, Utah and married 31 years ago in Wenatchee, Washington. Susan and Calvin, together and on their own, with very little help from others, built a beautiful home in the Uinta Mountains of Utah. They lived there for nearly 20 years before having to give it up due to their illnesses. They had lived there with their llamas and Australian Shepherd dogs. When they were able, they enjoyed traveling in their large trailer. They moved to and lived on the Rogue River in Grants Pass, Oregon, until moving to the Olympic Peninsula in Washington. They found and purchased a few acres of their own rain forest with a creek and pond where they enjoy the wildlife daily. Calvin enjoys gardening and remodeling their new home and Susan enjoys writing and genealogy research. They spend much of their time working on and researching for their Periodic Paralysis Network website and discussion board. Calvin and Susan continue to use their teaching and psychology skills on the discussion board helping others with Periodic Paralysis and by offering web cam support group sessions and sessions teaching about different aspects of living with Periodic Paralysis.

Appendix

Susan's Photographs

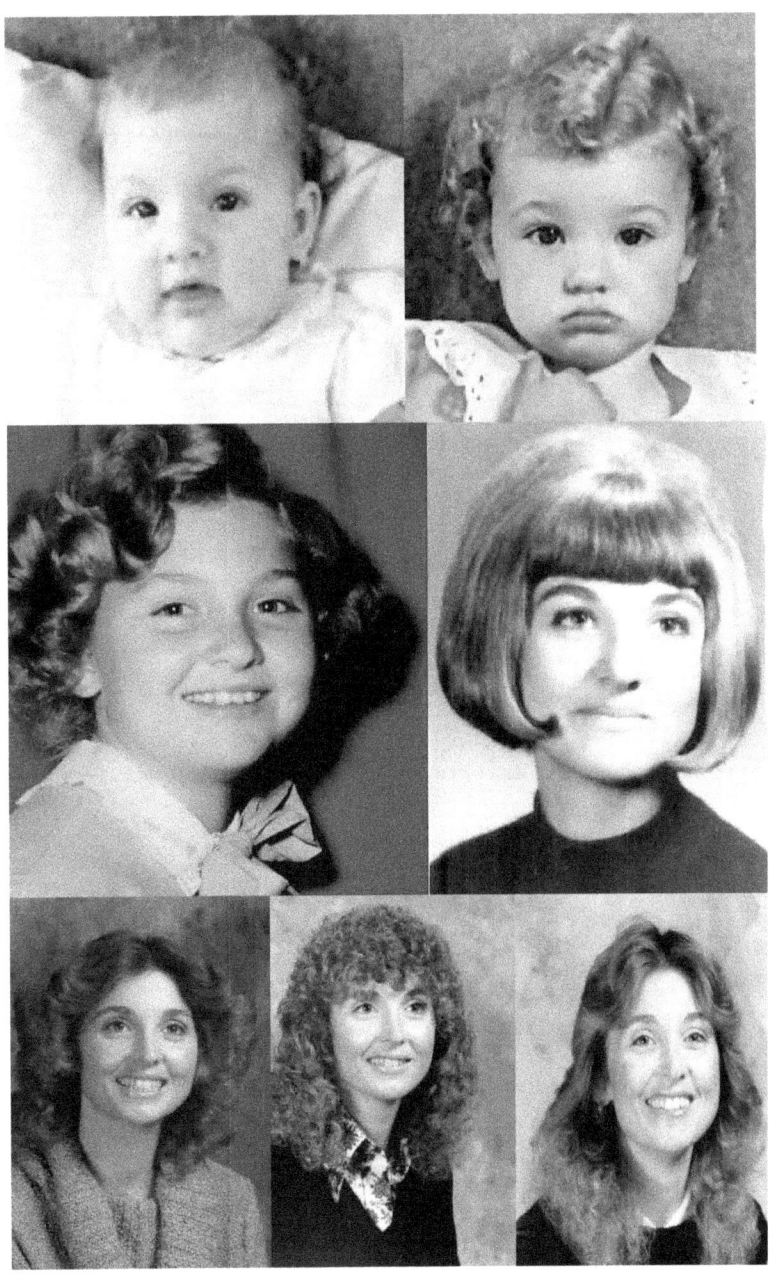

387

Due to a lack of a proper diagnosis and all of the wrong diagnoses, wrong medications and horrible treatment and malpractice by the doctors I have seen in the past several years, my physical condition had deteriorated drastically.

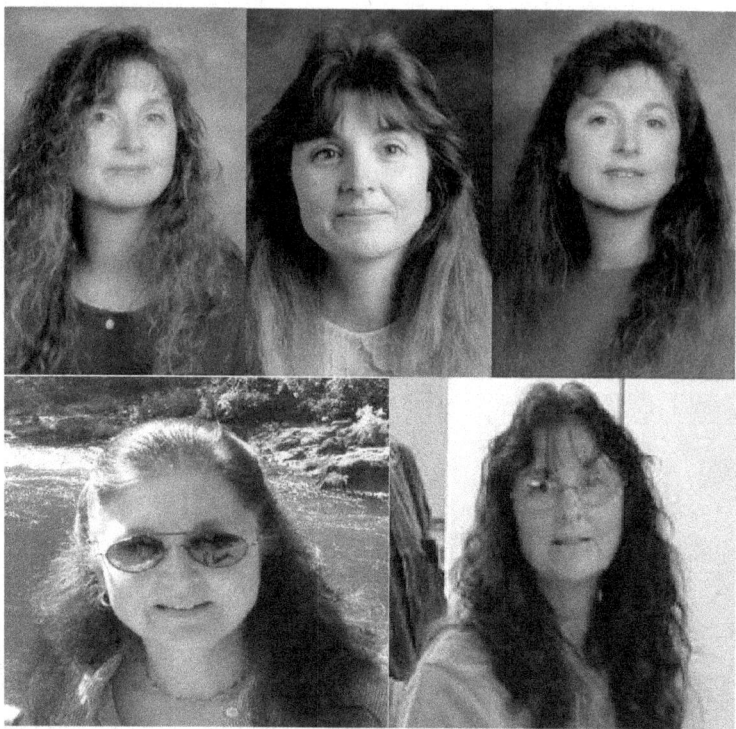

These two pictures were taken 2 months apart and only 7 months before the picture below.

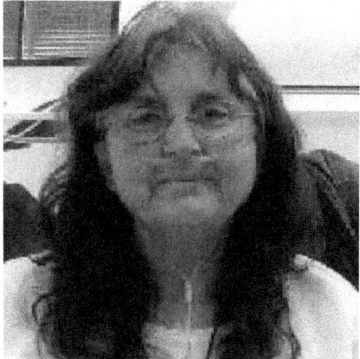

This picture was taken 6 months after I almost died and 4 months after I began oxygen.

Appendix

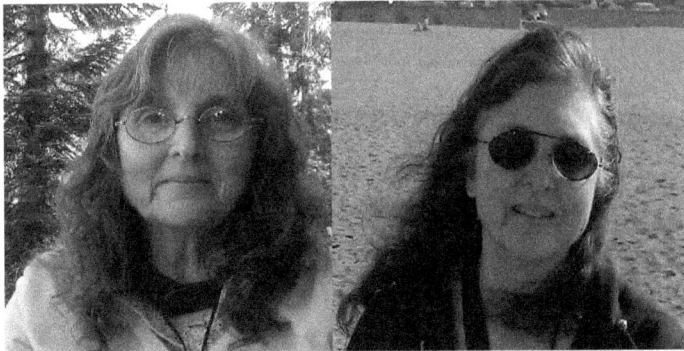

The picture on the left was taken 6 months after the previous one after following the "Plan"... eating a pH balanced diet, taking supplements and continued oxygen therapy. The one on the right
was taken one year later after continuing the "Plan".

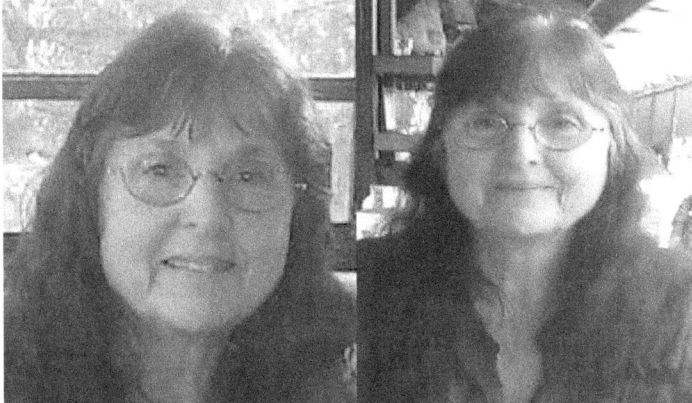

Susan November 2012 and March 2013. Still following the "Plan".

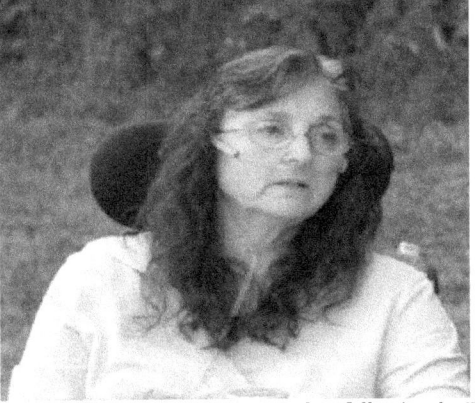

Susan going into paralysis. Even when following the "Plan", potassium will still shift and cause paralytic episodes.

Reality

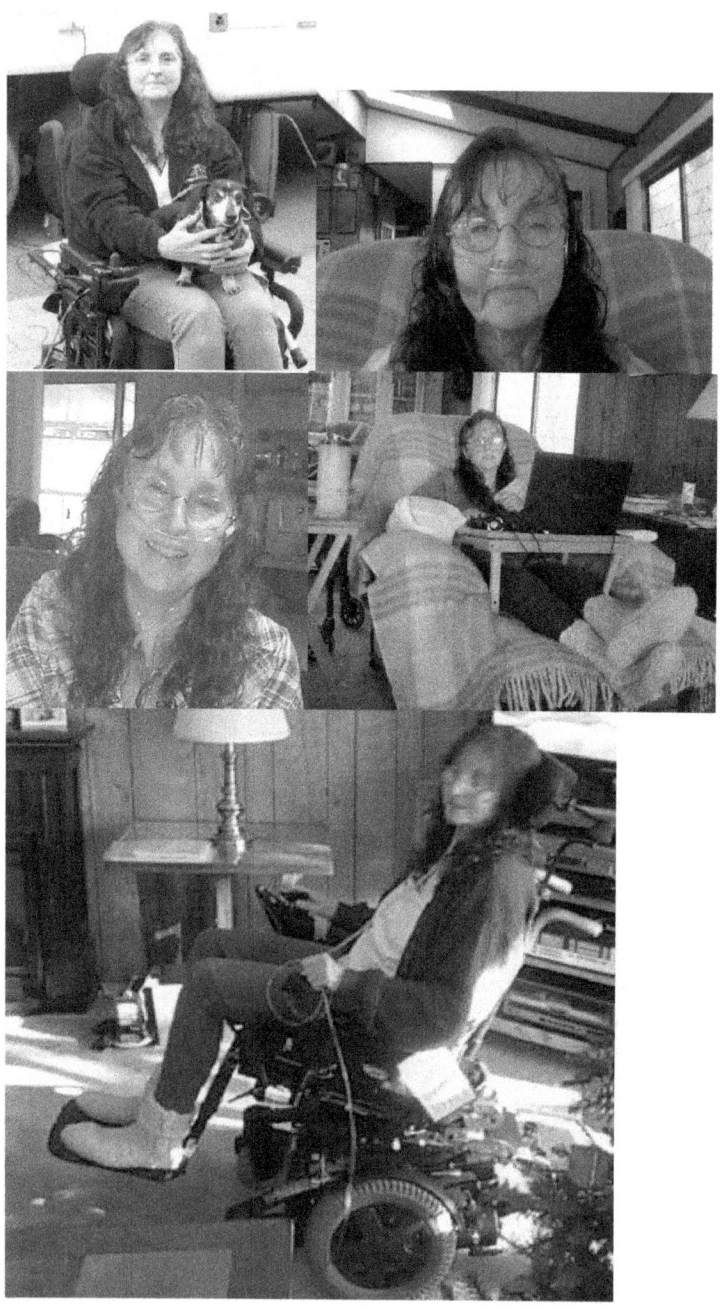

Episode Photos

Susan before the episode

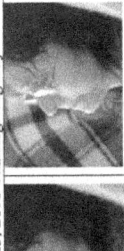
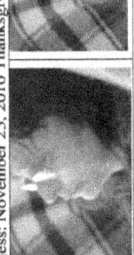
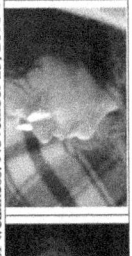
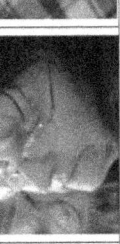
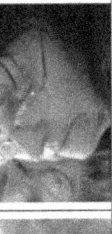
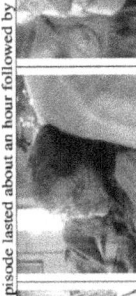
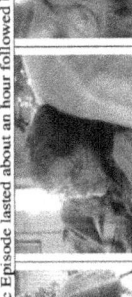
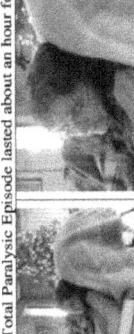
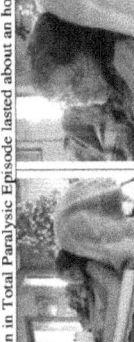

Susan in Total Paralysic Episode lasted about an hour followed by several hours of weakness: November 25, 2010 Thanksgiving Day

1. Totally paralyzed including eyes and mouth
2. About 15 minutes into episode
3. Drooping of mouth about 30 minutes into it
4. Trying to move mouth and speak as she was coming out of it
5. Still coming out of episode trying to keep eyes open

Susan was not asleep, she heard everything that was said and aware of everything that occurred during the episode.

Trigger Chart

Date	6am	7am	8am	9am	10am	11am	12pm	1pm	2pm	3pm	4pm	5pm	6pm	7pm	8pm	9pm	10pm	11pm	12am	1am	2am	3am	4am	5am
Food, Drink, Meds, Activity																								
Symptoms																								
Conditions																								
Total Paralysis																								
Partial Paralysis																								
Total Weakness																								
Partial Weakness																								
Numbness																								
Normal																								

Appendix

Emergency Information

Emergency Chart

My name is Susan. I am 64 years old and I have a very rare disease called Period Paralysis. The type I have is Andersen-Tawil Syndrome Type 2.

Potassium shifts in my body if I am hypokalemic, hyperkalemic or normokalemic. I become totally paralyzed when the potassium shifts from my organs and goes into my muscles. I am unable to move in any way and am not able to speak or open my eyes. I look like I am asleep, **BUT**, I can hear everything going on around me. I can hear everything being said.

I may be able to move my index finger on my right hand. If you ask "yes" or "no" questions, I may be able to answer. Up and down is "yes" and sideways is "no".

My husband, Calvin, knows exactly what to do for me, so listen carefully to what he says and follow his directions. If he is not with me or is unable to speak or help me please follow the outline below:

If I must go to a hospital take me to Valley Medical Center. My doctors are:

1. Dr. A   PCP   360-000-0000
2. Dr. B   Cardiologist   360-000-0000
3. Dr. C   Renal Specialist   360-000-0000
4. Dr. D   Endocrinologist   360-000-0000

- Please talk to me and tell me what you are doing to me and for me.
- Please make sure I am comfortable.
- Please make sure I am reclining but not lying flat.
- Please be sure my oxygen is on and working.
- Please cover me with a light sheet or blanket because I get cold.
- Please make sure my head and neck are supported. My head will fall to the side and can hurt a great deal.
- Please do not try to move me when I am paralyzed. Damage can occur to my muscles and joints.
- Please do not put me on an IV. I cannot have saline or glucose… if one must be used, mannitol may be ok.
- Please do not give me any medications of any kind to include antibiotics.
- Please do not give me any type of anesthesia, to include lidocaine.
- Please do not use a tourniquet if blood is to be taken to check my potassium levels.
- Please do not put any food or liquid in my mouth, I will choke because I cannot swallow.
- Please watch my breathing it may stop or be very shallow.
- Please watch my swallowing. I may choke.
- Please monitor my heart. I have a heart loop monitor in my chest. I have long QT interval beats, arrhythmias, tachycardia, bradycardia and my heart may stop beating. I may go into cardiac arrest.
- Please do not be alarmed if I have myoclonic jerks or fasciculations. It may mean that I am hyperkalemic, and is not a seizure.
- Please have patience. I will come out of it eventually. It may last 15 minutes to several hours or I may go in and out of it.
- Please be ready with a bedpan or be ready to help me to the bathroom. I will have to urinate urgently after I come out of it but will still be too weak to walk by myself to the bathroom.

Other conditions: Type 2 Diabetes; Fibromyalgia; severe osteoporosis (bone crush of spine);
Heart Arrythmias: PVC's, PAC's PJC's, Errants, ST Segment Abnormalities, Long QT interval, Non-conducted PAC's, Abnormal T waves and Angina;, Small Vessel Ischemia of the brain; Degenerative Disk Disease; Diverticulitis; Arthritis of the spine; Acid Reflux; Hiatal Hernia; High Cholesterol/Triglicerides; Restless Leg Syndrome; Muscle Myopathy

I have a Medtronic Reveal XT Heart LoopMonitor implanted in my chest…do not give me an MRI

My Medications: Mirapex , Potassium Bicarbonate as needed, Oxygen Therapy 2liters 24/7

Susan Quentine Knittle-Hunter
000 Summer Road
Small Town, Anywhere 12345
1-000-000-0000
Born January 00, 1900 64 years old
Emergency: Husband: Calvin Hunter : 1-000-000-0000

Flow Chart-1

Duggins-Critchfield & Alexander-Stevenson Family   **Italics= Family members who are symptomatic or have some characteristics.

*William
Periods of paralysis & heart
Died 59-paralysis & heart
&
Wife #1 Carrie

*William
Periods of paralysis
Died 59-heart
&
Wife #2 Mary

**Gr-Uncle Edward
(No children)
Died 41-heart stopped during paralysis
Periods of weakness and paralysis
Heart palpitations

** Gr-Aunt
(No children)
Periodic Paralysis symptoms

Sanderson and Harriet

William and Carrie

Gr-Uncle #1
(No children)
Died sudden heart age 57

Gr-Uncle #2
Died sudden heart age 69

Gr-Uncle #3
(No children)
Died sudden heart age 69

**Grandfather L
&
Sudden death due to heart age 67
#1 Grandmother

**Lahlee (mother)
*Sister #1 (aunt)
Grandfather L. & #2 Wife
*Sister #2 (aunt)
Grandfather L. & #3 Wife
*Sister #3 (aunt)
*Sister #4 (aunt)
*Sister #5 (aunt)

Flow Chart-2

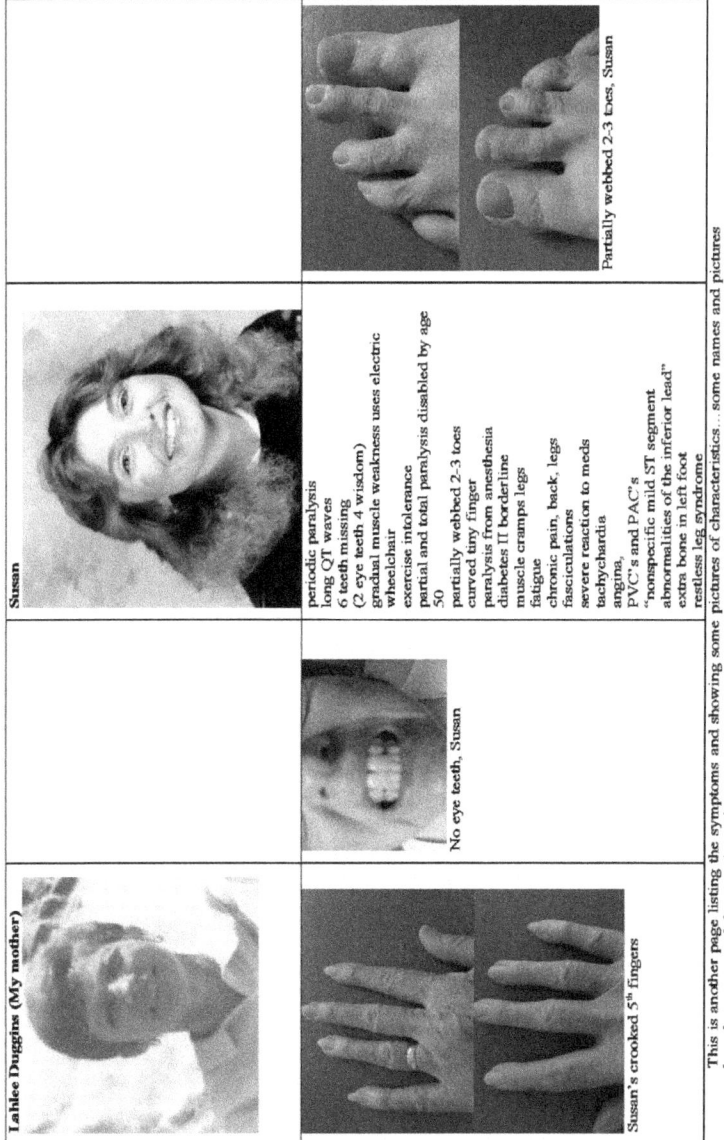

Partially webbed 2-3 toes, Susan

Susan

Lahlee Duggins (My mother)

No eye teeth, Susan

Susan's crooked 5th fingers

periodic paralysis
long QT waves
6 teeth missing
(2 eye teeth 4 wisdom)
gradual muscle weakness uses electric wheelchair
exercise intolerance
partial and total paralysis disabled by age 50
partially webbed 2-3 toes
curved tiny finger
paralysis from anesthesia
diabetes II borderline
muscle cramps legs
fatigue
chronic pain, back, legs
fasciculations
severe reaction to meds
tachycardia
angina,
PVC's and PAC's
"nonspecific mild ST segment abnormalities of the inferior lead"
extra bone in left foot
restless leg syndrome

This is another page listing the symptoms and showing some pictures of characteristics...some names and pictures

Works Cited

1. Wikipedia. (January 2013). Periodic Paralysis. Retrieved from: http://en.wikipedia.org/wiki/Periodic_Paralysis

2. Wikipedia. (February 2013) Ion Channel. Retrieved from: http://en.wikipedia.org/wiki/Ion_channel

3. Wikipedia. (February 2013). Metabolism. Retrieved from: http://en.wikipedia.org/wiki/Metabolism

4. Periodic Paralysis Network. (March 2011). What are the Periodic Paralysis Triggers? "AVOID AT ALL COST". Retrieved from: http://www.periodicparalysisnetwork.com/pdf/What are the Periodic Paralysis Triggers.pdf

5. U.S. National Library of Medicine. (December 2011). Hypokalemic periodic paralysis. Retrieved from: http://www.ncbi.nlm.nih.gov/pubmedhealth/PMH0001355/

6. U.S. National Library of Medicine. (December 2011). Hyperkalemic periodic paralysis. Retrieved from: http://www.ncbi.nlm.nih.gov/pubmedhealth/PMH0001359/

7. Smith, Andrew H. MD, Fish, Frank A. MD, and Kannankeril, Prince J. MD, MSCI (2006) Andersen-Tawil Syndrome. Retrieved from: http://www.ncbi.nlm.nih.gov/pmc/articles/PMC1501096/

8. Kelli Bosarge. (May 2012). The Battle Against Periodic Paralysis Spotlight on a Rare and Complex Disease. Yahoo Voices. Retrieved from: http://voices.yahoo.com/the-battle-against-periodic-paralysis-11282084.html?cat=70

9. Queen Square Centre for Neuromuscular Diseases (October 2012). TAPP: Therapeutic Trial Of Potassium And Acetazolamide In Andersen-Tawil Syndrome. Retrieved from: http://www.cnmd.ac.uk/research/clinical_trial/tapp

10. MedlinePlus. (April 2011). Malignant hyperthermia. Retrieved from: http://www.nlm.nih.gov/medlineplus/ency/article/001315.htm

11. Wikipedia. (February 2013). Malignant hyperthermia. Retrieved from: http://en.wikipedia.org/wiki/Malignant_hyperthermia

12. National Institute of Neurological Disorders and Stroke. (February 2007). Neuroleptic Malignant Syndrome. Retrieved from:

http://www.ninds.nih.gov/disorders/neuroleptic_syndrome/neuroleptic_s yndrome.htm

13. U.S. National Library of Medicine. (July 2012). Serotonin syndrome. Hyperserotonemia; Serotonergic syndrome. Retrieved from: http://www.ncbi.nlm.nih.gov/pubmedhealth/PMH0004531/

14. Wikipedia. (November 2012). Andersen–Tawil syndrome. Retrieved from: http://en.wikipedia.org/wiki/Andersen%E2%80%93Tawil_syndrome

15. Wikipedia. (December 2012). Channelopathy. Retrieved from: http://en.wikipedia.org/wiki/Channelopathy

16. WikiDoc. (August 2012). Metabolic disorder. Retrieved from: http://www.wikidoc.org/index.php/Metabolic_disorder

17. Wikipedia. (January 2013). ICD-10 Chapter VI: Diseases of the nervous system. Retrieved from: http://en.wikipedia.org/wiki/ICD-10_Chapter_VI:_Diseases_of_the_nervous_system

18. Wikipedia. (June 2012). Myopathy. Retrieved from: http://en.wikipedia.org/wiki/Myopathy

19. US National Library of Medicine. (2008). Pathological Conditions, Signs and Symptoms. Retrieved from: http://www.nlm.nih.gov/mesh/trees2008/C23.pdf

20. Medical Coding Reverence. (2013). ICD-10-CM Diagnosis Codes. Retrieved from: http://www.icd10data.com/ICD10CM/Codes/G00-G99/G70-G73/G72-/G72.3 2013

21. Kerry Brandis. ((1981). 'Acid-base pHysiology. Retrieved from: http://www.periodicparalysisnetwork.com/pdf/'Acid-base pHysiology' by Kerry Brandis.pdf

22. Genetics Home Reference. (February 2013). Hypokalemic periodic paralysis. Retrieved from: http://ghr.nlm.nih.gov/condition/hypokalemic-periodic-paralysis

23. Genetics Home Reference. (February 2013). Hyperkalemic periodic paralysis. Retrieved from: http://ghr.nlm.nih.gov/condition/hyperkalemic-periodic-paralysis

Works Cited

24. Korean Circulation Journal. (January 2013). Ventricular Tachyarrhythmias in a Patient with Andersen-Tawil Syndrome. Retrieved from: http://synapse.koreamed.org/DOIx.php?id=10.4070/kcj.2013.43.1.62

25. Medscape Reference. (March 2012). Myopathies. Retrieved from: http://emedicine.medscape.com/article/759487-overview#a0104

26. Livestrong. (March 2011). Degenerative Muscle Disease Symptoms. Retrieved from: http://www.livestrong.com/article/117083-degenerative-muscle-disease-symptoms/

27. Wikipedia. (March 2013). Muscle weakness. Retrieved from: http://en.wikipedia.org/wiki/Muscle_weakness

28. National Institute of Neurological Disorders and Stroke. (February 2013). What is Myopathy? Retrieved from: http://www.ninds.nih.gov/disorders/myopathy/myopathy.htm

29. Operational Medicine 2001. Health Care in Military Settings. Muscle weakness. Retrieved from: http://www.brooksidepress.org/Products/OperationalMedicine/DATA/operationalmed/SickCall/MuscleWeakness.htm

30. National Institute of Neurological Disorders and Stroke. (February 2013). Retrieved from: http://www.ninds.nih.gov/disorders/md/detail_md.htm

31. Livestrong. (March 2011). Degenerative Muscle Disease Symptoms. Retrieved from: http://www.livestrong.com/article/117083-degenerative-muscle-disease-symptoms/

32. Medscape. (February 2012). Types of Myopathies. Retrieved from: http://emedicine.medscape.com/article/1173338-overview#aw2aab6b3

33. Finsterer, J. (2008), Primary periodic paralyses. Retrieved from: Acta Neurologica Scandinavica, 117: 145–158. doi: 10.1111/j.1600-0404.2007.00963

34. Consultants in Neurology, S. C.. Myopathy. Skeletal Muscle Disorders Muscular Dystrophies. Retrieved from: http://www.consultantsinneurology.com/myopathy_81.html

35. Wikipedia. (March 2013). Exercise Intolerance. Retrieved from: http://en.wikipedia.org/wiki/Exercise_intolerance

36. US National Library of Medicine. (July-August 2003). Metabolic intolerance to exercise. Retrieved from: http://www.ncbi.nlm.nih.gov/pubmed/12838448

37. Wikipedia. (March 2013). Hypokalemia. Retrieved from: http://en.wikipedia.org/wiki/Hypokalemia

38. WebMD Heart Disease Health Center. (July 2012). Potassium and Your Heart. Retrieved from: http://www.webmd.com/heart-disease/potassium-and-your-heart

39. Wikipedia. (March 2013). Hyperkalemia. Retrieved from: http://en.wikipedia.org/wiki/Hyperkalemia

40. Wikipedia. (March 2013). ORS complex. Retrieved from: http://en.wikipedia.org/wiki/QRS_complex

41. US National Library of Medicine. (November, 2011). High potassium levels. Retrieved from: http://www.ncbi.nlm.nih.gov/pubmedhealth/PMH0002162/

42. U.S. National Library of Medicine. Genetics Home Reference. (April 2006). Andersen-Tawil syndrome. Retrieved from: http://ghr.nlm.nih.gov/condition/andersen-tawil-syndrome

43. National Heart, Lung, and Blood Institute. (January 2011). What Is Cardiomyopathy? Retrieved from: http://www.nhlbi.nih.gov/health/health-topics/topics/cm/

44. Wikipedia. (March 2013). Muscles of respiration. Retrieved from: http://en.wikipedia.org/wiki/Muscles_of_respiration

45. Wikipedia. (March 2013). Hyperventilation. Retrieved from: http://en.wikipedia.org/wiki/Hyperventilation

46. PubMed Health. (November 2011). Metabolic acidosis. Retrieved from: http://www.ncbi.nlm.nih.gov/pubmedhealth/PMH0001376/

47. Wikipedia. (February 2013). Hypoventilation. Retrieved from: http://en.wikipedia.org/wiki/Hypoventilation

48. Wikipedia. (March 2013). Metabolic Acidosis. Retrieved from: http://en.wikipedia.org/wiki/Metabolic_acidosis

Works Cited

49. Medscape Reference. (August 2011). Metabolic Acidosis. Retrieved from: http://emedicine.medscape.com/article/242975-overview

50. US National Library of Medicine. (June 2011). Lactic acid test. Retrieved from: http://www.ncbi.nlm.nih.gov/pubmedhealth/PMH0003978/

51. Wikipedia. (February 2013). Lactic acidosis. Retrieved from: http://en.wikipedia.org/wiki/Lactic_acidosis

52. Wikipedia. (March 2013). Acidosis. Retrieved from: http://en.wikipedia.org/wiki/Acidosis

53. Turin University Department of Medicine and Chirurgy. (February 2012). Hypokalemic Periodic Paralysis. Retrieved from: http://flipper.diff.org/app/items/info/3983

54. American Academy of Allergy, Asthma & Immunology. (April 2007), (March 2005), (September 2005). Epinephrine-induced hypokalemia. Retrieved from: http://www.aaaai.org/ask-the-expert/Epinephrine-induced-hypokalemia.aspx

55. Wikipedia. (February 2013). Hypokalemic periodic paralysis. Retrieved from: http://en.wikipedia.org/wiki/Hypokalemic_periodic_paralysis

56. Wikipedia. (March 2013). Epinephrine. Retrieved from: http://en.wikipedia.org/wiki/Epinephrine

57. WikiGenes Collaborative Publishing. (March 2013). Disease relevance of Hypokalemia. Retrieved from: http://www.wikigenes.org/e/mesh/e/9865.html

58. Healthline. (2002). Adrenal glands. Retrieved from: http://www.healthline.com/galecontent/adrenal-glands#1

59. Periodic Paralysis Network. (March 2013). Periodic Paralysis. Retrieved from: http://www.periodicparalysisnetwork.com

60. Wikipedia. (March 2013). Alkaline diet. Retrieved from: http://en.wikipedia.org/wiki/Alkaline_diet

61. Buhner, Stephen Harrod. *Herbal Antibiotics-2nd Edition*,

Massachusetts: Storey Publishing, 2012, Print.

62. Wikipedia. (March 2013). Potassium bicarbonate. Retrieved from:
http://en.wikipedia.org/wiki/Potassium_bicarbonate

63. Wikipedia. (February 2013). Potassium citrate. Retrieved from:
http://en.wikipedia.org/wiki/Potassium_citrate

64. Wikipedia. (March 2013). Potassium chloride. Retrieved from:
http://en.wikipedia.org/wiki/Potassium_chloride

65. Mayo Clinic. (November 2011). Potassium Supplement (Oral Route, Parenteral Route). Retrieved from:
http://www.mayoclinic.com/health/drug-information/DR602373

66. US National Library of Medicine. (August 1927). Acute Cardiac Dilatation. Retrieved from:
http://www.ncbi.nlm.nih.gov/pmc/articles/PMC407494/?page=1

67. US National Library of Medicine. (August 2006). Functional and clinical characterization of a mutation in *KCNJ2* associated with Andersen-Tawil syndrome. Retrieved from:
http://www.ncbi.nlm.nih.gov/pmc/articles/PMC2564587/

68. US National Library of Medicine. (April 2008). Practical aspects in the management of hypokalemic periodic paralysis. Retrieved from:
http://www.ncbi.nlm.nih.gov/pmc/articles/PMC2374768/

69. US National Library of Medicine. (May 1990). Pseudohyperkalemia caused by fist clenching during phlebotomy. Retrieved from:
http://www.ncbi.nlm.nih.gov/pubmed/2325722

70. The New England Journal of Medicine. (May 1990). Pseudohyperkalemia Caused by Fist Clenching during Phlebotomy. Retrieved from :
http://www.nejm.org/doi/full/10.1056/NEJM199005033221806

71. Psychology Today. (September 2011). The Challenges of Living with Invisible Pain or Illness. Retrieved from:
http://www.psychologytoday.com/blog/turning-straw-gold/201109/the-challenges-living-invisible-pain-or-illness

72. Statland, Jeffrey M. MD, Tawil, Rabi MD, and Venance, Shannon L. MD, PhD. (January 3, 2013) Andersen-Tawil

Works Cited

Syndrome. Retrieved from
:http://www.ncbi.nlm.nih.gov/books/NBK1264/

73. Genetics Home Reference. (March 2013). Conditions related to genes on Chromosome 17. Retrieved from: http://ghr.nlm.nih.gov/chromosome/17/show/Conditions

74. You Tube. (July 2012). Nutri Bullet Blender/Mixer System with David Wolfe. Retrieved from: http://www.youtube.com/watch?v=O-Bk10CQYCg

Bibliography

Akmal, Tayyaba. (March 2010). What is Weakness? A Comprehensive Review on Causes of Weakness. Retrieved from: http://www.healthgiants.com/2010/03/09/what-is-weakness-a-comprehensive-review-on-causes-of-weakness/

Answers. (2013). Hypokalemia. Retrieved from: http://www.answers.com/topic/hypokalemia

Answers. (2013). Metabolic Acidosis. Retrieved from: http://www.answers.com/topic/metabolic-acidosis

Baxamusa, Batul Nafisa. (January 2012). Lactic Acidosis: Symptoms. Causes and Treatment. Retrieved from: http://www.buzzle.com/articles/lactic-acidosis-symptoms-causes-and-treatment.html

Baxamusa, Batul Nafisa. (January 2011). Myopathy Symptoms. Retrieved from: http://www.buzzle.com/comments/509164-1.html

Baylor College of Medicine. (February 2013). KCNJ2 Mutation Analysis. Retrieved from: http://www.bcm.edu/pediatrics/cardiology/kcnj2

Benzer, Theodore I., MD, PhD. (June 7, 20120). Neuroleptic Malignant Syndrome in Emergency Medicine. Retrieved from: http://emedicine.medscape.com/article/816018-overview

Bernhard, Toni JD. (September 28, 2011). The Challenges of Living with Invisible Pain or Illness. Retrieved from: http://www.psychologytoday.com/blog/turning-straw-gold/201109/the-challenges-living-invisible-pain-or-illness

Bernstein, I. Leonard MD; Bloomberg, Gordon R. MD; Castells, Mariana C. MD. Phd; Mendelsen, Louis M. MD; and Weiss, Michael E. MD. (October 2010). Drug Allergy: An Updated Practice Parameter. Retrieved from: http://www.aaaai.org/Aaaai/media/MediaLibrary/PDF%20Documents/Practice%20and%20Parameters/drug-allergy-updated-practice-param.pdf

BMJ. (April 11, 1998). Neurological channelopathies. Retrieved from: http://www.ncbi.nlm.nih.gov/pmc/articles/PMC1112934/

Bora, Chandramita. (February 24, 2012). Metabolic Acidosis: Symptoms, Causes and Treatment. Retrieved from: http://www.buzzle.com/articles/metabolic-acidosis-symptoms-causes-

and-treatment.html

Boyers, Lindsay. (February 8, 2011). Potassium Supplements. Retrieved from: http://www.livestrong.com/article/376990-potassium-supplements/#ixzz2J67VHwql

Chinnery, Patrick F., PhD, MRCP, Walls, Timothy J., MD, FRCP, Hanna, Michael G., MD, MRCP, Bates, David, MA, FRCP, Fawcett, Peter R. W., BSc, FRCP. (June 23, 2002). Normokalemic periodic paralysis revisited: Does it exist?. Retrieved from: http://onlinelibrary.wiley.com/doi/10.1002/ana.10257/abstract

Cleveland Clinic. (March 12, 2012). Familial Periodic Paralysis. Retrieved from: http://my.clevelandclinic.org/disorders/hyperkalemia/hic_familial_period ic_paralyses.aspx

Cohen, Juliet. (2011). Hypokalemic Periodic Paralysis Treatment Information. Retrieved from: http://www.articlesnatch.com/Article/Hypokalemic-Periodic-Paralysis-Treatment-Information/292829#ixzz2DHyeqhdf

Coleman, Ruth, MD. (January 5, 2011). Calcium Carbonate and Kidney Stones. Retrieved from: http://www.livestrong.com/article/350557-calcium-carbonate-and-kidney-stones/

Danowski, T. S., Fisher, E. R., Vidalon, C., Vester, J. W., Thompson, R. Nolan, S., Stephan, T. and Sunder, J. H. (March 1975). Clinical and ultrastructural observations in a kindred with normo-hyperkalaemic periodic paralysis J Med Genet. 1975 March; 12(1): 20–28. Retrieved from: http://www.ncbi.nlm.nih.gov/pmc/articles/PMC1013227/

DaVita. (2013). Potassium and Chronic Kidney Disease. Retrieved from: http://www.davita.com/kidney-disease/diet-and-nutrition/diet-basics/potassium-and-chronic-kidney-disease/e/5308

Don, B.R., Sebastian, A., Cheitlin, M., Christiansen, M., Schambelan, M. (May 1990). Pseudohyperkalemia caused by fist clenching during phlebotomy. Retrieved from: http://www.ncbi.nlm.nih.gov/pubmed/2325722

EHow. (2013). Blood Potassium Levels. Retrieved from: http://www.ehow.com/blood-potassium-levels/#ixzz264rm9wPt

Bibliography

Encyclopedia Britannica. (2013). Neuromuscular Junction. Retrieved from: http://www.britannica.com/EBchecked/topic/410665/neuromuscular-junction

EquiMed Corporation. (2013). PACs Premature Atrial Contractions. Retrieved from: http://equimedcorp.com/rhythms/topic/39/#non-conducted

FM/CFS/ME Resources. (2013). CFS/ME Symptoms. Retrieved from: http://fmcfsme.d-3systems.com/cfs-symptoms.php

Fogoros, Richard N., MD. (December 2, 2003). Brief Review of Cardiac Arrhythmias. Retrieved from: http://heartdisease.about.com/cs/arrhythmias/a/cardarrhy.htm

The Free Dictionary. (2013). Dystophy. Retrieved from: http://www.thefreedictionary.com/dystrophy

The Free Dictionary. (2013). Metabolic Acidosis. Retrieved from: http://medical-dictionary.thefreedictionary.com/metabolic+acidosis

The Free Dictionary. (2013). Terminal Condition. Retrieved from: http://medical-dictionary.thefreedictionary.com/terminal+condition

The Free Dictionary. (2013). Terminal Illness. Retrieved from: http://medical-dictionary.thefreedictionary.com/Terminal+disease

GARD. (2011). Andersen-Tawil Syndrome. Retrieved from: http://rarediseases.info.nih.gov/GARD/Disease.aspx?PageID=4&DiseaseID=9453

GARD. (2010). Hyperkalemic periodic paralysis. Retrieved from: http://rarediseases.info.nih.gov/GARD/Condition/195/Hyperkalemic_periodic_paralysis.aspx

GARD. (2010). Hypokalemic periodic paralysis. Retrieved from: http://rarediseases.info.nih.gov/GARD/Disease.aspx?PageID=4&DiseaseID=6729

GARD. (2012). Normokalemic periodic paralysis. Retrieved from: http://rarediseases.info.nih.gov/GARD/Condition/4009/Normokalemic_periodic_paralysis.aspx

Garth, David MD. (April 25, 2012). Hypokalemia in Emergency

Medicine. Retrieved from:
http://emedicine.medscape.com/article/767448-overview

Georgia Health. (2013). Hyperventilation and Hypoventilation – Role of
the Lungs in Maintaining pH Balance in the Body. Retrieved from:
http://georgiahealth.edu/itss/edtoolbox/GeorgiaLabs/AcidBase/hyper_hy
poventilate/HyperHypoventilation.html

Godbole, Medha. (September 21, 2011). Normal Potassium
Levels. Retrieved from: http://www.buzzle.com/articles/normal-
potassium-levels.html

Goldenholz, Shira. (March 2011). Cardiac Effects of Hypokalemia.
Retrieved from: http://www.livestrong.com/article/212360-cardiac-
effects-of-hypokalemia/

Gregory, John. (September 2011). Six Signs of Exercise Intolerance.
Retrieved from: http://www.livestrong.com/article/532095-six-signs-of-
exercise-intolerance/#ixzz2DHzRcUgF

Gunnerson, Kyle J. (2013). Lactic Acidosis. Retrieved from:
http://misc.medscape.com/pi/android/medscapeapp/html/A167027-
business.html

Health Central. (2008). A.D.A.M. Medical Encyclopedia. Mineral
metabolism disorders. Retrieved from:
http://www.healthcentral.com/ency/408/007271.html?ic=506048

HeartPoint. (May 1999). Ventricular Arrhythmias. Retrieved from:
http://www.heartpoint.com/ventricular_arrhythmiasmore.html

Heller, Jane. (February 23, 2013). When Laughter is the Only Medicine.
Retrieved from: http://www.huffingtonpost.com/2013/02/23/caregiver-
support_n_2743363.html?ncid=edlinkusaolp00000003

Hoaks, Charlotte. (October 10, 2007). Caregivers for Disabled Adults.
Retrieved from: http://ezinearticles.com/?Caregivers-for-Disabled-
Adults&id=775804

Hypokalemia. (2013). Hypokalemia Symptoms. Retrieved from:
http://www.hypokalemia.net/symptoms.php

Hypokalemic Periodic Paralysis. (2012). A.D.A.M. Medical
Encyclopedia. Retrieved from:
http://www.nlm.nih.gov/medlineplus/ency/article/000312.htm

Bibliography

Knowledge of Medicine. (June 6, 2012). Multifocal Ectopic Purkinje-Related Premature Contractions A New SCN5A -Related Cardiac Channelopathy. Retrieved from: http://www.knowledgeofmedicine.com/cardiology/multifocal-ectopic-purkinje-related-premature-contractions-a-new-scn5a-related-cardiac-channelopathy/

Joel, T., MD, PhD, FACEP, FAAEM. (2012). ECG Diagnosis: Hypokalemia. Perm J. 2012 Spring; 16(2): 57. Retrieved from: http://www.ncbi.nlm.nih.gov/pmc/articles/PMC3383164/

John Hopkins Medicine. (November 16, 2009). Rapid, Erratic Heartbeats: Exercise-Linked Ventricular Tachycardia Is Not A Risk To Healthy Older Adults. Retrieved from: http://www.hopkinsmedicine.org/news/media/releases/rapid_erratic_heartbeats_exercise_linked_ventricular_tachycardia_is_not_a_risk_to_healthy_older_adults

Lederer, Eleanor, MD. (February 25, 2013). Hyperkalemia. Retrieved from: http://emedicine.medscape.com/article/240903-overview

Lederer, Eleanor, MD. (August 5, 2009). Hypokalemia. Retrieved from: http://emedicine.medscape.com/article/242008-overview

Livestrong. (2013). Blood Potassium Levels. Retrieved from http://www.livestrong.com/blood-potassium-levels/
Malignant Hyperthermia Association of the United States. (2011). What is MH? Retrieved from: http://www.mhaus.org/mhaus-faqs-healthcare-professionals/what-is-malignant-hyperthermia/

Maramattom, Bobby Varkey MD, DM, Wijdicks, Eelco F. M. (2006). Acute Neuromuscular Weakness In The Intensive Care Unit. Retrieved from: http://www.medscape.com/viewarticle/551288_2

Mayo Clinic. (May 2, 2012). Cardiomyopathy. Retrieved from: http://www.mayoclinic.com/print/cardiomyopathy/DS00519/DSECTION=all&METHOD=print

Mayo Clinic. (February 8, 2011). Serotonin syndrome. Retrieved from: http://www.mayoclinic.com/health/serotonin-syndrome/DS00860/DSECTION=causes

Mayr, F.B., Domanovits, H., Laggner, A.N. (August 25, 2011). Hypokalemic Paralysis in professional bodybuilder. Retrieved from:

http://www.ncbi.nlm.nih.gov/pubmed/21871759

McAtee, Martina. (August 18, 2010). Symptoms of Hyperkalemia.
Retrieved from: http://www.livestrong.com/article/209459-symptoms-of-
hyperkalemia/

McKusick, Victor A. (July 7, 1999). Sodium Channel, Voltage-Gated,
Type IV, Alph Subunit; SCN4A. Retrieved from:
http://www.omim.org/entry/603967

MDA. (2013). Inherited and Endrocrine Myopathies. Retrieved from:
http://www.mda.org/disease/inherited-and-endocrine-myopathies

MDA. (2009). Periodic Paralysis In Focus. Retrieved from:
http://www.mda.org/sites/default/files/In_Focus_Periodic_Paralysis.pdf

MedHelp. (2013). Hypokalemic Periodic Paralysis. Retrieved from:
http://www.medhelp.org/tags/show/123197/Hypokalemic-periodic-
paralysis

Medline Plus. (March 2013). Acidosis. Retrieved from:
http://www.nlm.nih.gov/medlineplus/ency/article/001181.htm

Medline Plus. (December 19, 2011). Hyperkalemic Periodic Paralysis.
Retrieved from:
http://www.nlm.nih.gov/medlineplus/ency/article/000316.htm

Medline Plus. (January 2013). Hypoventilation. Retrieved from:
http://www.nlm.nih.gov/medlineplus/ency/article/002377.htm

Medline Plus. (March 2013). Muscle Disorders: Also Called Myopathy.
Retrieved from:
http://www.nlm.nih.gov/medlineplus/muscledisorders.html

Medline Plus. (February 2012). Muscle Function Loss. Retrieved from:
http://www.nlm.nih.gov/medlineplus/ency/article/003190.htm

MedLine Plus. (March 19, 2013). Paralysis. Retrieved from:
http://www.nlm.nih.gov/medlineplus/paralysis.html

MedLine Plus. (May 30, 2011). Potassium test. Retrieved from:
http://www.nlm.nih.gov/medlineplus/ency/article/003484.htm

The Merck Manual Home Health Handbook. (2008). Long QT
Syndrome. Retrieved from:

Bibliography

http://www.merckmanuals.com/home/childrens_health_issues/chromoso
mal_and_genetic_abnormalities/long_qt_syndrome.html

The Merck Manual Home Health Handbook. (2008). Neuromuscular
Junction Disorders. Retrieved from:
http://www.merckmanuals.com/home/brain_spinal_cord_and_nerve_diso
rders/peripheral_nerve_disorders/neuromuscular_junction_disorders.html
?qt=&sc=&alt

The Merck Manual for Health Care Professionals (March 2013).
Metabolic Alkalosis. Retrieved from:
http://www.merckmanuals.com/professional/endocrine_and_metabolic_d
isorders/acid-base_regulation_and_disorders/metabolic_alkalosis.html

The Merck Manual for Health Care Professionals. (2013). Weakness.
Retrieved from:
http://www.merckmanuals.com/professional/neurologic_disorders/approa
ch_to_the_neurologic_patient/weakness.html

MitoAction. (2013). Fatigue and Exercise Intolerance. Retrieved from:
http://www.mitoaction.org/guide/fatigue-and-exercise-intolerance

Molecular Fitness. (2013). Potassium Supplements. Retrieved
from: http://www.molecularfitness.com/hcn1_0/potassium-
supplements.aspx

Morimoto, T. et al., Brown, M.J. et al., Kotelevtsev, Y. et al., Kaplan,
N.M. et al., Frokiaer, J. et al., et al. (2013). Hypokalemia. Retrieved
from: http://www.wikigenes.org/e/mesh/e/9865.html

National Center for Biotechnology Information. (August 1927). Acute
Cardiac Dilitation Can Med Assoc J. 1927 August; 17(8): 931. Retrieved
from: http://www.ncbi.nlm.nih.gov/pmc/articles/PMC407494/?page=1

National Institute of Neurological Disorders and Stroke. (September
2011). NINDS Congenital Myopathy Information Page. Retrieved from:
http://www.ninds.nih.gov/disorders/myopathy_congenital/myopathy_con
genital.htm

National Institute of Neurological Disorders and Stroke. (March 2012).
NINDS Familial Periodic Paralyses. Retrieved from:
http://www.ninds.nih.gov/disorders/periodic_paralysis/periodic_paralysis
.htm

National Institute of Neurological Disorders and Stroke. (February 14,

2012). NINDS Muscular Dystrophy: Hope Through Research. Retrieved from: http://www.ninds.nih.gov/disorders/md/detail_md.htm

Neuromuscular. (August 2012). Andersen Syndrome. Retrieved from: http://neuromuscular.wustl.edu/mtime/mepisodic.html#andersen

Neuromuscular. (August 2012). Episodic Muscle Weakness. Retrieved from: http://neuromuscular.wustl.edu/mtime/mepisodic.html#clinical

Neuromuscular. (August 2012). Hyperkalemic Periodic Paralysis. Retrieved from: http://neuromuscular.wustl.edu/mother/activity.html#hrpp

Neuromuscular. (August 2012). Hypokalemic Periodic Paralysis. Retrieved from: http://neuromuscular.wustl.edu/mtime/mepisodic.html#hhopp

News Medical. (April 4, 2005). New ion channel drug targets to emerge in pharmaceutical discovery. Retrieved from: http://www.news-medical.net/news/2005/04/04/8917.aspx

NIH. (September 21, 2011). What is Long QT Syndrome? Retrieved from: http://www.nhlbi.nih.gov/health/health-topics/topics/qt/

Nutritional Supplements Center. (2008) Potassium Deficiency Contributes to Poor Health. Retrieved from: http://www.nutritionalsupplementscenter.com/info/Minerals/potassiumdeficiency.html

Nutting, Pamela J. MS. (2005). Malignant Hyperthermia. Retrieved from: http://www.healthline.com/galecontent/malignant-hyperthermia-1

O'Brien, Jennifer. (January 27, 2010). Periodic paralysis study reveals gene causing disorder. Retrieved from: http://www.ucsf.edu/news/2010/01/4340/periodic-paralysis-study-reveals-gene-causing-disorder

O'Rourke, Brian, Cortassa, Sonia, and Aon, Miguel A. (October 2005). Mitochindrial Ion Channels: Gatekeepers of Life and Death. Retrieved from: http://physiologyonline.physiology.org/content/20/5/303.full

Orpha.net. (2006). Cardiodysrythmic potassium-sensitive periodic paralysis. Retrieved from: http://www.orpha.net/consor/cgi-bin/Disease_Search.php?lng=EN&data_id=10442&Disease_Disease_Sea

Bibliography

rch_diseaseGroup=Andersen-
Tawil&Disease_Disease_Search_diseaseType=Pat&Disease(s)/group of
diseases=Cardiodysrythmic-potassium-sensitive-periodic-paralysis--
Andersen-Tawil-syndrome-&title=Cardiodysrythmic-potassium-
sensitive-periodic-paralysis--Andersen-Tawil-syndrome-
&search=Disease_Search_Simple

Orpha.net. (2008). Hyperkalemic periodic paralysis. Retrieved from:
http://www.orpha.net/consor/cgi-
bin/Disease_Search.php?lng=EN&data_id=212&Disease_Disease_Searc
h_diseaseGroup=Hyperkalemic-periodic-
paralysis&Disease_Disease_Search_diseaseType=Pat&Disease(s)/group
of diseases=Hyperkalemic-periodic-paralysis&title=Hyperkalemic-
periodic-paralysis&search=Disease_Search_Simple

Orpha.net. (2008). Hypokalemic periodic paralysis. Retrieved from:
http://www.orpha.net/consor/cgi-
bin/OC_Exp.php?Lng=EN&Expert=681

Orpha.net. (2008). Normokalemic periodic paralysis. Retrieved from:
http://www.orpha.net/consor/cgi-
bin/Disease_Search.php?lng=EN&data_id=1224&Disease_Disease_Sear
ch_diseaseGroup=Periodic-
paralysis&Disease_Disease_Search_diseaseType=Pat&Disease(s)/group
of diseases=Normokalemic-periodic-paralysis--Periodic-paralysis-type-
3-&title=Normokalemic-periodic-paralysis--Periodic-paralysis-type-3-
&search=Disease_Search_Simple

Parker, Lolo. (2013). Definition of Lactic Acidosis. Retrieved from:
http://www.ehow.com/facts_5563238_definition-lactic-acidosis.html

Periodic Paralysis Research Library. (December 29, 2009).
Normokalemic Periodic Paralysis. Retrieved from:
http://www.pprl.org/Section_Article_View.asp?SECTION_ID=58&SUB
_SECTION_ID=0&CAT_ID=28&ARTICLE_ID=35

Plaster NM, Tawil R, Tristani-Firouzi M, Canún S, Bendahhou S,
Tsunoda A, Donaldson MR, Iannaccone ST, Brunt E, Barohn R, Clark J,
Deymeer F, George AL Jr, Fish FA, Hahn A, Nitu A, Ozdemir C,
Serdaroglu P, Subramony SH, Wolfe G, Fu YH, Ptácek LJ. (May 18,
2001). Mutations in Kir2.1 cause the developmental and episodic
electrical phenotypes of Andersen's syndrome. Retrieved from:
http://www.ncbi.nlm.nih.gov/pubmed/11371347

Princeton, Christine. (September 2008). High Potassium Levels and

Heart. Retrieved from: http://www.livestrong.com/article/237286-high-potassium-levels-and-heart/

Project Jessica. (2008). Project Jessica. Retrieved from: http://www.projectjessica.ca/index.html

PromiseO. (January 8, 2010). Renal Symptoms of Metabolic Acidosis. Retrieved from: http://www.livestrong.com/article/142492-renal-symptoms-metabolic-acidosis/

Ray, Linda. (2013). What are the causes of Adrenaline Rushes?. Retrieved from: http://www.ehow.com/how-does_4911638_what-causes-adrenaline-rushes.html

Reeves, Alexander G., M.D., Swenson, Rand DC, MD, PhD. (2008). Disorders of the Nervous System Chapter 12 – Evaluation of the Patient With Weakness. Retrieved from: http://www.dartmouth.edu/~dons/part_2/chapter_12.html

Right Diagnosis. (March 2013). Andersen-Tawil Syndrome. Retrieved from: http://www.rightdiagnosis.com/a/andersen_tawil_syndrome/symptoms.htm

Right Diagnosis. (March 2013). Hyperkalemic periodic paralysis. Retrieved from: http://www.rightdiagnosis.com/h/hyperkalemic_periodic_paralysis/intro.htm

Right Diagnosis. (March 2013). Hypokalemic periodic paralysis. Retrieved from: http://www.rightdiagnosis.com/h/hypokalemic_periodic_paralysis/intro.htm

Robinson, Richard. (2005). Channelopathies. Retrieved from: http://www.healthline.com/galecontent/channelopathies#2

Rosebush, Rose I., MD. (2011). Serotonin Syndrome. Retrieved from: http://www.nmsis.org/content.asp?type=education&src=pages/serotoninsyndrome.asp&title=Serotonin+Syndrome

Saguil, Aaron, CPT (P), MC, USA. (April 2005). Evaluation of the Patient with Muscle Weakness 71(7):1327-1336. Retrieved from: http://www.aafp.org/afp/2005/0401/p1327.html

Bibliography

Sandesara, Chirag M., MD, FACC. (November 2012). Atrioventricular Block. Retrieved from: http://emedicine.medscape.com/article/151597-overview

Sansone, V., Tawil, R. (April 2007). Management and treatment of Andersen-Tawil syndrome (ATS). Neurotherapeutics. 2007 Apr;4(2):233-7.. Retrieved from: http://www.ncbi.nlm.nih.gov/pubmed/17395133

Sarah, Naomi. (October 15, 2010). Lactic Acidosis. Retrieved from: http://www.buzzle.com/articles/lactic-acidosis.html

Scribd. (2013). List of ICD-10 codes. Retrieved from: http://www.scribd.com/doc/55405924/ICD-10

Socialstyrelsen. (April 13, 2011). Hyperkalemic periodic paralysis and Paramyotonia congenital. Retrieved from: http://www.socialstyrelsen.se/rarediseases/hyperkalemicperiodicparalysisa#anchor_18

Sripathi, Naganand, MD. (June 7, 2012). Periodic Paralyses Clinical Presentation. Retrieved from: http://emedicine.medscape.com/article/1171678-clinical

Sternberg, Damien MD, PhD, Tabti, Nacira MD, PhD, Hainque, Bernard PharmD, PhD, and Fontaine, Bernard MD, PhD. (April 28, 2009) Retrieved from: http://www.ncbi.nlm.nih.gov/books/NBK1338/

St. John, Tina M. M.D. (March 28, 2011). What Are the Symptoms of Potassium Deficiency?. Retrieved from: http://www.livestrong.com/article/92806-symptoms-potassium-deficiency/

Stoppler, Melissa Conrad, MD. (2013). Hyperkalemia. Retrieved from: http://www.medicinenet.com/hyperkalemia/page3.htm

SweetHaven Publishing Services. (2007). Cardia Rhythm Interpretation. Retrieved from: http://free-ed.net/sweethaven/MedTech/Cardiac/571.asp?iNum=0204

University of Florida, Department of Genetics and Metabolism. (2013). Facial Dysmorphology. Retrieved from: http://www.peds.ufl.edu/divisions/genetics/teaching/facial_dysmorphology.htm

University of Vienna. (July 14, 2011). Timothy syndrome mutations provide new insights into the structure of L-calcium channel. ScienceDaily. Retrieved from: http://www.sciencedaily.com/releases/2011/07/110714120718.htm

USLegal. (2013). Terminally Ill Law and Legal Definition. Retrieved from http://definitions.uslegal.com/t/terminally-ill/
Venance, S.L. Cannon, S.C. Fialho, Fontaine, D. B., Hanna, M. G., Ptacek, L.J., M. Tristani-Firouzi, M., Tawil, R., Griggs, R.C. and the CINCH investigators. (September 29, 2005). The primary periodic paralyses: diagnosis,pathogenesis and treatment. Retrieved from: http://brain.oxfordjournals.org/content/129/1/8.full.pdf

Waclawik, Andrew J., MD. (2011). Neuromuscular pathology: overview Muscle biopsy. Retrieved from: http://www.medmerits.com/index.php/article/neuromuscular_pathology_overview/P2

Wahl, Margaret. (July 2009). PP: It's All In The Muscles, Not The Head. Retrieved from: http://quest.mda.org/series/focus-periodic-paralysis/pp-it%E2%80%99s-all-muscles-not-head

Ward, Elizabeth M. MS, RD. (September 22, 2010). Are You Getting Enough Potassium? Retrieved from: http://www.webmd.com/food-recipes/features/potassium-sources-and-benefits

Washington University in St. Louis. (June 23, 2010). Epilepsy: Solving the puzzle of the BK ion channel. ScienceDaily. Retrieved from: http://www.sciencedaily.com /releases/2010/06/100623123355.htm

WebMD. (2008). Hyperkalemia. Retrieved from: http://www.webmd.com/a-to-z-guides/hyperkalemia

WebMD. (2008). Hypokalemia. Retrieved from: http://www.webmd.com/a-to-z-guides/hypokalemia

WebMD. (September 1, 2010). Potassium (K) in Blood. Retrieved from: http://www.webmd.com/a-to-z-guides/potassium-k-in-blood

WebMD. (2013). User Reviews & Ratings – Acetazolamide Oral. Retrieved from: http://www.webmd.com/drugs/drugreview-6755-acetazolamide+Oral.aspx?drugid=6755&drugname=acetazolamide+Oral

Wedro, Benjamin, MD, FACEP, FAAEM. (March 2012). Low

Bibliography

Potassium (Hypokalemia). Retrieved from:
http://www.medicinenet.com/low_potassium_hypokalemia/page3.htm#w
hat_are_the_symptoms_of_low_potassium

Wikipedia. (March 2013). Adrenaline. Retrieved from:
http://en.wikipedia.org/wiki/Adrenaline

Wikipedia. (March 2013). Adrenaline Rush. Retrieved from:
http://en.wikipedia.org/wiki/Adrenaline_Rush

Wikipedia. (March 2013). Sleep Paralysis. Retrieved from:
http://en.wikipedia.org/wiki/Sleep_paralysis

Wikipedia. (March 2013). Terminal Illness. Retrieved from:
http://en.wikipedia.org/wiki/Terminal_illness

Wikipedia. (March 2013). Weakness. Retrieved from:
http://en.wikipedia.org/wiki/Weakness

Zhang, Li, Benson, D. Woodrow, Tristani-Firouzi, Martin, Ptacek, Louis
J., Tawil, Rabi, Schwartz, Peter J., George, Alfred L., Horie, Minoru,
Andelfinger, Gregor, Snow, Gregory L., Fu, Ying-Hui, Ackerman,
Michael J., and Vincent G. Michael. (May 23, 2005).
Arrhythmia/Electrophysiology: Electrocardiographic Features in
Andersen-Tawil Syndrome Patients With *KCNJ2* Mutations:
Characteristic T-U–Wave Patterns Predict the *KCNJ2* Genotype.
Retrieved from: http://circ.ahajournals.org/content/111/21/2720.full.pdf

Index

A

Abortive attack: 66, 78, 112, 113

Acetazolamide (diamox): 152, 156, 158, 419

Acid: (see pH levels)

Acidosis: 21, 27, 36, 56, 59, 61, 91, 107, 115, 119, 120, 132, 135, 139, 143, 144, 151, 152, 153, 154, 155, 156, 157, 158, 159, 161, 162, 163, 164, 165, 166, 169, 171, 175, 176, 178, 213, 214, 220, 221, 230, 233, 235, 256, 266, 275, 312, 325, 330, 342, 343, 344, 402, 403, 407, 408, 409, 415, 416, 417

Acidosis (types):
Lactic acidosis: 56, 59, 91, 139, 143, 144, 154, 156, 157, 158, 159, 161, 162, 163, 325, 410, 415
Metabolic acidosis: ii, 21, 27, 36, 59, 61, 91, 107, 115, 119, 120, 132, 135, 143, 144, 151, 152, 153, 154, 155, 156, 157, 158, 159, 161, 162, 163, 164, 165, 166, 170, 172, 176, 178, 213, 214, 220, 221, 230, 233, 235, 256, 266, 275, 312, 330, 342, 343, 403, 407, 408, 409, 416

Acknowledgements:
Calvin Hunter: viii
Susan Q. Knittle-Hunter: vii

Adrenaline (epinephrine): 17, 126, 197, 203, 206, 414, 417

Afterword: 383

Aleksandr's Story: 290

Alkaline (see pH levels):

Alone in the dark: 9

Also by: vi

Ambulance: x, 42, 44, 47, 49, 50, 54, 133, 170, 229, 266, 270, 274, 275, 276, 277, 278,279, 280, 306, 309, 310, 311, 314, 332

Ambulance:
When to call: 272

Andersen-Tawil Syndrome (ATS):
ii, iv, 12, 15, 35, 36, 57, 59, 62, 63, 64, 65, 79, 81, 82, 85, 86, 87, 88, 91, 92, 93, 97, 98, 101, 104, 109, 117, 118, 128, 132, 134, 152, 153, 155, 157, 167, 190, 201, 227, 244, 249, 252, 259, 260, 263, 264, 266, 278, 280, 283, 287, 309, 321, 322, 323, 324, 331, 362, 363, 372, 405, 407, 411, 415, 422, 425
Cause: 83,
Characteristics: 12,15, 57, 62, 73,75, 77, 81, 82, 83, 84, 85, 86, 87, 90, 91, 93, 95, 105, 253, 316, 325, 358, 366, 367
Description: 12, 75, 84, 110
Diagnosis: 77, 84, 86, 251
Prognosis: 88, 110, 127
Symptoms: 77, 88, 110
Treatment: 79,
Triggers: 84,

Andersen-Tawil Syndrome (ATS) (types, forms): 81, 82, 251, 252
Andersen-Tawil Syndrome 1 (ATS1): 64, 77, 81, 82, 252
Andersen-Tawil Syndrome 2 (ATS2): 64, 65, 69, 79, 81, 82,251, 252

Anesthesia: 16, 19, 20, 21, 23, 30, 38, 46, 80, 84, 87, 88, 91, 93, 137, 265, 273, 322, 356, 362
Trigger: 87, 121, 125
Lidocaine: 56, 58, 62, 139, 140, 258, 260, 261, 275, 358, 364

Anesthetics: 125, 197

Anion gap: 156, 165, 166

Appendix: 387

Arrhythmias (see heart issues): 11, 59, 62, 63, 80, 81, 85, 88, 89, 90, 92, 114, 115, 116, 124, 131, 135, 139, 147, 148, 149, 153, 158, 164, 172, 178, 197, 209, 224, 231, 237, 256, 260, 267, 271, 275, 277, 279, 282, 285, 307, 308, 314, 315, 329, 333, 360, 373, 413

Arrhythmias (types):

Index

Index

IVs: 44, 45, 49, 50, 52, 55, 126, 196, 227, 256, 257, 267, 269, 271, 273, 274, 275, 276, 277, 278, 279, 280, 303, 305, 306, 307, 309, 310, 311, 354, 410
   Glucose (dextrose, sugar): 123, 196
   Mannitol: 126, 196
   Saline (sodium, salt): 125, 196

K
KCNJ2: 77
Kidney: 45, 92, 100, 127, 135, 152, 155, 174, 259, 260, 265, 318, 322, 408
Kidney (hyperkalemia): 109
Kidney (hypokalemia): 107
      Kidney stones: 92, 152, 155

L
Laboratory changes: 105, 107, 113
Laboratory changes (hyperkalemia): 107
Laboratory changes (hypokalemia): 105
Lactic acidosis (see acidosis):
Learning disabilities: 27, 85
Lidocaine (see anesthesia):
Lifestyle changes:
Liver: 107, 110, 184, 207
Liver (hyperkalemia): 110
Liver: (hypokalemia): 107
Long QT heart beat (see arrhythmias):
Low potassium (see hypokalemia) (see potassium levels)

M
Malingerer (see psychiatric disorders)
Malignant Hyperthermia: 87
Management of Periodic Paralysis (see treatment)
MDA (Muscular Dystrophy Association): 56, 57, 97, 128, 184, 238, 241, 242, 251, 262, 321, 322, 329, 338, 410
MDA doctors: 126,184, 242, 251, 262, 322
Medications: vii, viii, 2, 3, 4, 10, 16, 20, 21, 22, 27, 34, 35, 36, 38, 39, 44, 45, 46, 55, 61, 65, 70, 82, 86, 128, 129, 130, 133, 155, 158, 160, 176, 190, 196, 199, 200, 201, 207, 208, 213, 245, 251, 282, 306, 307, 310, 311, 312, 313, 321, 343, 346
      Adverse effects: 35, 38, 39, 40, 93, 95, 121, 123, 132, 308
      Cause of: Long QT interval: 126, 146, 147
   Cause of: Torsades de pointes: 126, 146, 147
      Over-the-counter: 84, 121, 123,124, 182, 206, 229, 360
      Paradoxal effect: 35, 40, 93, 95
Side effects (see adverse effects)
      To avoid (as) triggers: 39, 84, 121, 123
Meditation: 220
Mentally ill (see psychiatric disorders)
Metabolic acidosis (see acidosis)
Metabolic acidosis (technical): 163, 170
Metabolic disorders: 76, 81, 92, 95, 96, 98, 99, 103, 115, 154, 161, 183, 216, 225, 287, 289
Metabolic muscle myopathy: 11, 100
Mineral metabolic disorder: 96, 98, 99, 115, 154, 214
Mitochondrial disease: 11, 100
Monitor vitals: 223
      How to: 223

Index

427

Index

www.ingramcontent.com/pod-product-compliance
Lightning Source LLC
Chambersburg PA
CBHW051208170526
45166CB00005B/1812